# Rare Causes of Stroke

T0201410

# Rare Causes of Stroke

## A Handbook

Edited by

**Derya Uluduz**
Istanbul University

**Anita Arsovska**
University of Ss. Cyril and Methodius

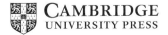

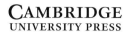

University Printing House, Cambridge CB2 8BS, United Kingdom

One Liberty Plaza, 20th Floor, New York, NY 10006, USA

477 Williamstown Road, Port Melbourne, VIC 3207, Australia

314–321, 3rd Floor, Plot 3, Splendor Forum, Jasola District Centre, New Delhi – 110025, India

103 Penang Road, #05–06/07, Visioncrest Commercial, Singapore 238467

Cambridge University Press is part of the University of Cambridge.

It furthers the University's mission by disseminating knowledge in the pursuit of education, learning, and research at the highest international levels of excellence.

www.cambridge.org
Information on this title: www.cambridge.org/9781108821254
DOI: 10.1017/9781108902793

© Cambridge University Press 2022

This publication is in copyright. Subject to statutory exception and to the provisions of relevant collective licensing agreements, no reproduction of any part may take place without the written permission of Cambridge University Press.

First published 2022

Printed in the United Kingdom by TJ Books Limited, Padstow Cornwall

*A catalogue record for this publication is available from the British Library.*

*Library of Congress Cataloging-in-Publication Data*
Names: Uludüz, Derya, editor. | Arsovska, Anita, 1970– editor.
Title: Rare causes of stroke : a handbook / edited by Derya Uluduz, Anita Arsovska.
Description: New York, NY : Cambridge University Press, [2022] | Includes bibliographical references and index.
Identifiers: LCCN 2021061756 (print) | LCCN 2021061757 (ebook) | ISBN 9781108821254 (paperback) | ISBN 9781108902793 (ebook)
Subjects: MESH: Stroke – etiology | Handbook
Classification: LCC RC388.5 (print) | LCC RC388.5 (ebook) | NLM WL 39 | DDC 616.8/1–dc23/eng/20220307
LC record available at https://lccn.loc.gov/2021061756
LC ebook record available at https://lccn.loc.gov/2021061757

ISBN 978-1-108-82125-4 Paperback

Cambridge University Press has no responsibility for the persistence or accuracy of URLs for external or third-party internet websites referred to in this publication and does not guarantee that any content on such websites is, or will remain, accurate or appropriate.

Every effort has been made in preparing this book to provide accurate and up-to-date information that is in accord with accepted standards and practice at the time of publication. Although case histories are drawn from actual cases, every effort has been made to disguise the identities of the individuals involved. Nevertheless, the authors, editors, and publishers can make no warranties that the information contained herein is totally free from error, not least because clinical standards are constantly changing through research and regulation. The authors, editors, and publishers therefore disclaim all liability for direct or consequential damages resulting from the use of material contained in this book. Readers are strongly advised to pay careful attention to information provided by the manufacturer of any drugs or equipment that they plan to use.

# Contents

*List of Contributors*   ix

*Preface*   xvii

## 1 Inflammatory Conditions

1.1   **Isolated Vasculitis of the Central Nervous System**   1
Bora Korkmazer, Osman Kızılkılıç

1.2   **Primary Systemic Vasculitis**   10
1.2.a.1   **Giant Cell Vasculitis: Temporal Arteritis**   10
Hrvoje Budinčević, Marija Sedlić, Marina Ikić Matijašević, Vedran Ostojić

1.2.a.2   **Giant Cell Vasculitis: Takayasu Arteritis**   17
Marialuisa Zedde, Rosario Pascarella

1.2.b.1   **Necrotizing Vasculitis: Polyarteritis Nodosa (PAN)**   24
Sezgin Sahin, Fatih Haslak, Kenan Barut, Ozgur Kasapcopur

1.2.b.2   **Necrotizing Vasculitis: Churg–Strauss Syndrome (Eosinophilic Granulomatosis with Polyangiitis) and Stroke**   28
Klearchos Psychogios

1.2.c.1   **Granulomatous Vasculitis: Wegener Granulomatosis**   34
Amra Adrovic, Mehmet Yildiz, Ayten Aliyeva, Ozgur Kasapcopur

1.2.c.2   **Granulomatous Vasculitis: Lymphomatoid Granulomatosis**   40

Phillip Ferdinand, Christine Roffe
1.2.d.1   **Vasculitis with Prominent Eye Movement: Susac Syndrome**   45
Bengi Gül Türk, Sabahattin Saip

1.2.d.2   **Vasculitis with Prominent Eye Movement: Vogt–Koyanagi–Harada Disease**   50
Cheryl Carcel

1.2.d.3   **Vasculitis with Prominent Eye Movement: Eales Disease**   54
Sabrina Anticoli, Francesco Motolese

1.2.d.4   **Vasculitis with Prominent Eye Movement: Cogan Disease**   60
Nikoloz Tsiskaridze, Alexander Tsiskaridze

1.3   **Vasculitis Secondary to Systemic Disease**   66
1.3.a   **Systemic Lupus Erythematosis**   66
Vildan Yayla, Hacı Ali Erdoğan, İbrahim Acır

1.3.b   **Behçet's Disease**   72
Uğur Uygunoğlu, Aksel Siva

1.3.c   **Sjögren Syndrome**   79
Marilena Mangiardi, Sabrina Anticoli

1.3.d   **Sarcoidosis**   85
Dilcan Kotan, Aslı Aksoy Gündoğdu

1.3.e **Inflammatory Bowel Disease** 92
Gökhan Kabaçam, Merhmet Arhan, Murat Törüner

1.3.f **Cerebral Amyloid Angiopathy-Related Inflammation** 99
Marialuisa Zedde, Rosario Pascarella, Jacopo C. De Francesco, Fabrizio Piazza

## 2 Infectious and Postinfectious Vasculitis

2.1 **Meningovascular Syphilis** 107
Thierry Adoukonou

2.2 **Neuroborreliosis** 112
Zeljko Zivanovic, Nikola Boban, Vladimir Galic

2.3 **Tuberculosis Meningitis** 119
Yared Z. Zewde, Seda Tadesse

2.4 **Bacterial Meningitis** 125
Marilena Mangiardi, Eytan Raz

2.5 **Neurocysticercosis** 132
Maria Cristina Bravi, Alfano Guido

2.6 **Varicella-Zoster Virus-Related: Cytomegalovirus (CMV) and Herpes Infections** 137
Asma Akbar Ladak, Mohammad Wasay

2.7 **HIV Infection** 141
Massimo Leone, Darlington Thole, Fausto Ciccacci, Maria Cristina Marazzi

2.8 **Chagas Disease** 147
Vinícius Viana Abreu Montanaro

## 3 Hypercoagulable Causes of Stroke

3.1 **Antiphospholipid Antibody Syndrome** 151
Luana Gentile, Danilo Toni

3.2 **Hyperhomocysteinemia** 157
Maria Cristina Bravi, Sabrina Anticoli

3.3 **Hyperviscosity Syndrome** 162
Francesca Romana Pezzella, Kateryna Antonenko, Larysa Sokolova

3.4 **Disseminated Intravascular Coagulation and Moschkowitz Syndrome** 168
Kateryna Antonenko, Valeria Caso, Andrea Blass, Andrea Fiacca

3.5 **Immunoglobulin A Vasculitis (Henoch Schönlein Purpura)** 174
Sarah M. Heldner, Barbara Goeggel Simonetti, Mirjam R. Heldner

3.6 **Stroke Associated With Cancer** 179
Christine Kremer, Olof Gråhamn

## 4 Drug-Related Stroke

4.1 **Medication-Related Stroke** 185
Francesca Romana Pezzella, Sabrina Anticoli, Antonella Urso

4.2 **Illicit-Drug-Related Stroke** 190
Francesca Romana Pezzella, Marilena Mangiardi

## 5 Hereditary and Genetic Causes of Stroke

5.1 **Genetic Collagen Disorders** 199
5.1.a **Ehlers–Danlos Syndrome** 199
Pietro Caliandro, Giuseppe Reale, Aurelia Zauli

5.1.b **Marfan Syndrome** 206
Turgay Demir, Filiz Koç

5.1.c **Fibromuscular Dysplasia** 212
Otgonbayar Luvsannorov, Baigali Gongor

5.1.d **Neurofibromatosis Type 1** 220
Zuhal Yapici, Çağla Turan, Oğuzhan Obuz

5.1.e **Hereditary Hemorrhagic Telangiectasia** 228
Paola Santalucia, Mariangela Piano

5.2 **Genetic Small-Vessel Diseases** 234

5.2.a **Cerebral Autosomal Dominant (Recessive) Arteriopathy with Subcortical Infarcts and Leukoencephalopathy: CADASIL and CARASIL** 234
Yasemin Akıncı, Adnan I. Qureshi

5.2.b **Retinal Vasculopathy with Cerebral Leukoencephalopathy and Systemic Manifestations (RVCL-S)** 240
Janika Kõrv

5.3 **Genetic Metabolic Diseases** 246

5.3.a **Fabry Disease** 246
Natan M. Bornstein, Yasemin Akıncı, Derya Uludüz

5.3.b **Mitochondrial Diseases** 253
Füsun Ferda Erdoğan, Duygu Kurt Gök, Halil Dönmez, İzzet Ökçesiz

5.3.c **Menkes Disease** 262
Linda Azevedo Kauppila, Mariana Fonseca, Ana Catarina Fonseca

5.3.d **Tangier Disease** 267
Fatih Süheyl Ezgü

5.3.e **Organic Acid Disorders** 271
Cristina Tiu, Vlad Eugen Tiu, Elena Oana Terecoasă

# 6 Rare Causes of Cardioembolism

6.1 **Paradoxical Embolism: Patent Foramen Ovale** 281
Hrvoje Budinčević, Petra Črnac Žuna, Edvard Galić, Vida Demarin

6.2 **Infective Endocarditis** 287
Filipa Dourado Sotero, Diana Aguiar de Sousa

# 7 Vasospastic Conditions and Other Vasculopathies

7.1 **Reversible Cerebral Vasoconstriction Syndrome** 293
Dejana R. Jovanović, Predrag Stanarčević

7.2 **Eclampsia and Strokes during Pregnancy and Postpartum** 299
Dejana R. Jovanović

7.3 **Migraines and Migraine-Like Conditions** 305
Yagmur Turkoglu Comert, Peter J. Goadsby

# 8 Other Non-inflammatory Vasculopathies

8.1 **Moyamoya Disease** 309
Bojana Žvan, Marjan Zaletel

8.2 **Cerebral Amyloid Angiopathy** 314
Matija Zupan

8.3 **Dolichoectasia and Fusiform Aneurysms** 321
Jernej Avsenik, Bojana Žvan

8.4 **Carotid Artery Dissection** 326
Füsun Mayda Domaç, Mustafa Ülker

# 9 Venous Occlusive Conditions

9.1 **Cerebral Venous Sinus Thrombosis** 331
Taşkın Duman, Derya Uludüz

# 10 Bone Disorders and Stroke

10.1 **Bone Disorders** 336
Milija Mijajlovic, Vuk Aleksic, Natasa Stojanovski, Natan M. Bornstein

10.2 **Eagle Syndrome** 343
Anita Arsovska, Vida Demarin, Patrik Michel

*Index* 349

# Contributors

## Editors

**Derya Uludüz**
Department of Neurology, Division of Vascular Neurology, Istanbul University-Cerrahpasa, Cerrahpasa Medical Faculty, Istanbul, Turkey

**Anita Arsovska**
University Clinic of Neurology, Faculty of Medicine, University of Ss. Cyril and Methodius, Skopje, North Macedonia

## Authors

**İbrahim Acır**
University of Health Sciences Bakırköy, Dr. Sadi Konuk Research and Training Hospital, Neurology Clinics, Istanbul, Turkey

**Thierry Adoukonou**
Department of Neurology, University of Parakou, Parakou, Benin; Clinic of Neurology, University Teaching Hospital of Parakou, Benin

**Amra Adrovic**
Istanbul University-Cerrahpaşa, School of Medicine, Department of Pediatric Rheumatology, Istanbul, Turkey

**Yasemin Akıncı**
Zeenat Qureshi Stroke Institute and Department of Neurology, University of Missouri, Columbia, MO, USA

**Vuk Aleksic**
Department of Neurosurgery, Clinical Hospital Center Zemun, Belgrade, Serbia

**Ayten Aliyeva**
Istanbul University-Cerrahpaşa, School of Medicine, Department of Pediatric Rheumatology, Istanbul, Turkey

**Sabrina Anticoli**
Stroke Unit, Head Neck and Neuroscience Department, S. Camillo Forlanini Hospital Rome, Italy

**Kateryna Antonenko**
National Bogomolets Medical University, Neurology Department, Kyiv, Ukraine

**Merhmet Arhan**
Gazi University School of Medicine, Department of Gastroenterology, Ankara, Turkey

**Jernej Avsenik**
Clinical Institute of Radiology, University Medical Centre Ljubljana, Slovenia

**Kenan Barut**
Istanbul University-Cerrahpaşa, School of Medicine, Department of Pediatric Rheumatology, Istanbul, Turkey

**Andrea Blass**
Santa Maria della Misericordia Hospital, University of Perugia, Department of Internal and Vascular Medicine, Perugia, Italy

**Nikola Boban**
Center for Radiology, Clinical center of Vojvodina, Novi Sad, Serbia

**Natan M. Bornstein**
Brain Division, ShaareZedek Medical
Center, Jerusalem, Israel

**Maria Cristina Bravi**
Department of Neuroscience, San Camillo
Forlanini Hospital Rome, Italy

**Hrvoje Budinčević**
Sveti Duh University Hospital,
Department of Neurology, Stroke
and Intensive Care Unit, Zagreb,
Croatia; Faculty of Medicine, J. J.
Strossmayer University of Osijek, Osijek,
Croatia.

**Pietro Caliandro**
Neurology Unit, Fondazione Policlinico
Universitario A. Gemelli IRCCS, Rome,
Italy

**Cheryl Carcel**
The George Institute for Global Health,
University of New South Wales, Sydney,
New South Wales, Australia

**Valeria Caso**
Santa Maria della Misericordia Hospital,
University of Perugia, Stroke Unit, Perugia,
Italy

**Fausto Ciccacci**
UniCamillus, Saint Camillus
International University of Health
Sciences, Rome, Italy

**Yagmur Turkoglu Comert**
NIHR-Wellcome Trust King's Clinical
Research Facility, King's College
Hospital, SlaM Biomedical
Research Centre; Institute of Psychiatry,
Psychology and Neuroscience, King's
College London, UK

**Vida Demarin**
International Institute of Brain Health,
Zagreb, Croatia

**Turgay Demir**
Cukurova University School of Medicine,
Adana, Turkey

**Füsun Mayda Domaç**
University of Health Sciences, Erenköy
Psychiatry and Neurological Diseases
Training and Research Hospital, Neurology
Department, Istanbul, Turkey

**Halil Dönmez**
Erciyes University, Faculty of Medicine,
Department of Neurology, Kayseri, Turkey

**Taşkın Duman**
Neurology Department, Hatay Mustafa
Kemal University, Hatay, Turkey

**Hacı Ali Erdoğan**
University of Health Sciences Bakırköy,
Dr. SadiKonuk Research and Training
Hospital, Neurology Clinics, Istanbul,
Turkey

**Füsun Ferda Erdoğan**
Erciyes University, Faculty of Medicine,
Department of Neurology, Kayseri,
Turkey

**Fatih Süheyl Ezgü**
Gazi University Faculty of Medicine,
Departments of Pediatric Metabolic and
Genetic Diseases, Ankara, Turkey

**Phillip Ferdinand**
Stroke Medicine, Neurosciences
Directorate, University Hospital North
Midlands, Stoke-on-Trent, UK

**Andrea Fiacca**
Santa Maria della Misericordia Hospital, University of Perugia, Neuroradiology Department, Perugia, Italy

**Ana Catarina Fonseca**
Stroke Unit, Hospital Santa Maria, Centro Hospitalar Universitário, Lisboa Norte, Portugal; Faculdade de Medicina da Universidade de Lisboa, Lisboa, Portugal; Instituto de Medicina Molecular, Faculdade de Medicina da Universidade de Lisboa, Lisboa, Portugal

**Mariana Fonseca**
Department of Paediatrics, North Middlesex University Hospital, London, United Kingdom

**Jacopo C. De Francesco**
Department of Neurology, ASST San Gerardo Hospital, University of Milano-Bicocca, Via Pergolesi, Monza, MB, Italy

**Peter J. Goadsby**
NIHR-Wellcome Trust King's Clinical Research Facility, King's College Hospital, SlaM Biomedical Research Centre; Institute of Psychiatry, Psychology and Neuroscience, King's College London UK; Department of Neurology, University of California, Los Angeles, CA, USA

**Fatih Haslak**
Istanbul University-Cerrahpaşa, School of Medicine, Department of Pediatric Rheumatology, Istanbul, Turkey

**Mirjam R. Heldner**
Department of Neurology, Inselspital, University Hospital and University of Bern, Bern, Switzerland

**Sarah M. Heldner**
Department of Pediatrics, Inselspital, University Hospital and University of Bern, Bern, Switzerland

**Edvard Galić**
Sveti Duh University Hospital, Department of Internal Medicine, Zagreb, Croatia

**Vladimir Galic**
Department of Neurology, Clinical center of Vojvodina, and Faculty of Medicine, University of Novi Sad, Serbia

**Luana Gentile**
Emergency Department Stroke Unit, Policlinico Umberto I Hospital – La Sapienza University, Rome, Italy

**Baigali Gongor**
Shastin Clinical Hospital, Neurology Center, Mongolia

**Duygu Kurt Gök**
Erciyes University, Faculty of Medicine, Department of Neurology, Kayseri, Turkey

**Olof Gråhamn**
Neurology Department, Skåne University Hospital, Department of Clinical Sciences, Lund University

**Alfano Guido**
Radiology Department of M.G. Vannini Hospital, Rome, Italy

**Aslı Aksoy Gündoğdu**
Neurology Department, Tekirdağ Namık Kemal University School of Medicine, Tekirdağ, Turkey

**Dejana R. Jovanović**
Neurology Clinic, Clinical Centre of Serbia; Medical Faculty, University of Belgrade, Serbia

**Gökhan Kabaçam**
Güven Hospital, Department of Gastroenterology, Ankara, Turkey

**Ozgur Kasapcopur**
Istanbul University-Cerrahpaşa, School of Medicine, Department of Pediatric Rheumatology, Istanbul, Turkey

**Linda Azevedo Kauppila**
Stroke Unit, Hospital Santa Maria, Centro Hospitalar Universitário Lisboa Norte, Portugal

**Osman Kızılkılıç**
Department of Radiology, Division of Neuroradiology, Istanbul University-Cerrahpasa, Cerrahpasa Medical Faculty, Istanbul, Turkey

**Filiz Koç**
Cukurova University School of Medicine, Adana, Turkey

**Bora Korkmazer**
Department of Radiology, Division of Neuroradiology, Istanbul University-Cerrahpasa, Cerrahpasa Medical Faculty, Istanbul, Turkey

**Dilcan Kotan**
Neurology Department, Sakarya University Medical Faculty, Sakarya, Turkey

**Janika Kõrv**
Department of Neurology and Neurosurgery, University of Tartu, Estonia

**Cristine Kremer**
Neurology Department, Skåne University Hospital, Department of Clinical Sciences, Lund University

**Asma Akbar Ladak**
Neurology Department, Aga Khan University, Karachi, Pakistan

**Massimo Leone**
Department of Neurology, Fondazione IRCCS Istituto Neurologico Besta Milano; Community of S. Egidio, DREAM Program, Rome, Italy

**Otgonbayar Luvsannorov**
Mongolian National University of Medical Sciences, School of Medicine, Neurology Department, Mongolia

**Marilena Mangiardi**
Stroke Unit Department, San Camillo-Forlanini Hospital, Rome, Italy

**Maria Cristina Marazzi**
LUMSA University, Rome, Italy

**Marina Ikić Matijašević**
Sveti Duh University Hospital, Department of Internal Medicine, Zagreb, Croatia

**Patrik Michel**
Centre Cerebrovasculaire, Service de Neurologie, Department des Neurosciences Cliniques, Lausanne, Switzerland

**Milija Mijajlovic**
Neurology Clinic, Clinical Center of Serbia, Faculty of Medicine University of Belgrade, Serbia

**Vinícius Viana Abreu Montanaro**
Department of Neurology, Sarah Network of Rehabilitation, Brasília, Brazil

**Francesco Motolese**
Neurology, Neurophysiology and
Neurobiology Unit, Department of
Medicine, Università Campus Bio-Medico,
Rome, Italy

**Oğuzhan Obuz**
Emar-Med Imaging Center, Istanbul,
Turkey

**Vedran Ostojić**
Sveti Duh University Hospital, Department
of Internal Medicine. Zagreb, Croatia

**İzzet Ökçesiz**
Erciyes University, Faculty of Medicine,
Department of Neurology, Kayseri, Turkey

**Rosario Pascarella**
Neuroradiology Unit, Department
od Diagnostic Imaging, Azienda
Unità Sanitaria Locale-IRCCS di Reggio
Emilia, Reggio Emilia (RE), Italy

**Mariangela Piano**
Neuroradiology Unit, Niguarda CàGranda
Hospital, Milan, Italy

**Adnan I. Qureshi**
Zeenat Qureshi Stroke Institute and
Department of Neurology, University of
Missouri, Columbia, MO, USA

**Francesca Romana Pezzella**
Stroke Unit Emergency Department, S.
Camillo-Forlanini Hospital, Rome, Italy

**Fabrizio Piazza**
Pharmaceutical Biotechnologist, PhD,
Professor of Translational Research,
Laboratory of CAA and AD Translational
Research and Biomarkers, School of
Medicine and Surgery, University of
Monza, Italy

**Klearchos Psychogios**
Metropolitan Hospital Stroke Unit, Athens,
Greece

**Eytan Raz**
Neurointerventional Radiology, NYU
Langone Hospital, USA

**Giuseppe Reale**
Department of Geriatrics, Neurosciences
and Orthopedics, Università Cattolica del
Sacro Cuore, Rome, Italy

**Christine Roffe**
Stroke Medicine, Neurosciences
Directorate, University Hospital North
Midlands, Stoke-on-Trent, UK; Faculty
of Medicine and Health Sciences, Keele
University, Stoke-on-Trent, UK

**Sabahattin Saip**
Department of Neurology, Division of
Vascular Neurology, Istanbul University-
Cerrahpasa, Cerrahpasa Medical Faculty,
Istanbul, Turkey

**Sezgin Sahin**
Istanbul University-Cerrahpaşa, School of
Medicine, Department of Pediatric
Rheumatology, Istanbul, Turkey

**Paola Santalucia**
Neurology and Stroke Unit, San Giuseppe
Hospital-Multimedica Group, Milan, Italy

**Marija Sedlić**
Sveti Duh University Hospital,
Department of Neurology. Stroke
and Intensive Care Unit, Zagreb, Croatia

**Barbara Goeggel Simonetti**
Neuropediatrics San Giovanni Hospital
Bellinzona, Bellinzona, Switzerland;

Department of Neurology, Inselspital, University Hospital and University of Bern, Bern, Switzerland

**Aksel Siva**
Department of Neurology, Division of Vascular Neurology, Istanbul University-Cerrahpasa, Cerrahpasa Medical Faculty, Istanbul, Turkey

**Larysa Sokolova**
National Bogomolets Medical University, Neurology Department, Kyiv, Ukraine

**Filipa Dourado Sotero**
Neurology, Department of Neurosciences and Mental Health, Hospital de Santa Maria, Centro Hospitalar Universitário Lisboa Norte, Lisbon, Portugal

**Diana Aguiar de Sousa**
Neurology, Department of Neurosciences and Mental Health, Hospital de Santa Maria, Centro Hospitalar Universitário Lisboa Norte, Lisbon, Portugal; Faculdade de Medicina, Universidade de Lisboa, Lisbon, Portugal

**Predrag Stanarčević**
Neurology Clinic, Clinical Centre of Serbia; Medical Faculty, University of Belgrade, Serbia

**Natasa Stojanovski**
Faculty of Medicine, University of Belgrade, Serbia

**Seda Tadesse**
Adama Hospital Medical College, Adama, Ethiopia

**Elena Oana Terecoasă**
Carol Davila University of Medicine and Pharmacy, Bucharest

**Darlington Thole**
DREAM Program, Balaka, Malawi

**Cristina Tiu**
Carol Davila University of Medicine and Pharmacy, Bucharest

**Vlad Eugen Tiu**
Carol Davila University of Medicine and Pharmacy, Bucharest

**Danilo Toni**
Emergency Department Stroke Unit, Policlinico Umberto I Hospital, La Sapienza University, Rome, Italy

**Murat Törüner**
Ankara University School of Medicine, Department of Gastroenterology, Ankara, Turkey

**Alexander Tsiskaridze**
Neurological Service, Pineo Medical Ecosystem, Tbilisi, Georgia; Department of Neurology, Ivane Javakhishvili Tbilisi State University, Tbilisi, Georgia

**Nikoloz Tsiskaridze**
Neurological Service, Pineo Medical Ecosystem, Tbilisi, Georgia

**Çağla Turan**
Istanbul University, Istanbul Faculty of Medicine, Department of Neurology, Istanbul, Turkey

**Bengi Gül Türk**
Department of Neurology, Division of Vascular Neurology, Istanbul University-Cerrahpasa, Cerrahpasa Medical Faculty, Istanbul, Turkey

**Antonella Urso**
Department of Health, Lazio Regional
Healthcare Government

**Uğur Uygunoğlu**
Department of Neurology, Division of
Vascular Neurology, Istanbul University-
Cerrahpasa, Cerrahpasa Medical Faculty,
Istanbul, Turkey

**Mustafa Ülker**
University of Health Sciences, Erenköy
Psychiatry and Neurological Diseases
Training and Research Hospital, Neurology
Department, İstanbul, Turkey

**Mohammad Wasay**
Neurology Department, Aga Khan
University, Karachi, Pakistan

**Zuhal Yapici**
Istanbul University, Istanbul Faculty of
Medicine, Department of Neurology,
Istanbul, Turkey

**Vildan Yayla**
University of Health Sciences Bakırköy,
Dr. Sadi Konuk Research and Training
Hospital, Neurology Clinics, Istanbul,
Turkey

**Mehmet Yildiz**
Istanbul University-Cerrahpaşa, School
of Medicine, Department of Pediatric
Rheumatology, Istanbul, Turkey

**Marjan Zaletel**
University Medical Centre Ljubljana,
Neurology Clinic, Clinical Department of
Vascular Neurology and Intensive
Therapy, Ljubljana, Slovenia

**Aurelia Zauli**
Department of Geriatrics, Neurosciences
and Orthopedics, Università Cattolica del
Sacro Cuore, Rome, Italy

**Marialuisa Zedde**
Neurology Unit, Stroke Unit, Department of
Neuromotor Physiology and Rehabilitation,
Azienda Unità Sanitaria Locale-IRCCS di
Reggio Emilia, Reggio Emilia, Italy

**Yared Z. Zewde**
Department of Neurology, College of
Health Science, Addis Ababa University,
Addis Ababa, Ethiopia

**Zeljko Zivanovic**
Department of Neurology, Clinical Center
of Vojvodina; Faculty of Medicine,
University of Novi Sad, Serbia

**Petra Črnac Žuna**
Sveti Duh University Hospital,
Department of Neurology, Stroke
and Intensive Care Unit, Zagreb, Croatia

**Matija Zupan**
University Medical Centre Ljubljana,
Department of Vascular Neurology,
Ljubljana, Slovenia

**Bojana Žvan**
University Medical Centre Ljubljana,
Neurology Clinic, Clinical Department of
Vascular Neurology and Intensive Therapy,
Ljubljana, Slovenia

# Preface

Stroke is the second leading cause of death and the major cause of long-term disability, directly impacting the quality of life, worldwide. Owing to the aging population, there has been a recent spike in the number of strokes, in both developed and developing countries. Unfortunately, strokes with rarer and unknown causes receive little or no attention due to the heterogeneity of disorders and a poor understanding of the clinical features. There are considerable variations in the etiology of this rare subcategory of stroke, requiring heightened clinical awareness for recognition, evaluation and treatment.

Many rare causes of stroke, such as infections and hypercoagulability, need specific treatments rather than standard therapies to prevent recurrences in patients. Early diagnosis is vital to understand the etiology of an acute cerebrovascular event, which could constitute the first manifestation of a systemic disease requiring different treatment.

Even though some rare causes are difficult to treat, a detailed evaluation and accurate diagnosis will allow better risk assessment and family counseling, for the future generations of doctors and patients, respectively.

We were motivated to create this book because we realized that there are limited recourses and a lack of available literature on rare causes of stroke. The majority of available books address the theoretical information behind stroke, rather than a more practical clinical approach.

We would like to emphasize the need for higher suspicion for a detailed etiological diagnosis of rare causes, to increase awareness and to provide practical clues with case presentations to improve knowledge and patient outcomes.

We have also realized the importance of early recognition and diagnosis of rare causes of stroke, and we wished to provide a serviceable guide for colleagues that would help them to recognize and treat stroke due to rare causes. This book looks at the topic in a new and pragmatic way, provides a workable model for management of strokes due to rare causes and covers all important aspects of rare causes of stroke. Also, it will allow readers to understand the subject in a new light; the information is topical, engaging and relevant for today's readers; and it is a useful tool for the diagnosis and treatment of rare causes of stroke.

This book provides a detailed practical, clinical and contemporary overview of rare causes of stroke. Through case reports, renowned authors describe concise and comprehensive approaches to the diagnosis and treatment of rare causes of stroke, from isolated vasculitis of the central nervous system, primary systemic vasculitis, vasculitis secondary to systemic disease, infectious and postinfectious vasculitis, hypercoagulable states, hereditary and genetic factors, rare causes of cardioembolism, vasospastic conditions and other vasculopathies, other non-inflammatory vasculopathies and venous occlusive conditions to bone disorders and Eagle's syndrome. This book is a user-friendly, useful and concise guide that will help the clinician to establish an accurate diagnosis through detailed evaluation of such patients. It represents a comprehensive and up-to-date clinical approach for the diagnosis and treatment of rare causes of stroke that will lead to increased awareness of this subject.

We would like to express our deepest appreciation and sincere gratitude to our families for their love and unwavering support that has helped us in finalizing this book.

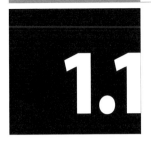

# Isolated Vasculitis of the Central Nervous System

Bora Korkmazer, Osman Kızılkılıç

## Case Presentation

A 53-year-old female was admitted to the emergency department with complaints of sudden facial paralysis and impaired speech. The patient's temperature was 36.7 °C, heart rate, 79 beats/min, blood pressure, 100/65 mm Hg and respiratory rate, 21 breaths/min with oxygen saturation of 99% on room air. Physical examination revealed no abnormalities in the head, neck, chest, abdomen or lymph nodes. On neurological exam, she demonstrated slightly decreased motor strength in her left side predominantly upper extremity. Fundoscopic examination was normal. Her medical and family history was unremarkable. No history of drug abuse or hormonal therapy was reported. Laboratory studies, including total peripheral blood count, biochemical screen, Fe, ferritin, HbA1c, vitamin B12, folic acid, thyroid function, and renal and hepatic functions, were normal. The erythrocyte sedimentation rate and C-reactive protein were slightly elevated. Inflammatory and coagulopathy panel antinuclear antibody, rheumatoid factor, antineutrophilic cytoplasmic autoantibody, HLAB27, serum angiotensin-converting enzyme (ACE), lupus anticoagulant, antithrombin, protein S, protein C, factor VIII levels, homocysteine levels, antiphospholipid antibodies, factor V Leiden mutation and activated protein C resistance were negative. Results of protein electrophoresis were within normal limits.

Diffusion magnetic resonance imaging (MRI) of the patient revealed an acute ischemic focus in the right basal ganglia and anterior limb of right internal capsule. Critical right middle cerebral artery stenosis was detected in MR angiography and CT angiography. The patient was hospitalized for further evaluation (Figure 1.1.1).

No pathological findings were detected in transthoracic echocardiography and 24-hour rhythm Holter, and transesophageal echocardiography reported a tunnel-type patent foramen ovale that did not show spontaneous passage.

Cerebrospinal fluid (CSF) analysis was normal except for slightly increased protein content and mild lymphocyctic leukocytosis.

The patient's complaints completely resolved spontaneously within a week. Digital subtraction angiography revealed an occlusion in the right anterior cerebral artery A1 segment and a 50% stenosis in the right middle cerebral artery M1 segment. In vessel-wall MRI (VWI MR) to examine the vascular wall, increased thickness and enhancement of the right internal carotid artery terminal segment and proximal segment of middle cerebral artery were detected (Figure 1.1.2).

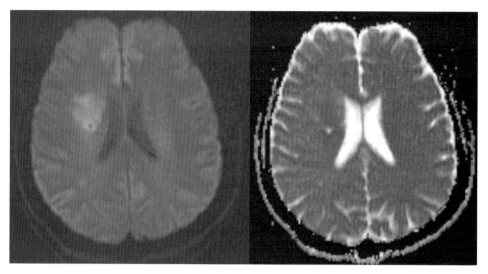

**Figure 1.1.1** DWI-ADC map images showing diffusion restriction in the right basal ganglia and anterior limb of the right internal capsule.

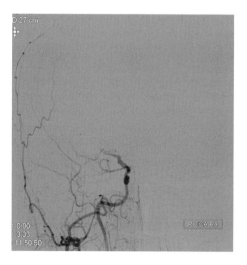

**Figure 1.1.2** DSA image demonstrating an occlusion in the right anterior cerebral artery A1 segment and a 50% stenosis in the right middle cerebral artery M1 segment.

She was diagnosed with isolated cerebral vasculitis of the central nervous system and treated with a combination of steroids and azathioprine. After an eight-month follow-up period, partial regression in stenosis in MR angiography, complete resolution in vessel-wall enhancement and partial resolution in wall thickening in VWI MR were observed (Figure 1.1.3).

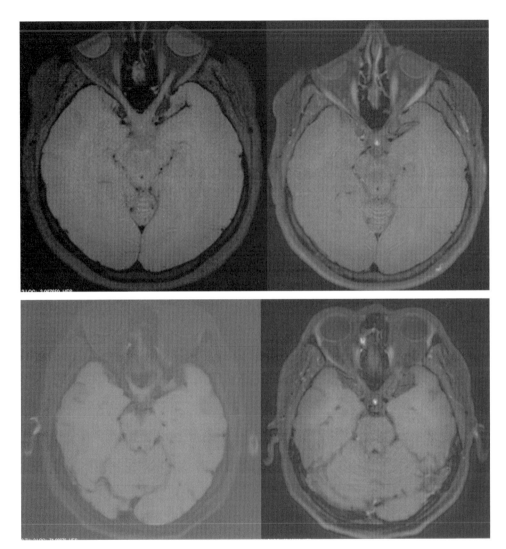

**Figure 1.1.3** Vessel-wall imaging showed active inflammation with contrast enhancement in the vascular wall of the M1 segment of the right middle cerebral artery. In follow-up VWI, complete resolution in vessel-wall enhancement and partial resolution in wall thickening were detected.

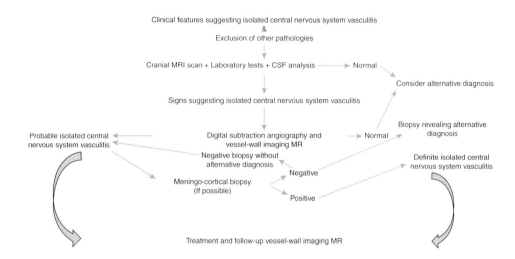

## Case Discussion

Isolated central nervous system vasculitis (ICNSV) is a rare and poorly understood vasculitis limited to the brain and spinal cord. The cause and pathogenesis of ICNSV have not yet been fully elucidated. Although spinal cord abnormalities are present in approximately 5% of patients, they are rarely seen alone. The thoracic spinal cord is the most frequently affected part of the spinal cord.[1] The annual incidence rate of ICNSV has been reported in the literature as 2.4 cases per 1,000,000 people.[2] Although ICNSV can be seen at any age, it is predominantly seen in the fourth to sixth decades and shows a similar frequency between the genders.[3]

Neurological symptoms in ICNSV can manifest in a broad spectrum, usually consisting of headache, cognitive dysfunction, focal neurological deficit or stroke. Although there is no definitive diagnostic laboratory/serological test for ICNSV, routine biochemical-serological testing and acute-phase reactants, antinuclear antibodies, antineutrophil cytoplasm antibodies and antiphospholipid antibodies should be sought in patients suspected of having ICNSV to exclude secondary causes.[4] CSF analysis is abnormal in 80–90% of pathologically documented ICNSV cases, often having a high protein content and lymphocytic pleocytosis.[5] However, the positive predictive value (37%) and specificity (40%) of abnormal CSF findings are found to be low in the diagnosis of ICNSV.[6]

Long-term survival in ICNSV is found to be decreased, and it has been demonstrated that increased mortality is associated with cerebral infarctions and the involvement of large vessels.[2]

## Imaging in Isolated Vasculitis of the CNS

Imaging findings are quite variable, ranging from small ischemic changes to large areas of infarction, hemorrhage, white matter edema and also contrast enhancement. Occlusion, various degrees of stenosis or contrast enhancement at the vessel wall can be detected in the cerebral arteries. Magnetic resonance (MR) imaging is the most common imaging modality in the work-up of patients with suspected ICNSV due to its high tissue contrast and the various sequences that can be used to visualize different pathological conditions in the context of ICNSV.[7] MRI should be performed with contrast media if possible, and diffusion-weighted imaging (DWI) is required for the detection of acute lesions and also for differentiating acute lesions from chronic lesions. It is also important to include susceptibility-weighted sequences in the MR examination, as susceptibility-weighted imaging (SWI) may demonstrate accompanying microhemorrhages and small vessel involvement.[8] MRI features similar to demyelinating diseases, including cases with bilateral diffuse white matter involvement, may result in diagnostic delay.[9-10] Therefore, if necessary, spinal MR examinations should be performed to exclude demyelinating pathologies such as neuromyelitis optica (NMO) and multiple sclerosis (MS) in terms of differential diagnosis.

Although many studies have reported a high sensitivity of MRI in histologically confirmed cases, MRI findings are not pathognomic.[6,11] In MRI, cortical-subcortical infarcts, parenchymal-leptomeningeal contrast enhancement, intracerebral-subarachnoid hemorrhage, tumor-like mass lesions, supratentorial-infratentorial white matter signal changes in T2-weighted and fluid-attenuated inversion recovery (FLAIR) sequences can be detected.[11,12] Multiple discrete infarcts are the most common MRI findings in ICNSV.[4] Less frequently in MRI, more specific findings can be detected, such as vessel-wall thickening and intramural contrast enhancement.

It has been demonstrated that the vessel-wall imaging (VWI) MR technique, which has been used frequently in recent years, is more successful in this regard.[13] It has been reported that VWI MR can play an important role in determining an accurate localization for biopsy by identifying inflamed intracranial vessels.[14] The main purpose of performing VWI MR is to differentiate pathologies such as dissection, which results in intramural hematoma, from vasculitis. However, it may not always be possible to distinguish vasculitis from the inflammatory changes in the vascular wall that accompany atherosclerosis.

Given that MRI is abnormal in most cases of ICNSV, the combination of normal MRI and CSF findings has a strong negative predictive value and will exclude the possibility of CNS vasculitis in most patients.[5]

If suspicious findings are detected in MR examination, it will be appropriate to perform MR angiography (MRA) and MR venography (MRV). Although natural findings in MRA do not rule out the diagnosis, it is recommended to perform MRA since vasculitic processes involving large vessels can be recognized by this examination. MRA has limitations, especially regarding the optimal visualization of posterior cerebral circulation and small vessels.[15]

In addition, serial MRI and MRA accompanied by neurological examinations can be used in the follow-up of patients who have been diagnosed with ICNSV.[4]

CT is abnormal in 33–66% of cases and due to its low sensitivity in ICNSV diagnosis, CT should be used only to exclude hemorrhage or when MRI cannot be performed.[5,16] CT angiography (CTA) is also useful for imaging large vessel involvement and may demonstrate stenosis, occlusion, aneurysm and concentric arterial wall thickening in ICNSV.[17] Cerebral digital subtraction angiography (DSA) is considered the most sensitive and is the gold standard imaging modality for the diagnosis of ICNSV, but the findings are not pathognomonic, similar to other radiological modalities.[18] The sensitivity of DSA in the diagnosis of ICNSV was reported to be between 50% and 90%; however, its specificity was found to be low.[4] Findings suggesting ICNSV in DSA include asymmetric narrowings and dilatations with a string of beads appearance along the vessel course, occlusions or stenoses in vascular structures, blurred vascular margins, accompanying aneurysms, formation of collaterals and delayed arterial emptying or prolonged circulation time along the involved vascular territories.[2,18] Although DSA has higher resolution than cross-sectional angiographic modalities, it does not allow direct evaluation of the vessel wall due to its focused intraluminal imaging.[7,19,20]

Since reversible cerebral vasoconstriction syndrome may simulate ICNSV findings in DSA, complete or nearly complete regression should be seen in control DSA or MRA within 12 weeks of onset of symptoms in cases suspected to have reversible cerebral vasoconstriction syndrome.[4] Flat detector CT angiography (FDCTA) is a novel modality that can be performed in DSA and has superior spatial resolution compared to DSA. FDCTA allows us to track small vascular structures in fine detail, and it is especially important in the evaluation of posterior circulation and brainstem lesions.[21] To avoid false positive results in the diagnosis of ICNSV, angiography and FDCTA results should always be interpreted alongside clinical, laboratory and MRI findings.

## Biopsy

Histological confirmation obtained with cerebral and meningeal biopsy samples is the gold standard for the definitive diagnosis of ICNSV.[22,23] In patients where angiography does not provide a diagnosis, biopsy is important, not only to confirm the diagnosis, but also to exclude mimickers of ICNSV.

In determining the accurate localization for biopsy, lesions that show contrast enhancement in MRI or areas with contrast enhancement in the vascular wall in VWI MR can be used, thereby increasing the sensitivity of the obtained specimen for the diagnosis of ICNSV.[14,19] In patients where focal findings have not been detected with radiological modalities, a random biopsy sample should be taken from the anterior tip of the non-dominant temporal lobe.[24] For optimal diagnostic sensitivity, the biopsy sample should include dural, leptomeningeal, cortical and subcortical tissues.[22] Detection of negative results on biopsy does not rule out the diagnosis of ICNSV, as in radiological modalities.

Histopathology is not uniform in biopsy samples obtained from ICNSV patients; however, granulomatous vasculitis is the most predominant histopathological form in ICNSV.[25]

## Diagnostic Criteria

ICNSV is a rare disease, and a high degree of clinical suspicion is of great importance for diagnosis. There are several criteria suggested by Mallek and Calabrese in the diagnosis of ICNSV:

1. A history or clinical findings of acquired neurological deficits which has remained unexplained after detailed initial examinations.
2. Classical angiographic findings or histopathological findings compatible with vasculitis within the central nervous system.
3. Lack of evidence showing that angiographic or pathological features are secondary to systemic vasculitis or any other condition.[26]

## Treatment

ICNSV is a disease in which clinical findings, radiological features and histopathological analysis results are not uniform, and there are no randomized clinical studies in terms of medical treatment.

As with other vasculitis, high-dose steroids and cytotoxic agents are used in the treatment of ICNSV.[4,27]

Aggressive medical therapy should be initiated rapidly in ICNSV patients with bilateral large vessel involvement, multiple and recurrent cerebral infarctions, and a progressive clinical course. Unfortunately, in these cases, response to treatment is poor and the disease usually leads to a grave prognosis.[28]

ICNSV cases who have small vascular involvement accompanied by leptomeningeal enhancement on MRI are generally diagnosed using brain biopsy, since there is no finding in DSA (Figures 1.1.4 and 1.1.5). In this subset of patients, the response to the medical treatment is better, and their clinical course is more favorable.[29,30]

# References

1. Abdel Razek AA, Alvarez H, Bagg S, Refaat S, Castillo M. Imaging spectrum of CNS vasculitis. *Radiographics.* 2014;**34**(4): 873–894.

2. Salvarani C, Brown RD Jr, Calamia KT, et al. Primary central nervous system vasculitis: Analysis of 101 patients. *Ann Neurol.* 2007;**62**(5): 442–451.

3. Moore P. Neurology of vasculitides and connective tissue diseases. *J Neurol Neurosurg Psychiatry.* 1998;**65**: 10–22.

4. Salvarani C, Brown RD Jr, Hunder GG. Adult primary central nervous system vasculitis. *Lancet.* 2012;**380**(9843): 767–777.

5. Calabrese LH, Duna GF, Lie JT. Vasculitis in the central nervous system. *Arthritis Rheum.* 1997;**40**(7): 1189–1201.

6. Duna GF, Calabrese LH. Limitations of invasive modalities in the diagnosis of primary angiitis of the central nervous system. *J Rheumatol.* 1995;**22**(4): 662–667.

7. Garg A. Vascular brain pathologies. *Neuroimaging Clin N Am.* 2011;**21**(4): 897–ix.

8. Poels MM, Ikram MA, Vernooij MW. Improved MR imaging detection of cerebral microbleeds more accurately identifies persons with vasculopathy. *Am J Neuroradiol.* 2012;**33**(8): 1553–1556.

9. Berger JR, Wei T, Wilson D. Idiopathic granulomatous angiitis of the CNS manifesting as diffuse white matter disease. *Neurology.* 1998;**51**: 1774–1775.

10. Finelli PF, Onykie HC, Uphoff DF. Idiopathic granulomatous angiitis of the CNS manifesting as diffuse white matter disease. *Neurology.* 1998;**49**: 1696–1699.

11. Pomper MG, Miller TJ, Stone JH, Tidmore WC, Hellmann DB. CNS vasculitis in autoimmune disease: MR imaging findings and correlation with angiography. *Am J Neuroradiol.* 1999;**20**: 75–85.

12. Cloft HJ, Phillips CD, Dix JE. Correlation of angiography and MR imaging in cerebral vasculitis. *Acta Radiol.* 1999;**40**: 83–87.

13. Obusez EC, Hui F, Hajj-Ali RA, et al. High-resolution MRI vessel wall imaging: spatial and temporal patterns of reversible cerebral vasoconstriction syndrome and central nervous system vasculitis. *Am J Neuroradiol.* 2014;**35**(8): 1527–1532.

14. Zeiler SR, Qiao Y, Pardo CA, Lim M, Wasserman BA. Vessel wall MRI for targeting biopsies of intracranial vasculitis. *Am J Neuroradiol.* 2018;**39**(11): 2034–2036.

15. Eleftheriou D, Cox T, Saunders D, et al. Investigation of childhood central nervous system vasculitis: Magnetic resonance angiography versus catheter cerebral angiography. *Dev Med Child Neurol.* 2010;**52**: 863–867.

16. Calabrese LH. Therapy of systemic vasculitis. *Neurologic Clinics.* 1997;**15**: 973–991.

17. O'Brien WT Sr, Vagal AS, Cornelius RS. Applications of computed tomography angiography (CTA) in neuroimaging. *Semin Roentgenol.* 2010;**45**(2): 107–115.

18. Alhalabi M, Moore P. Serial angiography in isolated angiitis of the central nervous system. *Neurology.* 1994;**44**: 1221–1226.

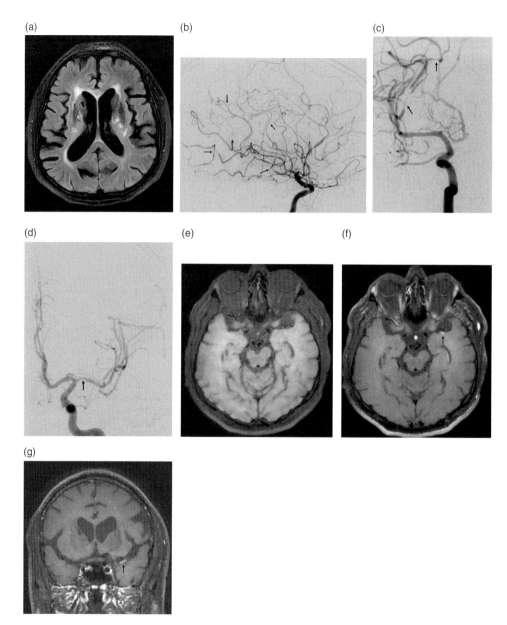

**Figure 1.1.4** (A) Axial FLAIR MRI shows multiple chronic ischemic lesions in the bilateral basal ganglia and periventricular white matter. (B–D) DSA images of the same patient. (B–C) demonstrate asymmetric involvement (black arrows) in the right middle and anterior cerebral artery branches. (D) shows asymmetric involvement (black arrow) in the M1 segment of the left middle cerebral artery. (E–G) Vessel wall imaging MR images of the same patient. (F) and (G) demonstrate active inflammation with contrast enhancement in the vascular wall of the M1 segment of the left middle cerebral artery (black arrows).

(a) 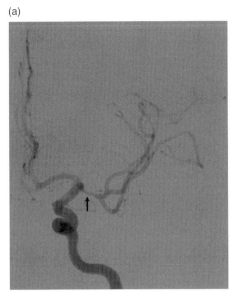 (b)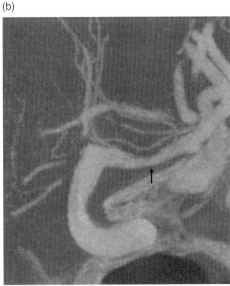

**Figure 1.1.5** (A) DSA image following left ICA injection shows the narrowing of the M1 segment of the left middle cerebral artery (black arrow). (B) Oblique maximum intensity projection image of left middle cerebral artery obtained with Flat Detector CT Angiography demonstrates the narrowing secondary to isolated CNS vasculitis (black arrow).

19. Rossi CM, Di Comite G. The clinical spectrum of the neurological involvement in vasculitides. *J Neurol Sci.* 2009;**285**(1–2): 13–21.

20. Drier A, Bonneville F, Haroche J, et al. Central nervous system involvement in systemic diseases: spectrum of MRI findings. *J Neuroradiol.* 2010;**37**(5): 255–267.

21. Alis D, Civcik C, Erol BC, et al. Flat-detector CT angiography in the evaluation of neuro-Behçet disease. *Diagn Interv Imaging.* 2017;**98**(11): 813–815.

22. Parisi JE, Moore PM. The role of biopsy in vasculitis of the central nervous system. *Semin Neurol.* 1994; **4**:341–348.

23. Miller DV, Salvarani C, Hunder GG, et al. Biopsy findings in primary angiitis of the central nervous system. *Am J Surg Pathol.* 2009;**33**(1): 35–43.

24. Siva A. Vasculitis of the nervous system. *J Neurol.* 2001;**248**(6): 451–468.

25. Lie JT. Primary (granulomatous) angiitis of the central nervous system: A clinicopathologic analysis of 15 new cases and a review of the literature. *Hum Pathol.* 1992;**23**(2): 164–171.

26. Calabrese LH, Mallek JA. Primary angiitis of the central nervous system: Report of 8 new cases, review of the literature, and proposal for diagnostic criteria. *Medicine.* 1988;**67**: 20–39.

27. Hajj-Ali RA, Calabrese LH. Primary angiitis of the central nervous system. *Autoimmun Rev.* 2013;**12**(4): 463–466.

28. Salvarani C, Brown RD Jr, Calamia KT, et al. Rapidly progressive primary central nervous system vasculitis. *Rheumatology.* 2011;**50**(2): 349–358.

29. Salvarani C, Brown RD Jr, Calamia KT, et al. Primary central nervous system vasculitis with prominent leptomeningeal enhancement: a subset with a benign outcome. *Arthritis Rheum.* 2008;**58**(2): 595–603.

30. Salvarani C, Brown RD Jr, Calamia KT, et al. Angiography-negative primary central nervous system vasculitis: a syndrome involving small cerebral vessels. *Medicine.* 2008; **87**(5): 264–271.

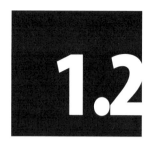

# Primary Systemic Vasculitis
## 1.2.a.1 Giant Cell Vasculitis: Temporal Arteritis

Hrvoje Budinčević, Marija Sedlić, Marina Ikić Matijašević, Vedran Ostojić

## Case Presentation

A 64-year-old male was admitted to the Department of Immunology, Rheumatology and Pulmonology of our hospital due to exacerbation of polymyalgia rheumatica that he was diagnosed with four months prior. His main complaints were severe pain and swelling of small and large joints for which he was treated with dexamethasone upon arrival. On the eighth day of hospitalization, the patient became abruptly confused and was examined by a neurologist.

The physical examination revealed no abnormalities, except erythematous skin changes and swelling of the right hand and the left ankle. The neurologic examination revealed incomplete left homonym hemianopsia and discrete dysmetria of the left arm. The patient was subjected to brain CT scanning, which revealed acute ischemic stroke in the posterior circulation. The patient was then transferred to the Department of Neurology (Figure 1.2.1).

Ultrasound examination of carotid and vertebral arteries showed atherosclerosis with stenosis of the right carotid internal artery and occlusion of the left vertebral artery (Figure 1.2.2).

There were no pathognomonic signs of temporal arteritis. However, the patient had already been receiving corticosteroids for two weeks. In further diagnostic assessment, CT angiography was performed. Subtotal stenosis of the right internal carotid artery and occlusion of the left vertebral artery were revealed (Figure 1.2.3).

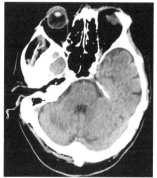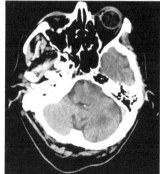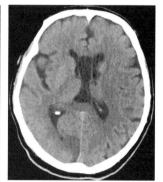

**Figure 1.2.1** Acute ischemic lesions in both cerebellar lobes and right occipital lobe showed by brain MSCT scan.

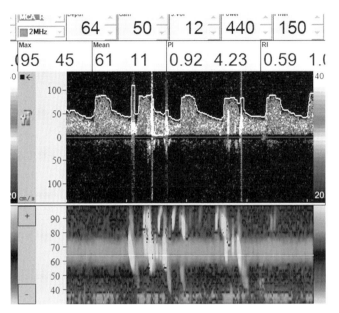

**Figure 1.2.2** Atherosclerosis with stenosis of the right carotid internal artery and occlusion of the left vertebral artery.

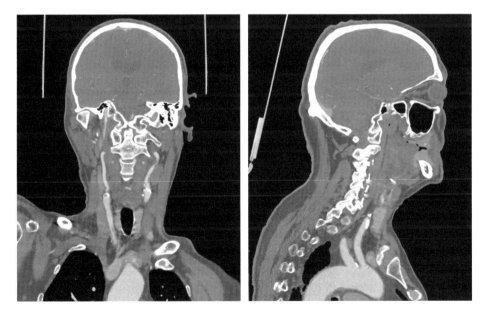

**Figure 1.2.3** Subtotal stenosis of the right carotid internal artery and occlusion of the left vertebral artery showed by brain MSCT scan.

Laboratory studies were performed, including total blood count, biochemical analysis, erythrocyte sedimentation rate (ESR) and C-reactive protein (CRP). Results showed normocytic anemia with decreased levels of iron and elevated ferritin levels, elevated levels of sedimentation rate and CRP. Results of onco-markers, thyroid functions and parathyroid hormone (PTH) were normal.

During the hospitalization, the patient was treated with acetylsalicylic acid (100 mg) and corticosteroids (prednisone in a daily dosage of 30 mg). The patient was then transferred to the Department of Vascular Surgery for surgical treatment of the subtotal stenosis of the right carotid internal artery.

# Diagnostic Algorithm

| Clinical suspicion of giant cell vasculitis (revised ACR criteria) |
| --- |
| 1. Entry criteria |
| Age at onset ≥50 years old |
| Absence of exclusion criteria: ear, nose and throat (ENT) and eye inflammation, kidney, skin and peripheral nervous system involvement, lung infiltration, lymphadenopathies, stiff neck and digital gangrene or ulceration |
| 2. Domain I |
| New-onset localized headache – 1 point |
| Sudden onset of visual disturbances – 1 point |
| Polymyalgia rheumatica (PMR) – 2 points |
| Jaw claudication – 1 point |
| Abnormal temporal artery – up to 2 points |
| 1. Domain II |
| Unexplained fever and/or anemia – 1 point |
| Erythrocyte sedimentation rate (ESR) ≥50 mm/hour – 1 point |
| Compatible pathology – up to 2 points |

(a) In the presence of 3 points or more out of 11 with at least one point belonging to domain I along with all entry criteria, the diagnosis of giant cell arteritis can be established.
(b) No other etiologies can better explain any one of the criteria.

| Diagnosis | |
| --- | --- |
| Clinical examination | The palpation of the temporal artery, auscultation of the arteries including the subclavian and axillary arteries, and bilateral blood pressure measurement |
| Laboratory testing | ↑ ESR and CRP, normocytic anemia, leukocytosis, thrombocytosis, antiferritin autoantibodies |
| CD sonography | Stenosis and occlusion, flow direction and velocity, inflammation of the walls – "halo sign" |
| MRI | Shows signs of wall inflammation (thickening, uptake of contrast agent) |
| PET | Accumulation of radioactive isotope in affected vessels |
| Biopsy | Patho-histological confirmation of the diagnosis |

(cont.)

**Corticosteroids**
**Dosage:**
- an initial dosage of prednisolone 1 mg/kg body weight per day (max. 60 mg)
- cerebral or ocular involvement, an initial intravenous high-dose treatment (methylprednisolone 250 to 1000 mg/day for 3 to 5 days and then conversion to oral therapy

**Alternatives:**

Methotrexate

Azathioprine

Tocilizumab

# Case Discussion

Giant cell arteritis (GCA) is a systemic vasculitis of unknown etiology that involves medium- and large-sized vessels and has a tendency to involve extracranial branches of the carotid arteries.[1] It has a reported annual incidence of 1/3,000–1/25,000 adults, and it is more frequent in populations of northern European background.[1] The age of onset is 50 years, and women are affected two to six times more often than men.[2] Diagnosis of GCA is based on symptoms, clinical findings, laboratory testing and diagnostic imaging. The symptoms of GCA can be divided into those caused by cranial vascular involvement (headache, loss of vision, jaw claudication, stroke), those due to arteritis of large vessels (claudication of extremities), those due to systemic inflammation (fever, weight loss, night sweats) and those due to polymyalgia rheumatica (PMR), mainly proximal myalgia and stiffness of the neck and shoulders.[3,4]

The physical examination includes palpation of the temporal artery, which can be stiff, tender to palpation or can have decreased/absent pulse. Measurement of blood pressure on both sides helps to detect unilateral vascular stenosis.[3,4] Levels of ESR and CRP are elevated. These tests are not very specific, but they show reasonable sensitivity (ESR: 77% to 86%; CRP: 95% to 98%).[5] In addition to raised ESR and CRP, normocytic anemia, leukocytosis and/or thrombocytosis can be found and are indicators of systemic inflammation.[5] Antiferritin autoantibodies are present in about 90% of patients with untreated GCA, but do not prove GCA since they can be present in other rheumatic diseases.[1,5]

Ultrasound examination of the carotid and vertebral arteries is a non-invasive tool that can reveal stenosis and occlusion of the affected vessels, flow direction and velocity, as well as hypoechoic wall thickening, known as a "halo" sign. It has a sensitivity of 85% and a specificity of over 90%.[1,6] A positive finding makes the diagnosis of GCA highly probable, but a negative finding does not rule it out.[6] High-resolution magnetic resonance imaging can reveal signs of wall inflammation (contrast enhancing, thickening of the vessel wall).[6,7] Positron emission tomography can visualize inflammatory processes in GCA through radioactive isotopes that accumulate in affected vessels.[6,8]

However, the gold standard for the diagnosis of GCA is a biopsy of the temporal artery, and although a positive result represents proof of GCA, a negative one does not rule it out. In 10–25% of cases, the biopsy result is a false negative, which may be because the biopsy was taken from a non-inflamed part of the vessel or because it was done too long after the beginning of the corticosteroid treatment.[9,10]

The treatment includes corticosteroids that can be given orally or intravenously, depending on the clinical picture.[11] In patients with GCA-related cerebral or visual symptoms, intravenous corticosteroid therapy should be considered.[12] However, those patients who have experienced a relapse or serious side-effects from corticosteroid therapy can be treated with methotrexate or azathioprine.[13,14] Tocilizumab is the first treatment that has shown efficacy in a large randomized prospective trial as a glucocorticoid sparing agent for GCA.[10,15] Recently, European League Against Rheumatism guidelines recommend the use of tocilizumab, which reduces cumulative glucocorticoid exposure and increases the rate of sustained remission.[13,15] In selected patients with GCA (refractory or relapsing disease, presence of an increased risk for glucocorticoid-related adverse events or complications), using tocilizumab as adjunctive therapy is a good treatment option.[15]

Ischemic complications of GCA occur generally in patients with as yet undiagnosed or uncontrolled disease.[16] The most common vascular complications are anterior ischemic optic neuropathy, large-artery stenoses and ischemia, and aortic aneurysms and dissections.[15] Ischemic complications may be due mostly to atherosclerosis, if the disease is fairly controlled.[16] Ophthalmic complications are most frequent and usually present as anterior ischemic optic neuropathy.

Acute cerebrovascular ischemic events are a rare and severe complication of giant cell arteritis.[17] Ischemic stroke is a rare but important complication that occurs in 2% to 20% of patients and is typically due to stenosis of carotid and/or vertebral or basilar arteries.[17–23] Patients with GCA and stroke are more often older and more frequently men compared to patients with GCA and no strokes.[17,24] The same study showed that cerebrovascular ischemic events were noted in 16% of GCA patients. However, GCA-related strokes can sometimes be difficult to distinguish from strokes of atherosclerotic origin.[17]

Patients with GCA are also at increased risk for multiple cardiovascular diseases and venous thromboembolism.[15] Monitoring for large-vessel involvement, particularly late manifestations like aortic aneurysms is important.[15]

Despite the fact that use of antithrombotic therapy is not recommended routinely, patients with increased cardiovascular risks should be taking antiplatelet therapy and should control risk factors.[12] Elective endovascular interventions or reconstructive surgery should be performed during stable remission.[12] However, arterial vessel dissection or critical vascular ischemia requires urgent referral to a vascular team.[12] Nevertheless, the treatment of acute stroke includes standard revascularization treatments in eligible patients (systemic thrombolysis and/or mechanical thrombectomy), as well as treatment in a stroke unit.[25] In patients with GCA who suffer stroke, secondary stroke prevention treatment is required, as well as control of modifiable stroke risk factors.[26] Antiplatelet therapy is the cornerstone of stroke prevention in the majority of these patients, except in patients with cardioembolic stroke (particularly atrial fibrillation), where an oral anticoagulant therapy is recommended.[27]

# References

1. Nesher G, Breuer GS. Giant Cell Arteritis and Polymyalgia Rheumatica: 2016 Update. *Rambam Maimonides Med J.* 2016; 7.

2. Gonzalez-Gay MA, Vazquez-Rodriguez TR, Lopez-Diaz MJ, et al. Epidemiology of giant cell arteritis and polymyalgia rheumatica. *Arthritis Rheum.* 2009; **61**:1454–1461.

3. Ness T, Bley TA, Schmidt WA, Lamprecht P. The diagnosis and treatment of giant cell arteritis. *Deutsches Arzteblatt Int.* 2013; **110**:376–385.

4. Ness T, Auw-Hadrich C, Schmidt D. [Temporal arteritis (giant cell arteritis). Clinical picture, histology, and treatment]. *Ophthalmologe*. 2006; **103**:296–301.

5. Gonzalez-Gay MA, Lopez-Diaz MJ, Barros S. Giant cell arteritis: laboratory tests at the time of diagnosis in a series of 240 patients. *Medicine*. 2005; **84**:277–290.

6. Schmidt WA, Kraft HE, Vorpahl K, et al. Color duplex ultrasonography in the diagnosis of temporal arteritis. *New Engl J Med*. 1997; **337**:1336–1342.

7. Bley TA, Reinhard M, Hauenstein C. Comparison of duplex sonography and high-resolution magnetic resonance imaging in the diagnosis of giant cell (temporal) arteritis. *Arthritis Rheum*. 2008; **58**:2574–2578.

8. Blockmans D. PET in vasculitis. *Ann New York Acad Sci*. 2011; **1228**:64–70.

9. Poller DN, van Wyk Q, Jeffrey MJ. The importance of skip lesions in temporal arteritis. *J Clin Pathol*. 2000; **53**:137–139.

10. Serling-Boyd N, Stone JH. Recent advances in the diagnosis and management of giant cell arteritis. *Curr Opin Rheumatol*. 2020; **32**:201–207.

11. Proven A, Gabriel SE, Orces C, O'Fallon WM, Hunder GG. Glucocorticoid therapy in giant cell arteritis: duration and adverse outcomes. *Arthritis Rheum*. 2003; **49**:703–708.

12. Hellmich B, Agueda A, Monti S, et al. 2018 Update of the EULAR recommendations for the management of large vessel vasculitis. *Ann Rheum Dis*. 2020; **79**:19–30.

13. Mahr AD, Jover JA, Spiera RF, et al. Adjunctive methotrexate for treatment of giant cell arteritis: An individual patient data meta-analysis. *Arthritis Rheum*. 2007; **56**:2789–2797.

14. Hocevar A, Jese R, Rotar Z, Tomsic M. Does leflunomide have a role in giant cell arteritis? An open-label study. *Clin Rheum*. 2019; **38**:291–296.

15. Kermani TA, Warrington KJ. Prognosis and monitoring of giant cell arteritis and associated complications. *Exp Rev Clin Immunol*. 2018; **14**:379–388.

16. Sailler L, Paricaud K. [Giant cell arteritis: Ischemic complications]. *Presse Med*. 2019; **48**:948–955.

17. Pariente A, Guedon A, Alamowitch S, et al. Ischemic stroke in giant-cell arteritis: French retrospective study. *J Autoimmun*. 2019; **99**:48–51.

18. Wilkinson IM, Russell RW. Arteries of the head and neck in giant cell arteritis: A pathological study to show the pattern of arterial involvement. *Arch Neurol*. 1972; **27**:378–391.

19. Gonzalez-Gay MA, Blanco R, Rodriguez-Valverde V, et al. Permanent visual loss and cerebrovascular accidents in giant cell arteritis: Predictors and response to treatment. *Arthritis Rheum*. 1998; **41**:1497–1504.

20. Reich KA, Giansiracusa DF, Strongwater SL. Neurologic manifestations of giant cell arteritis. *Am J Med*. 1990; **89**:67–72.

21. Salvarani C, Della Bella C, Cimino L, et al. Risk factors for severe cranial ischaemic events in an Italian population-based cohort of patients with giant cell arteritis. *Rheumatology (Oxford)*. 2009; **48**:250–253.

22. Nesher G, Berkun Y, Mates M, et al. Risk factors for cranial ischemic complications in giant cell arteritis. *Medicine*. 2004; **83**:114–122.

23. de Boysson H, Liozon E, Lariviere D, et al. Giant cell arteritis-related stroke: A retrospective multicenter case-control study. *J Rheumatol*. 2017; **44**:297–303.

24. Samson M, Jacquin A, Audia S, et al. Stroke associated with giant cell arteritis: A population-based study. *J Neurol Neurosurg Psychiatry*. 2015; **86**:216–221.

25. Powers WJ, Rabinstein AA, Ackerson T, et al. Guidelines for the early management of patients with acute ischemic stroke. 2019 update to the 2018 guidelines for the early management of acute ischemic stroke: a guideline for healthcare professionals from the American Heart Association/American

Stroke Association. *Stroke.* 2019; **50**: e344–e418.

26. O'Donnell MJ, Chin SL, Rangarajan S, et al. Global and regional effects of potentially modifiable risk factors associated with acute stroke in 32 countries (INTERSTROKE): A case-control study. *Lancet.* 2016; **388**:761–775.

27. Demarin V, Rundek T, Budincevic H. Kaj je novega v smernicahobravna veishemičnemožganskekapi/ What is new in the guidelines for ischemic stroke management? In: Žvan BMZ (Ed.) Akutnamožganskakap. Ljubljana: Društvozapreproč evanjemožganskih in žilnihbolezni. 2015:167–183.

# 1.2.a.2 Giant Cell Vasculitis: Takayasu Arteritis

Marialuisa Zedde, Rosario Pascarella

## Case Presentation

A 45-year-old woman was sent for neurological evaluation because of sudden onset of visual abnormalities in both eyes, slurred speech, confusion and temporal disorientation. She reported the occurrence of several transient monomorphic episodes over a few days. The past medical history was significant for smoking and treatment for arterial hypertension. The physical examination was unremarkable, and blood pressure values did not differ between the two upper limbs. Urgent brain CT revealed mild supratentorial leukoaraiosis. The ultrasound examination of extracranial and intracranial arteries showed widespread concentric wall thickening of the carotid arteries, with greater thickness on the left common carotid artery (CCA) and internal carotid artery (ICA), tight stenosis of the proximal left ICA, overall diameter reduction of the left CCA and ICA, mainly of the ICA over its entire course with stenosis of the terminal intracranial segment, bilateral stenosis of the V2 vertebral artery (VA) and right V1 VA. Vascular neuroimaging with computed tomography angiography (CTA), magnetic resonance angiography (MRA) and digital subtraction angiography (DSA) confirmed these findings, excluding arterial dissection; in particular, MR imaging found a concentric contrast enhancement in the left ICA wall from the origin to the intracranial course. Brain MRI showed multiple subacute ischemic lesions in the left MCA territory (Figure 1.2.4).

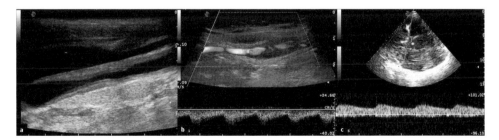

**Figure 1.2.4** Main neuroimaging findings of the presented clinical case.
Panel 1: Ultrasound examination of left CCA (a), showing vessel wall thickening with lumen narrowing, left ICA (b) with incomplete color-mode luminal filling and a demodulated velocity waveform with parvus-tardus post-stenotic pattern, as in severe stenosis, left middle cerebral artery (MCA) on transcranial color-coded sonography (TCCS) with a post-stenotic "dampened flow" waveform.
Panel 2: Brain MR with axial FLAIR (a,b) and corresponding DWI sequences (c,d), showing subacute and acute ischemic lesions in the left hemisphere in the ICA territory. The small lesions in the watershed internal zone are caused by a hemodynamic mechanism and the multiple small punctate cortical lesions are mainly caused by an embolic mechanism.
Panel 3: Vascular neuroimaging with CTA (a) and DSA (b) showing tight stenosis of the left ICA. MRA (c, d, e) of the extracranial and intracranial arteries with time-of-flight (TOF) reconstruction, showing multivessel involvement (right VA in V0 and V2 segments, left ICA, left VA in V2 segment).
Panel 4: High-resolution MRA with contract medium administration showing circumferential contrast enhancement of the left ICA wall from the origin to the intracranial course.

**17**

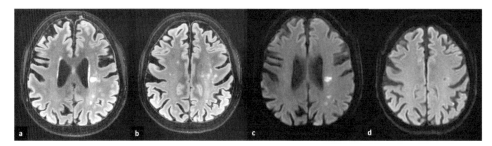

**Figure 1.2.4** (cont.)

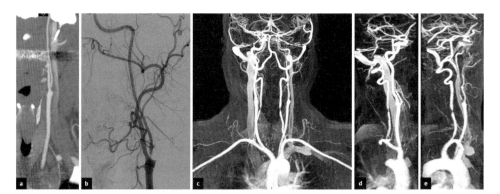

**Figure 1.2.4** (cont.)

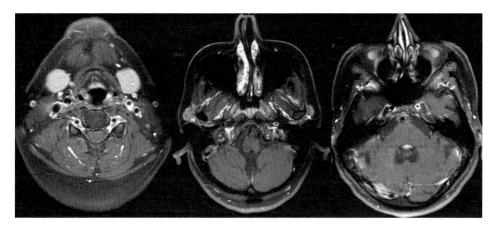

**Figure 1.2.4** (cont.)

Routine blood tests, including erythrocyte sedimentation rate (ESR) and C-reactive protein (CRP), were normal, and extensive immunological screening showed only antinuclear antibody (ANA) positivity at low titre (1:160). A lumbar puncture was performed with normal findings in the CSF. Meanwhile, antiplatelet drugs and a statin were started. Because neuroimaging findings raised the suspicion of large-vessel vasculitis (LVV), the other large vessels were evaluated using CTA, and in particular the thoraco-abdominal aorta and its main branches appeared normal. Moreover, fludeoxyglucose positron emission tomography-computerized tomography (FDG-PET/CT) was performed, excluding increased uptake of the tracer in the supra-aortic trunks and aorta. A close neuroimaging follow-up with MRA showed a slightly increased degree of left ICA stenosis with a persistent wall contrast enhancement in the same vessel.

A diagnosis of large-vessel vasculitis (LVV) was made on this basis and specifically Takayasu's arteritis (TAK). Oral steroid treatment was started, and intravenous cyclophosphamide was given for six months, followed by oral mycophenolate without stroke recurrences.

# Diagnostic Algorithm

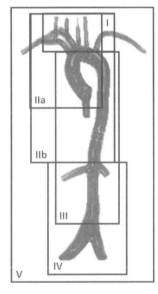

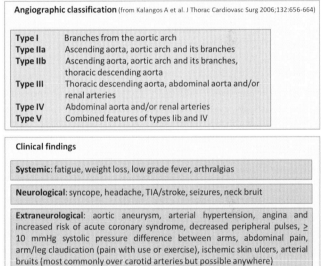

**Angiographic classification** (from Kalangos A et al. J Thorac Cardiovasc Surg 2006;132:656-664)

| | |
|---|---|
| **Type I** | Branches from the aortic arch |
| **Type IIa** | Ascending aorta, aortic arch and its branches |
| **Type IIb** | Ascending aorta, aortic arch and its branches, thoracic descending aorta |
| **Type III** | Thoracic descending aorta, abdominal aorta and/or renal arteries |
| **Type IV** | Abdominal aorta and/or renal arteries |
| **Type V** | Combined features of types IIb and IV |

**Clinical findings**

**Systemic**: fatigue, weight loss, low grade fever, arthralgias

**Neurological**: syncope, headache, TIA/stroke, seizures, neck bruit

**Extraneurological**: aortic aneurysm, arterial hypertension, angina and increased risk of acute coronary syndrome, decreased peripheral pulses, $\geq$ 10 mmHg systolic pressure difference between arms, abdominal pain, arm/leg claudication (pain with use or exercise), ischemic skin ulcers, arterial bruits (most commonly over carotid arteries but possible anywhere)

# Case Discussion

The two major variants of LVV are Takayasu arteritis (TAK) and giant cell arteritis (GCA). The 2012 International Chapel Hill Consensus Conference on the Nomenclature of Vasculitides (CHCC2012)[1] defines LVV as vasculitis affecting the aorta and its major branches, but any size artery may be affected. TAK is an arteritis, often granulomatous, predominantly affecting the aorta and/or its major branches. It usually occurs in patients younger than 50 years. The clinical, histopathological and pathogenetic features are similar to GCA; age at onset >50 years and coexistent polymyalgia rheumatica are the main clinical points to differentiate between TAK and GCA. Most TAK patients are women (up to 90%) in the 10–40 years age range,[2] with a greater prevalence in Asia, but recent surveys show that the disease can be seen in all ethnicities around the world with increasing prevalence rates.[3]

Immunohistopathology of aortic samples reveals tissue infiltration by cytotoxic lymphocytes in involved vessels. The first vascular lesion is usually reported in the left subclavian artery (SA) with a progression to the left CCA, VA, brachiocephalic trunk, right middle or proximal SA, right CCA, VA and aorta. Transmural inflammation of the vessel can lead to stenosis, occlusion or dilatation of involved arterial segments. Although involvement of the thoracic aorta and its branches is more common among females, males have a tendency toward limited involvement of the abdominal aorta and its branches.

Despite the availability of tools for disease definition (CHCC2012),[1] diagnostic criteria for clinical use[4,5] and classification criteria for research use[2] (see Diagnostic Algorithm), there is still a need for validated diagnostic criteria for systemic vasculitides.

The etiology of TAK is unknown, but several studies have demonstrated an association with human leukocyte antigen, suggesting a genetic predisposition for the immuno-mediated process. The clinical features of TAK are usually subacute, and a delay in diagnosis is commonly reported, ranging from months to years. At the time of diagnosis, approximately 20% of patients with TA are asymptomatic, with the disease being detected by abnormal vascular findings on examination. The most common findings at presentation are absence or asymmetry of peripheral pulses, claudication of arm or legs, transient visual disturbance, scotoma, blurring or diplopia.[3]

General constitutional symptoms include fatigue, weight loss and low-grade fever, and are common in the early phase of the disease. About one-half of patients report arthralgias or myalgias, both episodic and continuous. Up to 30% of patients have carotidynia. The main feature of TAK is absent or weak peripheral pulses, most common in radial arteries.[6] In rare cases the occlusion of limbs arteries can lead to gangrene; usually the progressive course of TAK allows the development of collateral circulation avoiding similar complications. Limb claudication more frequently affects the proximal SA with neurological symptoms in the VA territory because of subclavian steal syndrome; ultrasound is the preferred technique to evaluate this phenomenon, where retrograde flow through the VA supplies the SA distal to the stenosis, and vasodilation of the arterial bed in the upper limb with exercise compromises vertebrobasilar blood flow. Upper- or lower-extremity pain raised by mild physical activity is another claudication symptom and often limits functional activity in daily living. Reduced blood pressure in one or both arms is a common finding and sometimes pressures may be unmeasurable in arms. The correlative of progressive vessel stenosis is arterial bruit, and its location depends on the vascular territory in which stenosis is present. If renal arteries are involved, arterial hypertension can develop and accounts for about half of TAK patients. Coronary involvement (aortitis or coronary arteritis) may cause angina or myocardial infarction resulting in death. Mesenteric artery ischemia induces abdominal, particularly post-prandial, pain, diarrhea and gastrointestinal hemorrhage. Pulmonary arteritis is pathologically common, but pulmonary manifestations are relatively uncommon. Neurologic symptoms are common mainly because of the hemodynamic mechanism and range from light headedness, vertigo and orthostatic syncope to headache, seizures and strokes.

Laboratory abnormalities in patients with TAK are non-specific and generally reflect a chronic inflammatory process with increased levels of ESR and CRP. Chronic inflammation can cause normochromic normocytic anemia, as well as leukocytosis and/or thrombocytosis. However, it should be noted that none of these tests is a reliable indicator of the disease activity phase and results can be normal even in the active phase of the disease.

In many cases, diagnostic suspicion of TAK emerges from clinical data (e.g., constitutional symptoms, hypertension, diminished or absent pulses, and/or arterial bruits), although often belatedly, and is confirmed by vascular imaging techniques showing narrowing of the aorta and/or its primary branches. In other cases, the diagnosis from imaging is incidental in tests required for other suspects (e.g., cancer, aortic aneurysm) or histopathological on a surgically removed vessel sample.

After clinical suspicion, vascular imaging techniques play a fundamental role in the diagnosis and in determining the burden of vascular involvement. MRA and/or CTA are usually performed to evaluate the arterial lumen and wall in all large vessels. After the diagnostic phase, in which CTA is often more quickly executable and with greater anatomical detail and a more reliable grading of stenoses, the preferred technique for periodic checks of the disease is MRA for reasons of radiation protection. The main findings are almost the same for all involved vessels: smoothly tapered luminal narrowing or occlusion, sometimes associated with thickening of the vessel wall.[7] Ultrasound examination may directly image vessel wall thickening and luminal narrowing, from which the clinical suspicion can arise and may provide complementary information to MRA/CTA about hemodynamics. It has been shown that contrast-enhanced ultrasonography (CEUS) of CCAs could demonstrate neovascularization with significant correlation with vascular FDG uptake.[8,9] However, MR and CT guarantee greater anatomical coverage compared to ultrasonic techniques. DSA generally provides clear outlines of the lumen of involved arteries, but it does not allow arterial wall thickening to be assessed and is an invasive test which is usually used in anticipation of a revascularization.[7] Positron emission tomography (PET), often in combination with CT (PET-CT) or MR (PET-MR), is an increasingly utilized test to evaluate for possible LVV because it shows vascular inflammation even before any structural change. However, the persistence of FDG uptake has been described in clinically silent disease.[10]

According to EULAR (European League Against Rheumatism) recommendations on the role of imaging in the diagnosis and monitoring of patients with suspected LVV,[7] an early imaging examination is considered the preferred complement to clinical criteria in patients with suspected LVV. Preferably, imaging should take place before or as early as possible after the initiation of therapy, as the sensitivity is significantly reduced within a few days of treatment with glucocorticoids. In suspected TAK, MRI is recommended as the preferred diagnostic test if available to investigate luminal changes and mural inflammation. Alternatively, PET, CT and/or CCDS may be used for the assessment of inflammation processes or luminal changes in patients with TAK. At the moment, however, the diagnostic and prognostic value of enhancement of the vessel wall in MR or CT studies remains to be defined. For long-term monitoring of LVV, as well as the assessment of complications and structural damage, MRI/MRA, CTA and/or CCDS may be used.

The differential diagnosis of TAK includes atherosclerotic, inflammatory, infectious and hereditary diseases that affect the large arteries. The most difficult differential diagnosis is GCA because it involves the same vessels and is histopathologically indistinguishable. Age at onset and involved vessels may help in the differential diagnosis, but these criteria are arbitrary and TAK really overlaps with GCA in a continuum. The list of further differential diagnoses includes several other diseases associated with aortitis, such as Cogan's syndrome, relapsing polychondritis and spondyloarthropathies; however, they have other clinical features pathognomonic for the specific diagnosis. Behçet syndrome can involve medium- and large-sized arteries leading to dilatations and aneurysms. Moreover, IgG4-related disease may be associated with aortitis, usually without involvement of the other arteries. Patients with infectious aortitis can have constitutional symptoms similar to TAK, and usually the evolution of aortic involvement is infectious aneurysm with a typical CTA appearance. Another category of diseases in differential diagnosis are inherited connective tissue disorders, which predispose patients to aortic aneurysm and dissection, such as Marfan syndrome, vascular Ehlers–Danlos syndrome, Loeys–Dietz syndrome and Turner syndrome; these diseases usually lack systemic symptoms. For the same reasons, fibromuscular dysplasia must be considered in the differential diagnosis of TAK.

The main differential diagnosis is with atherosclerosis, but in young people it is easier because of the typical appearance of atheroma, even with associated inflammation. Furthermore, patients with large-vessel vasculitis can also develop atherosclerosis. Evaluation of all patients with TAK for risk factors and evidence of atherosclerosis is appropriate.

TAK is a chronic, relapsing and progressive disease; although about 20% of patients will have a self-limited condition, most patients will demonstrate a relapsing-remitting or progressive course, requiring long-term immunosuppression. Up to 20% will undergo surgical or endovascular revascularization.

The mainstay of therapy for TAK is systemic glucocorticoids, but, being a chronic relapsing disease, it is mandatory to avoid long-term steroid side effects and maintenance therapy for long-term disease control is usually prescribed. No specific agent has been well-proven to be effective, and it is common that patients are prescribed a series of medications, sometimes in combination (methotrexate, azathioprine, mycophenolate, cyclophosphamide, leflunomide, tocilizumab, rituximab). Sometimes, in patients with uncontrolled hemodynamic failure and critical ischemia because of irreversible arterial stenosis and aneurysms or failure of medical treatment, endovascular intervention and surgical procedures are performed.

# References

1. Jennette JC, Falk RJ, Bacon PA, et al. 2012 Revised international Chapel Hill consensus conference nomenclature of vasculitides. *Arthritis Rheum.* 2013; **65**(1):1–11.

2. Arend WP, Michel BA, Bloch DA, et al. The American College of Rheumatology 1990 criteria for the classification of Takayasu arteritis. *Arthritis Rheum.* 1990; **33**:1129.

3. Seyahi E. Takayasu arteritis: An update. *Curr Opin Rheumatol.* 2017; **29**(1):51–56.

4. Ishikawa K. Diagnostic approach and proposed criteria for the clinical diagnosis of Takayasu's arteriopathy. *J Am Coll Cardiol.* 1988; **12**:964e72.

5. Sharma BK, Jain S, Suri S, Numano F. Diagnostic criteria for Takayasu arteritis. *Int J Cardiol.* 1996; **54**:S141e7.

6. Serra R, Butrico L, Fugetto F, et al. Updates in pathophysiology, diagnosis and management of Takayasu arteritis. *Ann Vasc Surg.* 2016; **35**:210.

7. Dejaco C, Ramiro S, Duftner C et al. EULAR recommendations for the use of imaging in large vessel vasculitis in clinical practice. *Ann Rheum Dis.* 2018; 77:636–643.

8. Brkic A, Terslev L, Møller Døhn U. Clinical applicability of ultrasound in systemic large vessel vasculitides. *Arthritis Rheum.* 2019; **71**(11):1780–1787.

9. Germanò G, Monti S, Ponte C. The role of ultrasound in the diagnosis and follow-up

of large-vessel vasculitis: An update. *Clin Exp Rheumatol.* 2017; **35** Suppl 103(1): 194–198.

10. Grayson PC, Alehashemi S, Bagheri AA, et al. 18 F-fluorodeoxyglucose-positron emission tomography as an imaging biomarker in a prospective, longitudinal cohort of patients with large vessel vasculitis. *Arthritis Rheum.* 2018; **70**:439.

11. Hellmich B, Agueda A, Monti S. 2018 Update of the EULAR recommendations for the management of large vessel vasculitis. *Ann Rheum Dis.* 2020; **79**(1):19–30.

# 1.2.b.1 Necrotizing Vasculitis: Polyarteritis Nodosa (PAN)

Sezgin Sahin, Fatih Haslak, Kenan Barut, Ozgur Kasapcopur

## Case Presentation

A 17-year-old female was referred to our pediatric rheumatology outpatient clinic with a presumptive diagnosis of vasculitis. Over the past 3 years, she had a history of several neurological episodes with seizures, sudden vision loss and transient right- and left-sided hemiparesis. Increased acute-phase reactants had been associated with these episodes. A presumptive diagnosis of vasculitis was established after detection of fever, myalgia, abdominal pain, livedo reticularis and severe hypertension during the last episode. On admission, she was febrile (38.3 °C) and her blood pressure was 170/110 mmHg. Physical examination revealed livedo reticularis (Figure 1.2.5) on both lower and upper limbs with a normal neurologic and fundoscopic examination. Diffuse muscle tenderness and colicky abdominal pain without rebound tenderness were also observed.

The complete blood count showed a hemoglobin level of 8.7 g/dl (hematocrit: 28.0%, MCV: 55.6 fl), a platelet count of $352 \times 10^9/l$ and a total leukocyte count of $5.5 \times 10^9/l$. Elevated erythrocyte sedimentation rate (ESR) (41 mm/h) (normal <20 mm/h) and C-reactive protein (CRP) level (2.1 mg/dl) (normal <0.5 mg/dl) were present. Laboratory analyses of electrolyte, urine, coagulation tests, complement C3 and C4 levels, liver and renal function tests were all within normal ranges. The level of muscle enzymes was not suggestive of myositis (LDH: 180 IU/l, CK: 45 mg/dl, AST: 18 IU/l). Screening tests (antithrombin, protein S, protein C, factor VIII and homocysteine levels; factor V Leiden and prothrombin gene mutation; antiphospholipid antibodies including lupus anticoagulant, anticardiolipin antibodies and anti-β2-glycoprotein I antibodies) did not indicate any tendency towards thrombophilia. Antinuclear antibody (ANA), anti-dsDNA, anti-Sm, anti-RNP, anti-Ro, anti-La antibodies and rheumatoid factor were all negative. Asymmetrical axonal polyneuropathy was detected in a nerve conduction study. Electroencephalography, visual evoked potential and electroretinogram tests of both eyes were normal.

Cranial angiography was normal; however, higher signal intensity in bilateral parietal regions accompanied by parenchymal volume loss was observed in brain magnetic resonance imaging (MRI) (Figure 1.2.6A). Further investigation with conventional visceral angiography elicited multiple microaneurysms and segmental narrowings in branches of renal, hepatic and mesenteric arteries suggestive of vasculitis affecting primarily medium-sized arteries (Figure 1.2.6B).

The patient was diagnosed with polyarteritis nodosa (PAN), and all of the clinical manifestations including fever, myalgia, abdominal pain and hypertension were resolved by three types of antihypertensive medications (doxazosin, ramipril and amlodipine) and

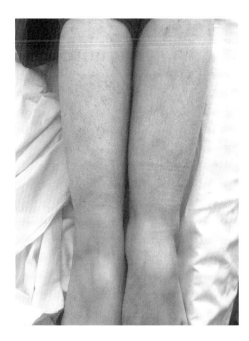

**Figure 1.2.5** Livedo reticularis on the lower extremities.

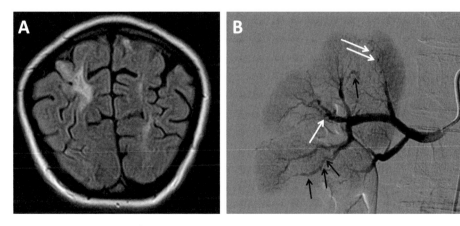

**Figure 1.2.6** (A) The coronal fluid-attenuated inversion recovery (FLAIR) image demonstrates increased signal intensities in the gray and white matters of bilateral parietal lobes accompanied by sulcal widening and parenchymal volume loss, which are suggestive of chronic ischemic stroke. (B) Conventional angiography demonstrating microaneurysms (white arrows) and segmental stenosis (black arrows) in branches of the right renal artery.

five days of pulse methylprednisolone (1 g/m$^2$/day). At discharge, oral methylprednisolone at a dose of 1 mg/kg/day and monthly intravenous cyclophosphamide infusions (1 g/m$^2$/month) for six months were planned for induction treatment. The patient no longer required antihypertensive medication by the second month after discharge and never had a recurrence of disease.

# Diagnostic Algorithm

| Clinical suspicion of PAN |
|---|
| Age = at any age but slightly frequent in individuals aged 6–12 and 45–65 years; Gender = F/M: 1–2/1; Type of onset = generally sudden onset of a severe multisystemic disease<br>Clinical manifestations:<br>a) Constitutional symptoms: fever, malaise, anorexia, weight loss.<br>b) Cutaneous involvement: livedo reticularis, livedo racemosa, skin nodules, cutaneous infarcts<br>b) Musculoskeletal manifestations: myalgia, muscle tenderness, arthralgia, arthritis<br>c) Renal involvement: proteinuria, hematuria, hypertension, perirenal hematoma<br>d) Neurologic manifestations: headache, hemiparesia, hemiplegia, visual loss, peripheral neuropathy<br>e) Other: abdominal pain, acute mesenteric ischemia and infarcts, testicular pain |

| Laboratory, imaging and histologic studies for diagnosis | Laboratory studies for differential diagnoses |
|---|---|
| Complete blood count: anemia of chronic diseases, thrombocytosis and lleucocytosis associated with vasculitides<br>C-reactive protein (CRP): elevated due to widespread inflammation of medium-sized arteries<br>Erythrocyte sedimentation rate: elevated due to widespread inflammation of medium-sized arteries<br>Urea, creatinine: occasionally increased<br>Urine analysis: hematuria and/or proteinuria<br>spot urine protein/creatinine ratio: proteinuria<br>Renal Doppler ultrasonography: aneurysms,, arterial wall thickening and irregularity: aneurysms, arterial thickening and irregularity<br>Computed tomography angiography or magnetic resonance angiography or conventional angiography (gold standard): microaneurysms, stenosis, occlusions in splanchnic and renal arteries<br>Electromyography (EMG) and nerve conduction studies (NCS): asymmetric axonal nerve involvement<br>Biopsy of an accessible involved tissue (skin, muscle, nerve: fibrinoid necrosis within walls of medium or small arteries with marked inflammatory cells within or surrounding the vessel wall | **Other types of vasculitides: granulomatosis with polyangiitis (GPA), microscopic polyangiitis (MPA), eosinophilic granulomatosis with polyangiitis (EGPA), Cryoglobulinemic vasculitis (CPV)** |
| | c-ANCA (immunofluorescence), p-ANCA (immunofluorescence), MPO-ANCA (ELISA), PR3-ANCA (ELISA), cryoglobulins |
| | **Antiphosholipid syndrome** |
| | Lupus anticoagulant, anticardiolipin antibodies and anti β2-glycoprotein I antibodies |
| | **Systemic lupus erythematosus** |
| | Complement C3 and C4 levels, antinuclear antibody (ANA), anti-dsDNA, anti-Sm, anti-RNP, anti-Ro, anti-La antibodies |
| | **Thrombophilic conditions** |
| | Antithrombin, protein S, protein C, factor VIII and homocysteine levels; factor V leiden and prothrombin gene mutation |

| Confirmed diagnosis of PAN: Treatment options | | |
|---|---|---|
| **Induction therapy**<br>• Pulse methylprednisolone 1 g/m²/day (for three to five days), followed by oral corticosteroid at a dose of 1–2 mg/kg/day<br>• Cyclophophamide 500–1000 mg/m²/monthly infusions for six months<br>**Maintenance therapy (for 12–18 months)**<br>• Daily or alternate-day corticosteroid at a dose of 0.2–0.4 mg/kg<br>• Azathioprine at a dose of 1–2 mg/kg/day | **Adjunctive and/or alternative therapies (for severe disease)**<br>• Plasma exchange<br>• Biologic agents:<br>  o Anti–tumor necrosis factor-α (anti-TNFα) agents<br>  o Rituximab<br>  o Mycophenolate mofetil (MMF) | **Therapies for prevention or management of complications and underlying etiologies**<br>• Acetylsalicylic acid<br>• Antiviral drugs for hepatitis B associated PAN<br>• Anti-TNFα agents and/or haematopoietic stem cell transplantation (HSCT) for Deficiency of Adenosine Deaminase-2 (DADA–2)-associated PAN |

# Case Discussion

Polyarteritis nodosa is a systemic vasculitis characterized by necrotizing inflammation of medium- or small-sized arteries.[1] Unlike antineutrophil cytoplasmic antibodies (ANCA)-associated vasculitis, autoantibodies are not present and there is no vasculitis in arterioles, venules and capillaries. Thus, glomerulonephritis and pulmonary hemorrhage are not observed in patients with PAN. The typical histologic feature of PAN is fibrinoid necrosis within the vessel walls of the medium or small arteries, sometimes accompanied by thrombosis inside the lumen.[1,2]

Although infectious triggers such as streptococci, hepatitis B and C have been implicated in the etiopathogenesis, the cause of PAN seems to be heterogeneous. Hepatitis-B-associated PAN has almost disappeared with the aid of vaccination programs. In 2004, deficiency of adenosine deaminase-2 (DADA-2), a novel monogenic PAN-like vasculopathy associated with early-onset ischemic/hemorrhagic strokes, has been described by two international groups in several families, including multiple members with a PAN-like vasculopathy.[3–5]

The Ankara 2008 classification criteria have been widely used for childhood-onset PAN cases. Histopathological demonstration of necrotizing vasculitis or radiologic demonstration of microaneurysms, occlusion or stenosis by angiography in medium or small arteries is a mandatory criterion for Ankara 2008. In addition, the presence of at least one of the following items is required to classify the patient as having PAN:[1]

- Cutaneous features including livedo reticularis, nodules, infarcts
- Myalgia or muscle tenderness
- Hypertension (>95th percentile for height)
- Peripheral neuropathy
- Renal involvement.

The manifestations depend on the location of the arteries affected by vasculitis. Frequently, a constellation of long-standing constitutional symptoms precedes the development of organ-specific manifestations such as livedo reticularis, myalgia, hypertension and focal neurologic deficits.

High-dose corticosteroids and cyclophosphamide for six months are the mainstays of induction treatment. Additional therapies, including plasma exchange and biologic agents should be reserved for severe disease at any time during the disease course. Mycophenolate mofetil (MMF) has been suggested as a less-toxic alternative to cyclophosphamide, with similar efficacy in recent clinical trials.

# References

1. Barut K, Sahin S, Kasapcopur O. Pediatric vasculitis. *Curr Opin Rheumatol*. 2016;**28**: 29–38.

2. Sönmez HE, Armağan B, Ayan G, et al. Polyarteritis nodosa: lessons from 25 years of experience. *Clin Exp Rheumatol*. 2019;**37** Suppl 117(2): 52–56.

3. Navon Elkan P, Pierce SB, Segel R, et al. Mutant adenosine deaminase 2 in a polyarteritis nodosa vasculopathy. *N Engl J Med*. 2014;**370**(10): 921–931.

4. Sahin S, Adrovic A, Barut K, et al. Clinical, imaging and genotypical features of three deceased and five surviving cases with ADA2 deficiency. *Rheumatol Int* 2018;**38**(1): 129–136.

5. Sahin S, Adrovic A, Kasapcopur O. A monogenic autoinflammatory disease with fatal vasculitis: deficiency of adenosine deaminase 2. *Curr Opin Rheumatol*. 2020;**32**(1): 3–14.

# 1.2.b.2 Necrotizing Vasculitis: Churg–Strauss Syndrome (Eosinophilic Granulomatosis with Polyangiitis) and Stroke

Klearchos Psychogios

## Case Presentation

A 65-year-old female was admitted to the emergency department due to right arm paresis of sudden onset. The patient's medical history was remarkable for asthma, treated for more than seven years, and hypothyroidism.

On presentation her temperature was 36.6°C, heart rate, 75 bpm and blood pressure, 130/80 mmHg. Neurological examination revealed a psychomotor retardation, mild dysarthria, right mild central facial paresis, severe paresis of the right arm and mild paresis of the right leg (NIHSS 6). Brain MRI revealed acute embolic infarcts affecting multiple vascular territories (bilateral anterior, middle and posterior cerebral arteries) (Figure 1.2.7) and chronic sinusitis (Figure 1.2.8).

MR and CT angiography of intracranial vessels was normal. High-sensitivity troponin-T was increased at 958.7 (<14 pg/ml). Transthoracic echocardiography (TTE) and transoesophageal echocardiography (TEE) were normal. A coronary angiography was performed and revealed no stenoses. Due to the continuous elevation of the cardiac enzymes (troponin reached 1558 pg/ml) during the next day, we performed a cardiac MRI, which showed signs of myocarditis. The white blood cell count was $20.6 \times 10^9$/l with remarkable eosinophilia ($9 \times 10^9$ cells/l), which continued to rise over the next two days. There were also elevated ESR (57mm/1 h) and IgE at 752 (<100 IU/ml). A lumbar puncture was performed with a normal CSF examination. Blood and stool cultures screening for parasites were negative. Toxocariasis and human immunodeficiency serology were negative. Antiphospholipid antibodies, antinuclear antibodies, P-ANCA and C-ANCA were also negative. Bone marrow aspiration and biopsy showed immunomorphological findings compatible with idiopathic hyper-eosinophilic syndrome (HES). Peripheral blood fluorescent in situ hybridization for PDGFRA, PDGFRB, FGFR1 and karyotype were negative. A CT scan of the lungs showed only signs of atypical pneumonic infiltration. During the hospitalization, our patient experienced a painful rash over both lower limbs (Figure 1.2.9).

Considering the coexistence of acute brain infarction in multiple arterial territories, eosinophilia, skin rash and heart involvement, the differential diagnosis includes idiopathic hyper-eosinophilic syndrome (HES) and autoimmune disease (Churg–Strauss syndrome). These two syndromes have many overlapping features,[1] and a careful differential diagnosis is necessary in patients with multiorgan dysfunction in the presence of sustained eosinophilia (>1500 cells/mm$^3$) for more than six consecutive months. However, HES is mostly a diagnosis of exclusion. The simultaneous presence of a long-standing history of asthma

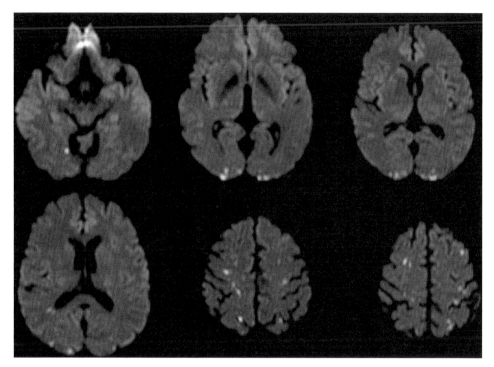

**Figure 1.2.7** Diffusion-weighted magnetic resonance imaging revealed cortical and subcortical acute infarcts in multiple arterial territories of both hemispheres (bilateral anterior, middle and posterior cerebral arteries).

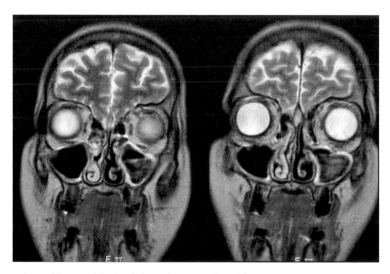

**Figure 1.2.8** Coronal T2 MRI of the head showed sinusitis of the left maxillary sinus as well as thickening of the nasal mucosa.

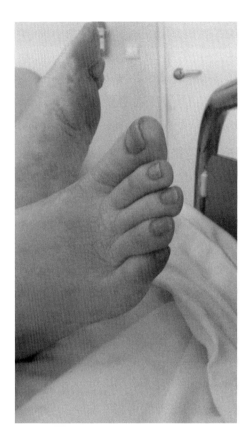

**Figure 1.2.9** Purpuric rash over the fourth and fifth toe of both lower limbs.

and chronic sinusitis made Churg–Strauss syndrome the most possible diagnosis, and this was further confirmed by the results of a skin biopsy, which revealed small-vessel eosinophilic vasculitis.[2] The patient was treated with anticoagulants, corticosteroids (1 g methylprednisolone iv for three days followed by per os prednisolone 1mg/kg/d which was then slowly tapered down), and monthly infusions of cyclophosphamide (700 mg/m²). The eosinophil count immediately returned to normal, and the patient had a good neurological recovery.

## Case Discussion

Eosinophilic granulomatosis with polyangiitis (EGPA, previously named Churg–Strauss syndrome) is a form of necrotizing vasculitis occurring in patients with asthma and eosinophilia. Histopathology of tissue biopsy specimens consists of three main elements: fibrinoid necrosis of small- to medium-sized vessel walls, eosinophil-rich infiltrates and granuloma formations in connective tissue and vessel walls; even so, these types of lesions are found simultaneously in less than 20% of EGPA patients.

EGPA shares clinicopathological features with other ANCA-vasculitides like microscopic polyangiitis (MPA) and granulomatosis with polyangiitis (GPA–Wegener granulomatosis). However, ANCA are positive in almost 30–40% of EGPA patients, with a perinuclear (p-ANCA) fluoroscopic staining pattern caused by antibodies directed against myeloperoxidase (anti-MPO) on enzyme-linked immunosorbent assay (ELISA). New insights into the disease tend to further separate EGPA into two major subsets according to the ANCA status[3]: a subset of ANCA-positive patients sharing features of vasculitis (with the most prominent clinical features being glomerulonephritis and mononeuritis multiplex), and a subset of ANCA-negative patients clinically characterized by tissue eosinophilic infiltration, resulting in fibrotic organ damage (especially cardiomyopathy). Recent genome-wide association studies have lent genetic support to this distinction.[4]

EGPA has traditionally been described to evolve in three phases: a prodromal phase with asthma and rhinitis-sinusitis that may last many years, an eosinophilic phase characterized by marked eosinophilia and organ involvement and finally a vasculitic phase. Clinical manifestations range from general symptoms like fever, arthralgias, myalgias and loss of weight to involvement of virtually any organ system in the body. Nervous system involvement is usual and mainly concerns the peripheral nerves in 50–75% of EGPA patients. Mononevritis multiplex is the most frequent finding, followed by peripheral neuropathy. Mononevritis presentation typically involves the common peroneal, internal popliteal, ulnar and, to a lesser degree, radial and median nerves. The central nervous system is affected in almost 5% of patients. A large French study[5] has grouped EGPA-related CNS manifestations into four neurological pictures: cerebral ischemic lesions, intracerebral/subarachnoid hemorrhages, cranial palsies and loss of visual acuity. Optic nerve and central retinal artery involvement may be a specific characteristic of EGPA compared to GPA and MPA.

Ischemic stroke is the most frequent CNS complication of the disease. In all reported cases, three possible mechanisms of stroke have been proposed: cardioembolism, a vasculitic process and direct eosinophilic infiltration. Cardiac endothelial injury results in fibrosis and thrombosis of endocardiac surfaces.[6] In the early stages of this process, multiple microthrombi lead to a multifocal distal field, and subcortical (border-zone) and cortical embolization of the brain, even though echocardiography may not confirm any highly embolic cardiac source. In such patients it is important to perform a cardiac MRI, as it seems to be a more sensitive tool for assessing heart involvement. Several types of cardiac complications have been described: eosinophilic vasculitis, pericarditis, myocarditis, cardiomyopathies, conduction abnormalities and intracavitary thrombus.[7] One other possible mechanism is a microscopic in situ thromboembolism due to the thrombogenic potential of the eosinophils. Eosinophilic cationic protein (ECP) has been shown to activate the intrinsic coagulation pathway through binding to the Hageman factor. Other studies have also demonstrated that ECP could interfere with endogenous heparan sulfate and reduce antithrombin III activity.[8] Cerebral vasculitis has long been hypothesized, but only recently was there an autopsy study[9] of an EGPA patient that documented vasculitis accompanied by eosinophil infiltration of the parenchymal small arteries, in the setting of systemic eosinophilic polyangiitis that included the brain. This study confirms that all the aforementioned mechanisms may coexist in the same patient.

Diagnosis of EGPA remains mostly clinical. Organ biopsy is not always helpful, because the simultaneous presence of the characteristic types of lesions is uncommon. At least four of the six classification criteria of the American College of Rheumatology criteria[2] are needed in order to establish a diagnosis: 1. asthma, 2. eosinophilia (>10% of white blood cell count), 3. mononeuropathy or polyneuropathy, 4. non-fixed pulmonary infiltrates, 5. paranasal sinus abnormality and 6. extravascular eosinophils demonstrated in tissue biopsies (Table 1.2.1). Differential diagnosis comprises primary CNS angiitis, other systemic

**Table 1.2.1** American College of Rheumatology classification criteria for Churg–Strauss Syndrome[2]

| Criterion | Definition |
| --- | --- |
| Asthma | History of wheezing or diffuse high-pitched rales on expiration |
| Eosinophilia | Eosinophilia >10% on white blood cell differential count |
| Mononeuropathy or polyneuropathy | Development of mononeuropathy, multiple mononeuropathies or polyneuropathy (i.e., glove/stocking distribution) attributable to systemic vasculitis |
| Pulmonary infiltrates, non-fixed | Migratory or transitory pulmonary infiltrates on radiographs (not including fixed infiltrates), attributable to systemic vasculitis |
| Paranasal sinus abnormality | History of acute or chronic paranasal sinus pain or tenderness or radiographic opacification of the paranasal sinuses |
| Extravascular eosinophils | Biopsy including artery, arteriole or venule showing accumulations of eosinophils in extravascular areas |

**Table 1.2.2** Five-Factor-Score (FFS) for assessment of prognosis of eosinophilic granulomatosis with polyangiitis (EGPA)

| FFS (Guillevin 1996) | FFS (2009 revision) |
| --- | --- |
| Proteinuria greater than 1 g/day | Age >65 years |
| Gastrointestinal bleeding, perforation, infarction and/or pancreatitis | Gastrointestinal involvement: bowel perforation, bleeding and pancreatitis |
| Renal insufficiency (with creatinemia >1.58 mg/dl or 140 μmol/l) | Renal insufficiency (with creatinemia > 150 μmol/L) |
| Central nervous system involvement | Myocardial involvement |
| Cardiomyopathy | Ear, nose and throat (ENT) involvement |
| Each item is accorded +1 point. Scores of 0, 1 and 2 were associated with five-year mortality rates of 12, 26 and 46%, respectively | Each of the first four items is accorded +1 point. ENT manifestations are associated with a better outcome (−1 point). An FFS of 0, 1 or 2 is associated with five-year mortality rates of 9, 21 or 40%, respectively |

vasculitides (especially polyarteritis nodosa and GPA) and hypereosinophilic syndrome, as highlighted in the present case report.

CNS involvement in EGPA patients was among the poor prognostic factors in the original Five-Factor Score (FFS) (Table 1.2.2), which is a useful tool for guiding treatment decisions. A more recent univariate analysis of prognostic factors in a large cohort of systemic necrotizing vasculitides patients, which included 230 EGPA patients, did not confirm a statistically significant association of nervous system involvement with poorer outcomes. Consequently, nervous system involvement was excluded from the revised 2009 FFS criteria (Table 5.2).[10] However, this result could be due to the small sample size of patients with CNS manifestations. Given the rarity and the detrimental impact on quality of life and mortality, stroke (especially in association with cardiomyopathy) should be considered a negative prognostic factor and therefore treatment in these cases should be more aggressive in order to achieve clinical remission as quickly as possible.

EGPA is not an absolute contraindication for intravenous thrombolysis administration in the acute setting, even though vessel-wall abnormalities due to vasculitis could predispose for secondary hemorrhagic conversion. In the case of large-vessel occlusion there is a paucity of literature data. Mechanical thrombectomy should be considered carefully after balancing the risk:benefit ratio. Secondary stroke prevention may include antiplatelets or anticoagulants, whereas the mainstay of treatment is the combination of corticosteroids and immunosuppressants. Corticosteroids are very effective in rapidly achieving a decrease in the eosinophilia burden and tissue infiltrates. A three-day pulse of intravenous methylprednisolone may be followed by 1 g/kg/d prednisone per os. Induction therapy with cyclophosphamide pulses (600 to 750 mg/m$^2$) for 6–12 months is the preferred choice because of the high efficacy and fewer side effects compared to oral administration. After remission, maintenance therapy with a less-toxic immunosuppressant like azathioprine or methotrexate is important. In refractory cases, plasma exchange, intravenous immunoglobulin (IV-IG), tumor necrosis factor (TNF) inhibitors and rituximab could be an alternative therapeutic choice.

# References

1. Thomson CC, Tager AM, Weller PF. More than your average wheeze. *N Engl J Med.* 2002;**346**: 438–442.

2. Masi AT, Hunder GG, Lie JT, et al. The American College of Rheumatology 1990 criteria for the classification of Churg-Strauss syndrome (allergic granulomatosis and angiitis). *Arthritis Rheum.* 1990;**33**: 1094–1100.

3. Sinico RA, DiToma L, Maggiore U, et al. Prevalence and clinical significance of antineutrophil cytoplasmic antibodies in Churg–Strauss syndrome. *Arthritis Rheum.* 2005;**52**: 2926–2935.

4. European Vasculitis Genetics Consortium, Lyons PA, Peters JE, Alberici F, et al. Genome-wide association study of eosinophilic granulomatosis with polyangiitis reveals genomic loci stratified by ANCA status. *Nat Commun.* 2019;**10**(1): 5120.

5. French Vasculitis Study Group (FVSG), André R, Cottin V, Saraux JL, et al. Central nervous system involvement in eosinophilic granulomatosis with polyangiitis (Churg-Strauss): Report of 26 patients and review of the literature. *Autoimmun Rev.* 2017;**16**(9): 963–969.

6. Sarazin M, Caumes E, Cohen A, Amarenco P. Multiple microembolic border zone brain infarctions and endomyocardial fibrosis in idiopathic hypereosinophilic syndrome and in *Schistosoma mansoni* infestation. *J Neurol Neurosurg Psychiatry.* 2004;**75**(2): 305–307.

7. Bhagirath KM, Paulson K, Ahmadie R, et al. Clinical utility of cardiac magnetic resonance imaging in Churg-Strauss syndrome: case report and review of the literature. *Rheumatol Int.* 2009;**29**(4): 445–449.

8. Ames PR, Roes L, Lupoli S, et al. Thrombosis in Churg-Strauss syndrome: Beyond vasculitis? *Br J Rheumatol.* 1996;**35**: 1181–1183.

9. Hira K, Shimura H, Kamata R, et al. Multiple cerebral infarction diagnosed as Eosinophilic Granulomatosis with Polyangiitis by autopsy. *BMC Neurol.* 2019;**19**(1): 288.

10. French Vasculitis Study Group (FVSG), Guillevin L, Pagnoux C, Seror R, et al. The Five-Factor Score revisited: assessment of prognoses of systemic necrotizing vasculitides based on the French Vasculitis Study Group (FVSG) cohort. *Medicine (Baltimore).* 2011;**90**(01): 19–27.

# 1.2.c.1 Granulomatous Vasculitis: Wegener Granulomatosis

Amra Adrovic, Mehmet Yildiz, Ayten Aliyeva, Ozgur Kasapcopur

## Case Report

A 16-year-old female patient was admitted to hospital due to fatigue, myalgia, weight loss and night sweats lasting for 10 days. First, she was seen by a family medicine specialist who prescribed an antipyretic and antibiotics, but there was no response. In the control evaluation the patient appeared pale with livedo reticularis of the lower extremities. In the laboratory examination, she had elevated acute phase markers: CRP 15 mg/dl, ESR 96 mm/h. She had leukocytosis (WBC 14,000/mm$^3$) with a left shift, mild anemia (Hgb 10.8 g/dl), thrombocytosis (PLT 460,000/mm$^3$) and normal biochemical parameters, including markers of renal function. The patient was referred to pediatric rheumatology.

At the time of admission, the patient was subfebrile (37.4 °C), with mild tachycardia (110 beats/min). Due to a history of systemic symptoms, elevated acute phase markers and cutaneous signs of vasculitis (livedo reticularis), the patient was hospitalized for further evaluation and treatment. On the second day of hospitalization, she developed acute right hemiparesis, dysarthria and right facial droop. Cranial computerized tomography was performed, which revealed multiple bilateral lesions consistent with acute intracranial hemorrhage. The cranial MRI showed restricted diffusion in the left internal capsule which was in concordance with clinical signs of acute stroke.

When the detailed medical history of the patient was obtained, it revealed recurrent attacks of bronchitis, which were treated with single doses of steroids and bronchodilator inhalers.

Together with the previously mentioned acute phase markers and routine biochemical parameters, a work-up for possible antineutrophil cytoplasm antibodies (ANCA)-associated vasculitis (AAV) was performed. It revealed significantly high c-ANCA (1:1560) and proteinase 3 antibody titers (> 8.0, reference: 0.0–0.3 AI), whereas myeloperoxidase antibody was negative. Chest X-ray and high-resolution computerized tomography (HRCT) revealed lesions that were compatible with granulomas located in both lungs (Figures 1.2.10–1.2.12).

A diagnosis of granulomatosis with polyangiitis (GPA) was confirmed and treatment with high doses of glucocorticoids in combination with cyclophosphamide was started. The glucocorticoids (30 mg/kg/day for five days) were given as the induction part of the treatment together with pulse doses of cyclophosphamide (1 g/m$^2$/month for six months). Rituximab was added to the treatment (375 mg/m$^2$/week for four weeks) since the patient was considered to have life-threating complications from the

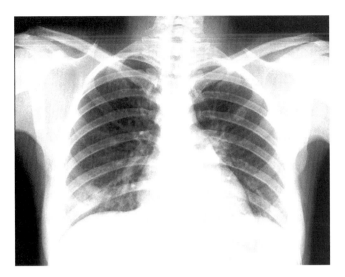

**Figure 1.2.10** Thoracic X-ray of patient with granulomatosis with polyangiitis.

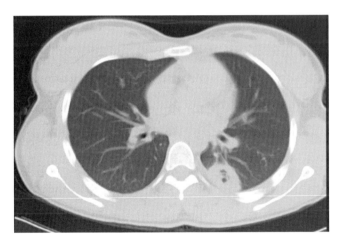

**Figure 1.2.11** Thoracic high-resolution computerized tomography of patient with granulomatosis with polyangiitis (granulomatous lesion in the left lung of patient).

underlying disease. The patient responded promptly with regression of neurological findings, decline in acute phase markers and significant improvement in the patient's general condition. A hematologist was consulted and aspirin 100 mg/day p.o. was added.

After remission was achieved, a low dose of glucocorticoids in combination with azathioprine was continued as a maintenance phase of treatment.

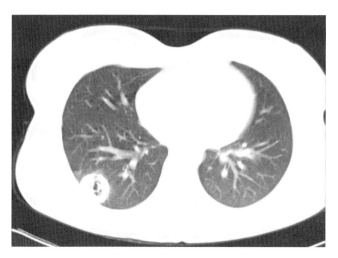

**Figure 1.2.12** Thoracic high-resolution computerized tomography of patient with granulomatosis with polyangiitis (granulomatous lesion in the right lung of patient).

**Patient with signs or a history of unexplained systemic inflammation**

Pyrexia of unknown origin
Vasculitic skin rash
PNS or CNS involvement
Unexplained arthritis, myalgia, serositis
Unexplained pulmonary, gastrointestinal, cardiovascular or renal disease

**Work up**

**Specific organ involvement**

**Tissue biopsy** (e.g. skin, nasal or sinus, kidney, sural nerve, lung, liver, gut, temporal artery, brain)

**Neuropathy:** nerve conduction studies

**Cerebral involvement:** MRI/MRA of brain and cerebral contrast angiography

**Organ-specific auto-antibodies** (e.g. ASCAs, brain/neuronal specific auto-antibodies)

**Differential Diagnosis–Infection**

Tuberculosis screen
PCR for viral infection (e.g. CMV, EBV, enterovirus, adenovirus, VZV, HBV, HCV)
Serology for HIV, Rickettsiae, Borrelia burgdorferi, Mycoplasma
Viral serology for HBV, HCV, Parvovirus B19

**GPA**

ELISA for ANCA (MPO and PR3) (IFA not sufficient)
Histopathological confirmation highly diserable
Target tissue biopsy for diagnosis and staging
Sinus imaging (CT/MRI) helpful/Chest X-ray/HRCT indicated
Pulmonary function test (including DLCO) in lung involvement
Cranial MRI/MRA in case of neurological symptoms

*Haematology and acute phase reactants:*
Full blood count, ESR, CRP,
Peripheral blood smear

*Basic biochemistry:*
Renal function, liver function, CPK, LDH
Urine dipstick test of urine

*Infection:*
Routine infection screen
Anti-streptolysin O antibody titre
and/or anti DNase
VZV antibody status

*Immunological tests:*
ANA, ENA antibodies, ANCA, antiphospholipid
antibodies
Immunoglobulins IgG/IgA/IgM/IgE
Complement (C3, C4)
RF (if nephritis or interstitial lung disease)
GBM-antibody

*Radiological/other:*
Chest X-ray
Doppler ultrasound scan
ECG; echocardiography
Digital clinical photography of lesions
Cranial MRI/MRA

## Case Discussion

Granulomatosis with polyangiitis (GPA), eosinophilic granulomatosis with polyangiitis and microscopic polyangiitis represent the main conditions classified as antineutrophil cytoplasm antibodies (ANCA)-associated vasculitis (AAV). GPA, previously known as Wegener's granulomatosis, is a necrotizing vasculitis, predominantly affecting small vessels. The annual incidence of GPA is considered to be 0.2 to 1.2 per 100,000. Although pretty rare in the pediatric population, GPA shows peaks in adolescence and middle age (40–60 years), predominantly appearing among females.[1,2]

The disease is characterized by the triad of granulomatous inflammation in the both the upper and lower respiratory tracts and pauci-immune necrotizing glomerulonephritis. Non-specific systemic complaints, including fatigue, weight loss, fever and malaise, are common at disease onset. Otolaryngologic, pulmonary and renal findings are most common in the physical examination.[1,2] In a study by Bohm et al.,[3] nasal septum perforation, saddle nose, ear chondritis, subglottic stenosis, coarsening and stridor are the most frequent otorhinolaryngological findings. Signs of lower respiratory tract involvement include wheezing, expiratory dyspnea, and pulmonary nodules and cavities.

Peripheral nervous system involvement is the most common type of neurologic complication. Central nervous system (CNS) disorders are rare, with stroke being an unexpected complication. Different studies from the literature have reported the frequency of neurological involvement to be 22–34% of GPA patients, with cerebrovascular events accounting approximately 4%.[4] CNS involvement is extremely rare in the pediatric population, compared to adults. According to A Registry for Childhood Vasculitis:e-entru (ARChiVe), CNS features were present in 16/65 (24%) of pediatric patients with GPA, severe headache in 9/65 (13.8%) and dizziness 8/65 (12.3%) patients. None of the patients in this cohort had signs of an acute vascular event or stroke.[5]

The disease prognosis depends on timely diagnosis and appropriate treatment. If untreated, the disease is characterized by a mortality rate as high as 90%.[1,2] The main treatment modality consists of intensive immunosuppression for the induction of disease remission, followed by long-term maintenance treatment.

Glucocorticoids in combination with cyclophosphamide and rituximab have proven to be effective in the induction of remission. A combination of lower doses of glucocorticoids and disease-modifying antirheumatic drugs (azathioprine) is reserved for the maintenance phase aimed to prevent relapses of disease.[1,2] There is no particular treatment for CNS involvement in GPA. The routine treatment algorithm proposed for GPA is considered appropriate since CNS involvement represents an organ-threating manifestation (including stroke). Antiplatelet agents and/or anticoagulation may be indicated in the case of a vascular event.

## Conclusion

Stroke represents an unexpected but significant complication of GPA. Prompt diagnosis and treatment are essential to prevent further sequelae. Patients with signs of upper/lower respiratory tract inflammation, renal involvement and newly developed neurological signs require urgent evaluation for a diagnosis of GPA.

# References

1. Barut K, Sahin S, Kasapcopur O. Pediatric vasculitis. *Curr Opin Rheumatol.* 2016;**28**: 29–38.

2. De Graeff N, Groot N, Brogan P, et al. European consensus-based recommendations for the diagnosis and treatment of rare paediatric vasculitides – The SHARE initiative. *Rheumatology (Oxford).* 2019;**58**: 656–671.

3. Bohm M, Gonzalez Fernandez MI, Ozen S, et al. Clinical features of childhood granulomatosis with polyangiitis (Wegener's granulomatosis). *Pediatr Rheumatol Online J.* 2014;**12**: 18.

4. De Luna G, Terrier B, Kaminsky P, et al. Central nervous system involvement of granulomatosis with polyangiitis: clinical–radiological presentation distinguishes different outcomes. *Rheumatology.* 2015;**54**: 424–432.

5. Morishita K, Li SC, Muscal E, et al. Assessing the performance of the Birmingham Vasculitis Activity Score at diagnosis for children with antineutrophilcytoplasmic antibody-associated vasculitis in A Registry for Childhood Vasculitis (ARChiVe). J *Rheumatol.* 2012;**39**: 1088–1094.

# 1.2.c.2 Granulomatous Vasculitis: Lymphomatoid Granulomatosis

Phillip Ferdinand, Christine Roffe

## Case Presentation

A 50-year-old male presented to the emergency department with a four-month history of progressive confusion, right-sided weakness and problems walking. On examination he was confused but alert. He knew his age, but not the month. He had mild right hemiparesis affecting the arm and leg, and gait apraxia. His temperature, blood pressure, oxygenation and pulse rate were all within normal range. Full blood count, renal, liver and bone profiles were unremarkable. C-reactive protein was slightly elevated at 8 mg/l and erythrocyte sedimentation rate was increased at 32 mm/h. Chest radiography was normal.

Computed tomography (CT) and subsequent magnetic resonance imaging (MRI) of the head with contrast showed multiple T2 and fluid-attenuated inversion recovery (FLAIR) lesions with surrounding edema, together with numerous punctate and linear enhancing regions in the white matter in bilateral frontal and parietal lobes and also the basal ganglia. There were also bilateral lacunar infarcts.

A lumbar puncture was performed and cerebrospinal fluid (CSF) analysis showed an elevated protein count at 185 mg/dl and 250 white blood cells on microscopy with 98% lymphocytes. Polymerase chain reaction (PCR) for adenovirus, varicella, Epstein–Barr virus (EBV), cytomegalovirus, acid fast bacilli and CSF culture were all negative. CT of the thorax, abdomen and pelvis showed no evidence of primary malignant disease or widespread lymphadenopathy. Given the negative systemic results and potential differential diagnosis that included lymphoproliferative disease, malignancy, sarcoidosis and vasculitis, a brain biopsy was performed.

Histological analysis revealed an angiocentric and angiodestructive T cell infiltrate with large areas of necrosis. Many atypical cells were seen and greater than 50 were Epstein–Barr virus-encoded small RNAs (EBERs) positive by in-situ hybridization leading to a diagnosis of grade 3 lymphomatoid granulomatosis. He was referred to the local hem-oncologist for specialist treatment and ongoing management.

# Diagnostic Algorithm

Lymphomatoid Granulomatosis

EBV-mediated lymphoproliferative disorder; angiocentric and angiodestructive features on histology

**Age** = 4th–6th decade; Gender = M:F 2:1

**Systems affected:** Lung (>90%), skin, liver, CNS, upper respiratory tract, GI tract (isolated disease possible)

**Presenting CNS features:** confusion, dementia, ataxia, paresis, seizures or cranial nerve signs. Often normal blood investigations

**CSF examination:** may show increased protein, lymphocytosis. EBV PCR result does not diagnose or rule out.

**CT and MRI with contrast:**

- Multiple T2/FLAIR parenchymal lesion (cerebral/cerebellar white matter, basal ganglia, brainstem, corpus callosum)
- Punctate and linear enhance suggestive of vessel wall/perivascular space involvement.
- Leptomeningeal cranial nerve enhancement
- Large masses/aneurysms

**Differential Diagnosis**

- Other lymphoproliferative disorder
- Disseminated malignancy
- Sarcoidosis
- Vasculitis

- Consider CT thorax, abdomen and pelvis to exclude primary lesion and widespread lymphadenopathy
- If normal (or no easy biopsy target) – proceed to brain biopsy

**Histology** – angiocentric and angiodestructive infiltrate; atypical B cells; in situ hybridization to prove EBERs positivity

**Grading:** Grade 1: <5 EBERs positive cells; Grade 2: 5–50; Grade 3: >50 with necrosis

**Treatment:** requires specialist haemo-oncologist input; high grade treated with chemo/immunotherapy; success reported with interferon and steroid at lower grades; reports of spontaneous resolution.

M: Male; F: Female; CNS: Central nervous system; GI: Gastrointestinal; CSF: Cerebrospinal fluid; EBV: Epstein Barr virus; PCR: polymerase chain reaction; CT: Computed tomography; MRI: Magnetic resonance imaging; FLAIR: fluid-attenuated inversion recovery; EBERs: Epstein–Barr virus-encoded small RNAs

# Case Discussion

First described by Liebow in 1972,[1] lymphomatoid granulomatosis (LG) is an angiocentric and angiodestructive lymphoproliferative disease[2] that is an extremely rare cause of stroke. Presentation is usually within the fourth to sixth decades with a median age of 46–48 years. Males are affected more than females in a 2:1 ratio.[3,4] Paediatric cases have been described but this is uncommon. Risk factors include impaired immune function including high-dose chemotherapy, immunomodulatory therapy (including methotrexate and azathioprine), post solid-organ transplant, HIV and Wiskott–Aldrich syndrome.[4,5,6] If there is no clear suggestion in the history then work-up should be performed to look for evidence of immunocompromise. However, the majority of cases do not report or are not found to have any evidence of overt immunodeficiency.

The disorder is driven by EBV, with which 90% of the world is infected.[7] The gamma herpesvirus has two phases of infection, firstly an acute lytic phase (productive phase) during which B lymphocytes are infected via binding to the CD 21 surface receptor and HLA Class II molecules.[7] This phase is asymptomatic in most subjects. In the subsequent latent or non-productive phase the virus is regulated and controlled by cytotoxic T lymphocytes and natural killer cells. EBV is able to evade this immune response by restricting is genomic expression to a limited number of nuclear antigens, latent membrane proteins and small non-coding RNAs. There are three well-defined latency patterns according to the pattern of expression, with LG reported to show type II or III patterns.[2,5,7]

Histological analysis shows angiocentric and angiodestructive infiltration of mainly reactive T-lymphocytes and histiocytes and occasionally plasma cells. These are interspersed with neoplastic EBV-positive B cells. EBV-positive cells are large, atypical and express CD20, LMP-1 and EBERs.[7] Intimal thickening and necrosis are also seen alongside the hallmark angiocentric and angiodestructive changes. Despite the name LG is not a granulomatous disorder.[8]

LG has three grades based on the number of EBV-positive large B cells found in histology. Grade 1 LG encompasses an angiocentric polymorphous lymphohistiocytic infiltrate with minimal atypia, very few large atypical lymphoid cells and no necrosis. Rarely there may be no EBV-positive cells. The number of EBV-positive cells detected by EBER is less than five per high-power field (HPF). Grade 2 LG contains occasional large atypical cells and more necrosis, with 5–50 EBER-positive cells per HPF. Grade 3 LG shows many large atypical cells and necrosis. More than 50 EBER-positive cells are detected.[3,6] In large necrotic lesions the number of positive cells may be low as a result of the necrosis, thus this staging method is considered inaccurate by some in such histological samples.[9,10]

The main organ affected is the lungs in well over 90% of cases. Coexisting extra-pulmonary disease occurs in up to a third, with the skin in up 50%, kidneys in up to 40%, central nervous system (CNS) in up to a third and the liver in up to 29%.[11] Upper respiratory tract, gastrointestinal tract and peripheral nervous system involvement has also been reported. The bone marrow, lymph nodes and spleen are rarely affected and involvement of these areas should prompt the clinician to consider an alternative lymphoproliferative disorder. There are several case reports of isolated extra-pulmonary disease, including the central nervous system, but these are rare in the context of the spectrum of presentation of the disease.

The lungs are generally the site of initial symptoms, which include cough, dyspnoea and chest pain.[2,4,5] Skin manifestations include cutaneous and dermal nodules, maculopapular rashes, macular erythema and ulcers.[8]

CNS involvement may present with any one or a combination of confusion, dementia, ataxia, paresis, seizures or cranial nerve signs.[5,12] Parkinsonism has also been reported.[13] Any clinical suspicion of LG should prompt examination and radiological investigation of lungs and skin for evidence of disease there.

Lymphopenia or leukocytosis may be seen, but the full blood count is normal in over 50% of cases. Half of the cases show polyclonal hypergammaglobulinemia.[3,9,14] CSF analysis may show raised protein count and lymphocytosis. Whilst a positive EBV PCR may add weighting to a diagnosis, it is not specific and a negative result does not exclude LG. Thus any suspicion of LG or any other CNS lymphoproliferative disorder should prompt further assessment.

Most knowledge of the radiological CNS manifestations of the disease comes from MRI imaging.[8] The commonest findings are small (with potential to coalesce), multiple focal parenchymal lesions, which have increased signal on FLAIR/T2 sequences and were located in at least one of the cerebral/cerebellar white matter, basal ganglion (BG), midbrain, brainstem and corpus callosum. Multiple punctate and linear enhancements can also be seen, which is thought to represent involvement of the vessel wall and peri-vascular spaces, as on follow up in one study these areas progressed to lacunar infarcts with cavities. Other findings include leptomeningeal and cranial nerve enhancement, intracranial masses and aneurysm formation.[8,15] Some of the imaging features are shared with sarcoidosis, lymphoma, or CNS vasculitis and, thus, in the absence of systemic disease and in a suitable patient, a biopsy should be performed to confirm diagnosis. PET/CT imaging may be useful in identifying disease as well, suitable biopsy targets and surveillance is not well established, however.[16]

Management must be in the hands of a hemo-oncologist with expertise in the treatment of lymphoproliferative disorders. Treatment over the years has varied – there are reports of subjects with minimal clinical symptoms, low-grade disease or on cessation of immunotherapy undergoing spontaneous remission.[17,18] Grade 1 or grade 2 lesions have been managed with interferon and corticosteroids, although the latter has the potential for aggressive rebound disease later in the clinical course. As Grade 3 closely resembles diffuse large B-cell lymphoma chemo/immunotherapy is often preferred.[6] Older studies have suggested poor prognostic features, including leukopenia, fever, young age and CNS involvement,[19,20] however reports suggest isolated CNS disease may have better outcomes than CNS disease as a result of systemic spread.[11]

# References

1. Liebow AA, Carrington CR, Friedman PJ. Lymphomatoid granulomatosis. *Hum Pathol.* 1972;**3**(4): 457–558.

2. Dunleavy K, Roschewski M, Wilson WH. Lymphomatoid granulomatosis and other Epstein-Barr virus associated lymphoproliferative processes. *Curr Hematol Malig Rep.* 2012;**7**(3): 208–215.

3. Song JY, Pittaluga S, Dunleavy K, et al. Lymphomatoid granulomatosis – a single institute experience: pathologic findings and clinical correlations. *Am J Surg Pathol.* 2015;**39**(2): 141–156.

4. Sukswai N, Lyapichev K, Khoury JD, Medeiros LJ. Diffuse large B-cell lymphoma variants: an update. *Pathology.* 2020;**52**(1): 53–67.

5. Dojcinov SD, Fend F, Quintanilla-Martinez L. EBV-positive lymphoproliferations of B-T-and NK-cell derivation in non-immunocompromised hosts. *Pathogens.* 2018;**7**(1): 28.

6. Melani C, Jaffe ES, Wilson WH. Pathobiology and treatment of lymphomatoid granulomatosis, a rare EBV-driven disorder. *Blood.* 2020;**135**(16): 1344–1352.

7. Roschewski M, Wilson WH. EBV-associated lymphomas in adults. *Best Pract Res Clin Haematol.* 2012;**25**(1): 75–89.

8. Patsalides AD, Atac G, Hedge U, et al. Lymphomatoid granulomatosis: abnormalities of the brain at MR imaging. *Radiology.* 2005;**237**(1): 265–273.

9. Katzenstein AL, Doxtader E, Narendra S. Lymphomatoid granulomatosis: insights gained over 4 decades. *Am J Surgical Pathol.* 2010;**34**(12): e35–e48.

10. Rezk SA, Weiss LM. EBV–associated lymphoproliferative disorders: update in classification. *Surg Pathol Clin.* 2019;**12**(3): 745–770.

11. Kim JY, Jung KC, Park SH, Choe JY, Kim JE. Primary lymphomatoid granulomatosis in the central nervous system: A report of three cases. *Neuropathology*. 2018;**38**(4): 331–336.

12. Koeller KK, Shih RY. Extranodal lymphoma of the central nervous system and spine. *Radiol Clin North Am*. 2016;**54** (4): 649–671.

13. Oliveras C, D'Olhaberriague L, Garcia J, Matias-Guiu X. Parkinsonism as first manifestation of lymphomatoid granulomatosis. *J Neurol Neurosurg Psychiatry*. 1988;**51**(7): 999.

14. Borie R, Wislez M, Antoine M, Cadranel J. Lymphoproliferative disorders of the lung. *Respiration*. 2017;**94**(2): 157–175.

15. Tateishi U, Terae S, Ogata A, et al. MR imaging of the brain in lymphomatoid granulomatosis. *Am J Neuroradiol*. 2001;**22** (7): 1283–1290.

16. Yang M, Rosenthal AC, Ashman JB, Craig FE. The role and pitfall of F18-FDG PET/ CT in surveillance of high grade pulmonary lymphomatoid granulomatosis. *Curr Probl Diagn Radiol*. 2021;**50**(3): 443–449.

17. Zhang YX, Ding MP, Zhang T, et al. Lymphomatoid granulomatosis with CNS involvement can lead to spontaneous remission: case study. *CNS Neurosci Ther*. 2013;**19**(7): 536.

18. Aiko N, Sekine A, Umeda S, et al. The spontaneous regression of grade 3 methotrexate-related lymphomatoid granulomatosis: a case report and literature review. *Intern Med*. 2018;**57**(21): 3163–3167.

19. Tang VK, Vijhani P, Cherian SV, et al. Primary pulmonary lymphoproliferative neoplasms. *Lung India*. 2018;**35**(3): 220–230.

20. Katzenstein AL, Carrington CB, Liebow AA: Lymphomatoid granulomatosis: a clinicopathologic study of 152 cases. *Cancer*. 1979;**43**: 360–373.

# 1.2.d.1 Vasculitis with Prominent Eye Movement: Susac Syndrome

Bengi Gül Türk, Sabahattin Saip

## Case Presentation

A 35-year-old man was referred with the complaints of gait instability and hearing loss. In August 2012, he had sudden hearing loss in the right ear. A few months later he developed gait instability. Considering the acute onset of the complaints, diffusion-weighted cranial imaging was performed to rule out any cerebrovascular events. Diffusion-weighted imaging was normal. However, his cranial MRI revealed multiple non-contrast-enhancing, T2-hyperintense lesions, mainly in the corpus callosum and periventricular-subcortical areas (Figure 1.2.13).

An audiogram was performed to explore the type of hearing loss, and sensorineural hearing loss was detected bilaterally. Lumbar puncture was performed for the differential diagnosis. Cerebrospinal fluid (CSF) total protein level was 173.2 mg/dl. Analysis of CSF showed a normal IgG index and absence of oligoclonal IgG bands. Susac syndrome (SS) or multiple sclerosis (MS) was suggested for the initial diagnosis. The patient was treated with intravenous methylprednisolone (IVMP) 1 g/day for five days, with continuation of oral prednisolone treatment for the following four weeks and a mild improvement was observed.

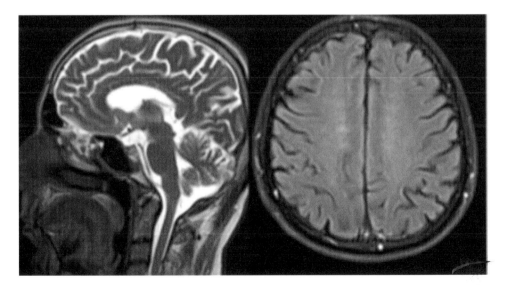

**Figure 1.2.13** Cranial MRI images revealing multiple non-contrast-enhancing, T2-hyperintense lesions in the corpus callosum and periventricular-subcortical areas.

One year after the first admission, he presented with hearing loss in the left ear. Cranial MRI revealed new contrast-enhancing lesions in the corpus callosum (Figure 1.2.14).

Sudden onset hearing loss in a young patient with callosal involvement suggested a diagnosis of SS. Therefore, fundus fluorescein angiography (FFA) was performed and branch retinal artery occlusion was detected (Figure 1.2.15).

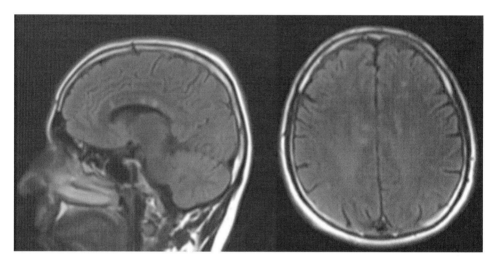

**Figure 1.2.14** Cranial MRI images revealing new T2-hyperintense, non-contrast-enhancing lesions in the corpus callosum.

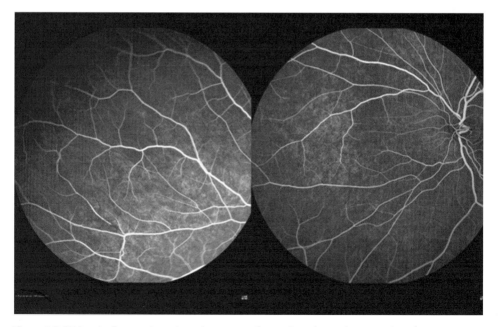

**Figure 1.2.15** Fundus fluorescein angiography images reflecting branch retinal artery occlusion.

Seven days of IVMP (1 g/day) treatment was initiated and the symptoms improved. In addition, 100 mg/day acetylsalicylic acid was administered against thrombosis. The patient was relapse-free for seven years without long-term maintenance therapy till the last follow-up.

# Diagnostic Algorithm

### Clinical suspicion of Susac syndrome/differential diagnosis

Age = 20–40 years; gender = F:M 3:1; classic triad = CNS involvement (60–100%), visual symptoms (40–50%), auditory symptoms (40–50%)

o **Cranial MRI**: In T2-weighted images; small, roundish, multifocal hyperintense lesions in the periventricular, subcortical and deep white matter areas, with at least one centrally located in the corpus callosum ("snowball" appearance). The callosal lesions are important for the diagnosis and they are accepted as pathognomonic signs for SS

o **Audiometry**: Bilateral sensorineural hearing loss, especially at low frequencies

o **Fundus fluorescein angiography (FFA)**: The gold standard for detecting "branch retinal artery occlusion (BRAO)" is FFA. BRAO is detected in 95% of patients.

# Case Discussion

Susac syndrome (SS) is an occlusive arteriolar disease, leading to infarcts in the retina, cochlea and brain. The classic triad of the disease consists of subacute encephalopathy, visual disturbances and hearing loss. Although the disease is most common in women between the ages of 20–40, it can be seen in both sexes between the ages of 10–60. It is observed three times more frequently in women than in men.[1,2]

Though the underlying etiological factors are not precisely known, it is accepted as an autoimmune disease causing endoteliopathy disturbing the microvasculature of the inner ear, retina and brain. Immune reactions, coagulopathy and vasospastic events are accepted as possible underlying factors that are implicated in the etiology of SS. It is hypothesized that antibodies against antiphospholipid and/or antiendothelial cells may have a part in endothelial cell injury. On the other hand, the presence of previous infections that could be triggering has also been proposed as the underlying cause.[3]

SS is classified as "monocyclic, polycyclic or chronic" according to the course of the disease. The most common is the monocyclic type.[2] The disease can manifest in many different clinical pictures. Loss of vision alone or with hearing loss can be the initial complaints. When there is CNS involvement, headache, change in personality, ataxia, confusion and dysarthria can be seen in the patients. Symptoms such as blind spots, light disturbance or visual field defects may appear due to obstruction of the retinal vessels in the eye. Branch retinal artery occlusion causes loss of vision, and is a very specific feature of the disease. In most patients, even without visual complaints, branch retinal artery occlusions were detected. Hearing loss, tinnitus, peripheral vertigo and sometimes dizziness occur as a result of obstruction of the inner ear vessels. Hearing loss may be sudden. Encephalopathy can sometimes mask the visual and auditory symptoms; therefore, it is not easy to catch the classic triad in all cases.[1,2,4,5]

The rarity and the clinical diversity of the disease can make cases challenging for clinicians to diagnose. Since there is a wide range of symptoms, it is essential to emphasize the importance of making a differential diagnosis with other neuropsychiatric, ophthalmologic and ear-related diseases.

There are no defined criteria for the diagnosis of SS. Diagnosis can be made based on the findings of brain magnetic resonance imaging (MRI), fundus fluorescein angiography (FFA) and audiometry.[6] On the audiogram, bilateral sensorineural hearing loss, especially at low frequencies, can be detected. FFA is useful to detect any obstruction of the branches of the retinal artery.[6] Brain MRI is one of the essential tools for SS diagnosis. In T2-weighted images, small, roundish, multifocal hyperintense lesions in the periventricular, subcortical and deep white matter areas with at least one centrally located in the corpus callosum ("snowball" appearance) can be observed. Callosal lesions are important for the diagnosis and are accepted as pathognomonic signs for SS. However, according to literature data, about 20% of patients do not have callosal lesions.[7]

There are no standardized treatment protocols for SS, as yet. Treatment is mainly based on expert recommendations. The symptoms of SS generally have a tendency to recover spontaneously. However, the course of the disease is not homogenous for each patient and cannot be predicted. There are cases in the literature where delayed treatment caused permanent neurological symptoms and severe hearing loss. Therefore, it is recommended to start treatment as soon as the diagnosis is made.

In the acute phase of the disease, high-dose corticosteroids (1000 mg/day IV methylprednisolone) for three to five days and oral prednisolone treatment for the following four weeks are recommended.[2] For patients who do not respond to this first-line treatment, plasmapheresis or IVIG can be chosen as an alternative in the acute phase.[8] If these treatment steps also fail, more aggressive immunosuppression with agents such as cyclophosphamide and rituxumab can be considered for appropriate cases.[5] It is also unclear how long immunosuppressive therapy should be continued. After providing clinical improvement at the acute stage of the disease, it is recommended to decrease prednisolone treatment over two- to four-week intervals and to switch to agents such as mycophenolate mofetil, methotrexate or azathioprine for long-term treatment.[4-9] If clinical stability has been maintained for about two years, discontinuation of treatment can be considered. The use of anti-aggregant agents such as acetylsalicylic acid is also recommended for all patients with SS to decrease the risk of thrombosis.[9]

# References

1. Dörr J, Krautwald S, Wildemann B, et al. Characteristics of Susac syndrome: a review of all reported cases. *Nat Rev Neurol.* 2013;9(6): 307–316.

2. Karahan SZ, Boz C, Saip S, et al. Susac syndrome: clinical characteristics, diagnostic findings and treatment in 19 cases. *Mult Scler Relat Disord.* 2019;33: 94–99.

3. García-Carrasco M, Jiménez-Hernández C, Jiménez-Hernández M, et al. Susac's syndrome: an update. *Autoimmun Rev.* 2011;10(9): 548–552.

4. Mateen FJ, Zubkoc AY, Muralidharan R, et al. Susac syndrome: clinical characteristics and treatment in 29 new cases. *Eur J Neurol.* 2012;**19**(6): 800–811.

5. Vodopivec I, Venna N, Rizzo 3rd JF, Prasad S. Clinical features, diagnostic findings, and treatment of Susac syndrome: a case series. *J Neurol Sci.* 2015;**357**(1–2): 50–57.

6. European Susac Consortium (EuSaC), Kleffner I, Dörr J, Ringelstein M, et al. Diagnostic criteria for Susac syndrome. *J Neurol Neurosurg Psychiatry.* 2016;**87**(12): 1287–1295.

7. Susac JO1, Murtagh FR, Egan RA, et al. MRI findings in Susac's syndrome. *Neurology.* 2003; **61**(12): 1783–1787.

8. Fox RJ, Costello F, Judkins AR, et al. Treatment of Susac syndrome with gamma globulin and corticosteroids. *J Neurol Sci.* 2006;**251**: 17–22.

9. Vishnevskia-Dai V, Chapman J, Sheinfeld R, et al. Susac syndrome: clinical characteristics, clinical classification, and long-term prognosis. *Medicine.* 2016;**95**(43): e5223.

# 1.2.d.2 Vasculitis with Prominent Eye Movement: Vogt–Koyanagi–Harada Disease

Cheryl Carcel

## Case Presentation

A 42-year-old Asian woman was admitted to the emergency department with doubling of vision. She reported a four-day history of fever, neck stiffness and dizziness.

On arrival, the patient was drowsy but easily rousable. Ear temperature was 39.2°C, heart rate, 86 beats/min, blood pressure, 120/60 mmHg, respiratory rate, 24 breaths/min with an oxygen saturation of 97% on room air. The chest was clear to percussion and auscultation. No murmurs were found on cardiac examination. The abdomen was soft and non-tender. The skin and hair showed no vitiligo, alopecia or poliosis. Visual and fundoscopic examinations were normal. Neurologic findings included cranial nerve III palsy and positive Brudzinski sign. The patient was pre-hypertensive and was on a low fat and low salt diet. There was no history of ocular trauma or surgery. The family history was positive for diabetes and hypertension.

Because an infectious etiology was entertained, a cranial computed tomography (CT) scan was performed to rule out increased intracranial pressure. The CT brain was normal. Cerebrospinal fluid (CSF) analysis showed 35 nucleated cells/mm$^3$ (89% lymphocytes), glucose 80 mg/dl, and protein 257 mg/dl. CSF flow cytometry did not reveal monoclonal lymphoproliferation. All infectious serologies were negative.

The patient was admitted and provided with supportive therapy. Two days later she complained of sudden bilateral blurring of vision. An ophthalmology consult was requested. Visual acuity was "counting fingers" on both eyes. Fundoscopic examination showed optic disc swelling and hyperemia with multiple yellowish deep round lesions and exudative retinal detachment. Further imaging studies: (1) fluorescein angiography (FA) found pinpoints and optic disc hyperfluorescence in the early phase with eventual coalescing of pinpoints, hyperfluorescence and contrast pooling in exudative retinal detachment areas, (2) FLAIR and T2-weighted imaging on magnetic resonance imaging (MRI) showed choroidal thickening and retinal detachment. The patient was diagnosed with incomplete Vogt–Koyanagi–Harada (VKH) disease and started on intravenous (IV) methylprednisolone 1000 mg per day, for three days, followed by a slow tapering of oral corticosteroids for three to six months. The doubling of vision and visual acuity improved after IV methylprednisolone. The patient will be closely followed up by the ophthalmology service.

# Diagnostic Algorithm

## Clinically Suspicious of VKH

- 20–50 years old
- Female
- Asian, Middle Eastern, Hispanic or Native American
- Flu-like symptoms with meningismus preceding acute blurring of vision
- Ocular disease, recurrent aseptic meningitis with or without focal neurologic findings
- Sunset glow fundus
- Poliosis, vitiligo, alopecia
- No history of ocular trauma or surgery

## Diagnostic Findings

- CSF pleocytosis
- MRI findings: bilateral, symmetric choroidal thickening, and retinal detachment with abnormal choroidal enhancement. The brain may have small, non-specific periventricular white matter[1]
- Fundus FA in acute phase: subretinal pooling, disc hyperfluorescence, window defects
- Ultrasonography: thickening of the posterior choroid, retinal detachment, vitreous opacity[2]

## Treatment[3]

- Consults with specialists: ophthalmologists, neurologists and dermatologists
- Early and aggressive treatment with systemic corticosteroids then continue with oral prednisolone for three to six months, occasionally up to one year
- Immunomodulatory therapy when systemic corticosteroids fail. For example, cyclosporine, tacrolimus, mycophenolate mofetil, azathioprine, cyclophosphamide or chlorambucil
- For anterior uveitis, topical corticosteroids are advised
- Ocular complications are common in the late stages. These include glaucoma, cataract and choroidal neovascularization. Close follow up with an ophthalmologist to manage these complications.

# Case Discussion

VKH disease is an idiopathic autoimmune disease primarily manifesting as bilateral, chronic and diffuse granulomatous panuveitis associated with auditory, neurological and integumentary findings. It has an acute onset that causes inflammation of organs with high melanocyte concentrations such as the eye, meninges, ear and skin.[4] VKH disease is uncommon, but is mostly seen in Asians, Middle Easterners, Hispanics and Native Americans. Most reports have found that women are affected more frequently than men. Most patients will be in the second to fifth decades of life at the onset of the disease; however, it can occur at any time between the first and eighth decades of life.[3]

There are four clinical stages described in VKH disease:[3]

1. *Prodromal or early stage* lasts up to 10 days and is characterized by flu-like symptoms, meningismus, vertigo, orbital pain, tinnitus and hearing loss. Cranial nerve palsies, hemiparesis and transverse myelitis are uncommon neurological manifestations.

2. *Uveitic or acute stage* occurs within three to five days after the prodromal stage and lasts for several weeks. Most patients experience sudden bilateral blurring of vision but in 30% of patients, involvement of the fellow eye occurs in a few days. Other symptoms at this stage are eye pain, eye swelling and irritation, and dark floaters that indicate retinal detachment.

3. *Convalescent stage* follows the uveitic stage a few months later. It is characterized by depigmentation of the choroid, hair and skin. The findings include "sunset glow fundus" where there is an exaggerated reddish glow of the fundus, vitiligo, alopecia and poliosis.

4. *Recurrent or chronic stage* usually occurs in the first six months and most often in those with rapid tapering of corticosteroids. Patients may develop recurrent or chronic anterior uveitis or other ocular complications, such as glaucoma and cataract.

The International Nomenclature Committee put forth Revised Diagnostic Criteria (RDC) in 2001.[3,5] The RDC classifies VKH disease into three categories: complete, incomplete and probable (see Table 1.2.3). Complete VKH disease must have criteria 1–5. Incomplete VKH disease must have criteria 1–3 and either 4 or 5. Probable VKH disease or isolated ocular disease must have criteria 1–3.

The emergency or primary-care physician may be the point of first contact with a patient with VKH disease. The key components of managing this disease are awareness of symptoms that lead to early diagnosis and a multidisciplinary approach. For patients with severe visual loss and bilateral serous retinal detachments, systemic prednisolone at 1–2 mg/kg/day should be started. For more severe cases, pulsed methylprednisolone up to 1 g/day for three

**Table 1.2.3** Revised diagnostic criteria for Vogt–Koyanagi–Harada disease

| Number | Criteria |
| --- | --- |
| 1 | No history of penetrating ocular trauma or surgery preceding the initial onset of uveitis |
| 2 | No clinical or laboratory evidence suggestive of other ocular diseases |
| 3 | Bilateral ocular involvement |
| 4 | Neurological/auditory findings which may resolve by time of evaluation: |
| | Meningismus |
| | Tinnitus |
| | Cerebrospinal fluid pleocytosis |
| 5 | Integumentary findings (not preceding onset of central nervous system or ocular disease): |
| | Alopecia, or |
| | Poliosis, or |
| | Vitiligo |

to five days before starting oral prednisone at 1 mg/kg/day is suggested.[4] For those who fail to respond to systemic corticosteroids, immunomodulators or immunosuppressors have been used. Gradual tapering of the corticosteroid dose, with regular follow-up eye examinations, is necessary to prevent the recurrence of posterior segment inflammation or the development of anterior segment problems.[3]

# References

1. Shruthi P, Sridhar A, Sharath Kumar G. Case of the week: Vogt-Koyanagi-Harada syndrome (VKH). *Am J Neuroradiol.* 2018. www.ajnr.org/content/cow/12062018 (accessed January 2022).

2. Yang P, Ren Y, Li B, et al. Clinical characteristics of Vogt-Koyanagi-Harada syndrome in Chinese patients. *Ophthalmology.* 2007;**114**: 606–614.

3. Lavezzo MM, Sakata VM, Morita C, et al. Vogt-Koyanagi-Harada disease: Review of a rare autoimmune disease targeting antigens of melanocytes. *Orphanet J Rare Dis.* 2016;**11**: 29.

4. Patil YB, Garg R, Rajguru JP, et al. Vogt-Koyanagi-Harada (VKH) syndrome: A new perspective for healthcare professionals. *J Family Med Prim Care.* 2020;**9**: 31–35.

5. Yang P, Zhong Y, Du L, et al. Development and evaluation of diagnostic criteria for Vogt-Koyanagi-Harada disease. *JAMA Ophthalmol.* 2018;**136**: 1025–1031.

# 1.2.d.3 Vasculitis with Prominent Eye Movement: Eales Disease

Sabrina Anticoli, Francesco Motolese

## Case Presentation

A 38-year-old male presented to the emergency department with headache, confusion and left hemiparesis. Symptoms had started the day before, his medical history was unremarkable and he was not taking any medications. In addition, the patient denied illicit drug use. On examination, he was afebrile and had normal vital signs. Neurologic review of systems showed mild dysarthria, left-sided hemiparesis, cognitive slowing and blurred vision in his left eye.

Basic laboratory tests, including electrolytes, complete blood count, and liver function tests, gave normal results. A brain computerized tomography (CT) scan did not show hemorrhages or acute signs of stroke. Brain magnetic resonance imaging (MRI) was performed, revealing multiple lesions with restricted diffusion both at cortical and subcortical levels in the right hemisphere, indicative of acute stroke. MRI also showed diffuse leukoencephalopathy and MRI angiography highlighted irregular brain vessel stenosis involving diffusely anterior and posterior circulation (Figure 1.2.16). The patient did not receive intravenous thrombolytic therapy with

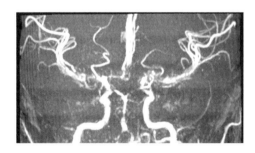
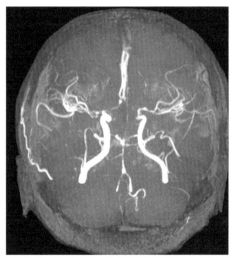

**Figure 1.2.16** MRI angiography showed multiple irregular stenosis of cerebral vessels involving both anterior and posterior circulation

recombinant tissue plasminogen activator (rTPA) because of the timing ($\geq$ 4.5 hours). He was then admitted to the stroke unit.

Other laboratory tests were ordered, including metabolic panel, autoantibodies – among others, antineutrophil cytoplasmic antibodies (ANCA) and antinuclear antibodies (ANA) – inflammatory markers, the Venereal Diseases Research Laboratory (VDRL) test and coagulation profile. All these tests were normal except for a slightly abnormal renal function (i.e., creatinine values 1.4 mg/dl).

Because of blurred vision in his left eye, a neuro-ophthalmological evaluation was performed. Fundus examination of the left eye revealed vitreous hemorrhage and sheathing of peripheral veins without macular edema. Accordingly, retinal vasculitis was suspected and oral prednisolone 75 mg per day was given with a gradual tapering off. In light of the neuro-ophthalmological findings, a diagnosis of Eales disease was established. The patient's condition progressively improved over the next three weeks and he was then discharged to a rehabilitation facility. On follow-up one month later, no signs of active retinal inflammation were found and he had partially recovered from the motor impairment.

# Diagnostic Algorithm

## Clinical suspicion of Eye / CNS Vasculitis

Young male complaining of sudden blurring of vision in one eye ± floaters ± neurological deficits

### Brain CT scan + multiphase CT angiography

*CT may show signs of acute infarction (e.g. loss of grey-white matter differentiation, hypoattenuation of deep nuclei) or gliosis. CTA may show segmental narrowing or occlusions of both small and medium-sized intracranial vessels.*

### Brain MRI (including DWI, FLAIR and post-contrast sequences)

*MRI may show multiple infarctions in various territories and in various stages of healing. Meningeal enhancement and hemorrhages may be present too. MRA is equivalent to CTA. Vessel-wall MRI may be useful to distinguish atherosclerotic stenosis vs vasculitis.*

### Lab tests

*Peripheral blood count, iron, ferritin, urea, creatinine, metabolic panel (including TSH), liver enzymes, ACE, thyroid antibodies, erythrocyte sedimentation rate, CRP, HCG test, ANA, ENA screen, antiphospholipid antibody, lupus anticoagulant, anticardiolipin, anti beta2 glycoprotein-1 antibody, ANCA, activated protein C, prothrombin time, activated partial thromboplastin time, HLAB27, pathergy test, syphilis testing, tuberculin skin testing/QuantiFERON Gold, hemoglobin A1c, Lyme disease testing, HIV testing*

### Ophthalmological assessment (including slit lamp, gonioscopy, fundoscopy)

*Examination may reveal vitreous hemorrhages, macular edema, perivascular venous sheathing and exudate, venous tortuosity, venous obstruction, capillary non-perfusion, sclerosed vessels, intraretinal hemorrhages, retinal neovascularization.*

### ± OCT ± Fluoroangiography

*Leakage of dye surrounding veins indicates active inflammation. Venous staining without leakage indicates sclerosed vessels or resolved inflammation.*

### Additional tests *(to exclude other diagnoses)*

*Vascular ultrasound, ocular ultrasound, chest X-ray, full-body CT scan, CT angiography, echocardiography, temporal artery biopsy*

## TREATMENT

### CORTICOSTEROIDS

*Systemic and/or local/periocular*

*Corticosteroid (prednisolone 1-2 mg/kg body weight) is the mainstay of treatment for the inflammatory stage.*

### PHOTOCOAGULATION

*It is the mainstay of the proliferative phase.*

### SURGICAL TREATMENT

*In some cases (e.g. vitreous haemorrhage, tractional retinal detachment, rhegmatogenous retinal detachment) vitrectomy may be indicated.*

### Other treatments

*Intravitreal injection of antivascular endothelial growth factor (Anti-VEGF)*
*Antitubercular treatment (only for patients who have positive test for TB)*

Legends: CT: Computerized tomography; CTA: CT angiography; MRI: Magnetic resonance imaging; DWI: Diffusion weighted imaging; FLAIR: Fluid Attenuated Inversion Recovery; MRA: MR angiography; OCT: Optical Coherence Tomography; CRP: C-reactive protein; ACE: angiotensin-converting enzyme; HCG: human chorionic gonadotropin; ANA: Antinuclear antibodies; ENA: extractable nuclear antigens; ANCA: Antineutrophil cytoplasmic antibodies; HIV: Human immunodeficiency virus; TB: Tuberculosis

# Case Discussion

Vasculitis is a heterogeneous group of diseases causing inflammation of vessel walls, eventually leading to necrosis and occlusion of the vessel and then ischemia of the end organ. Vasculitis may be idiopathic or secondary to other diseases and the clinical picture is heterogeneous too, depending on the organs involved; accordingly, they can present as a systemic disorder or as a local disease involving a specific organ. In this regard, ocular involvement is pretty common and it is sometimes the first manifestation of systemic disorders. However, although rarely, a primary form of vasculitis affecting only retinal vessels can occur. Table 1.2.4 reports a classification of eye vasculitis.[1]

The differential diagnosis of primary and secondary vasculitis is mandatory since treatment consists of immunosuppressive therapy in cases of autoimmune disorders that must be avoided if an infection is suspected. There are several causes of secondary retinal vasculitis (i.e., secondary to a systemic condition) such as Behçet's disease, sarcoidosis, systemic lupus erythematosus (SLE), granulomatosis with polyangiitis, polyarteritis nodosa and other rheumatologic conditions. Infectious agents may also cause retinal vasculitis, such as syphilis, tuberculosis (TB) and Lyme disease. In addition, paraneoplastic syndromes can also occur.[2,3]

Among primary forms of eye vasculitis, Eales disease – also known as retinal periphlebitis or retinal perivasculitis – is a rare inflammatory venous occlusive disease. It is an idiopathic condition affecting primarily young male adults and it is often bilateral. Rarely, it has been associated with neurological symptoms. It is named after Henry Eales, a British ophthalmologist who, in the nineteenth century described a clinical condition affecting young man with recurrent vitreous hemorrhages – in some cases associated with a positive

**Table 1.2.4** Classification of eye vasculitis (according to Chapel Hill nomenclature)

| | |
|---|---|
| Eye vasculitis without systemic involvement | Single-organ– retinal vasculitis, pars planitis, birdshot chorioretinopathy, idiopathic retinal vasculitis, aneurysm and neuroretinitis syndrome, Eales disease |
| Eye vasculitis with primary systemic vasculitis | Small vessel vasculitis, microscopic polyangiitis, granulomatosis with polyangiitis (Wegener's), eosinophilic granulomatosis with polyangiitis (Churg–Strauss syndrome), medium vessel vasculitis, polyarteritis nodosa, Kawasaki disease, large vessel vasculitis, Takayasu arteritis, giant cell arteritis |
| Eye vasculitis with autoimmune disorders | Variable vessel vasculitis, Behçet's disease, Cogan's syndrome, vasculitis associated with systemic disease, sarcoid vasculitis, lupus vasculitis, spondyloarthropathies |
| Eye vasculitis associated with probable infectious etiology | Vasculitis secondary to infection, endogenous endophthalmitis, viral retinitis, tuberculosis, acquired syphilis, Lyme disease, toxoplasmosis, toxocariasis, vasculitis with masquerade syndromes, paraneoplastic vasculitis, drug-associated vasculitis |

Modified by Azad et al.[1]

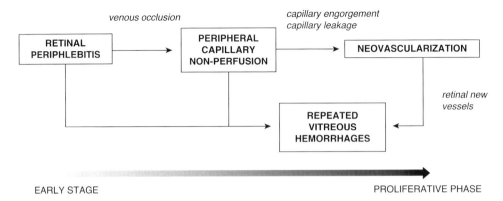

**Figure 1.2.17** Eales disease is characterized by three overlapping stages of periphlebitis (i.e., vessel inflammation), vessel occlusion and neovascularization.

history of epistaxis, headache or gastrointestinal motility problems. Although the first cases were reported in Europe or North America, Eales disease is now more common in developing countries, probably because of public health issues.[4]

The etiopathogenesis of Eales disease is yet unclear; indeed, it is considered a primary vasculitis of unknown etiology in young adults. The pathological hallmark of the disease is the involvement of peripheral retinal vessels with a first stage of inflammation (i.e., acute phlebitis) that eventually leads to ischemia, hemorrhages into the vitreous body and then neovascular proliferation due to circulatory deficiency. Neovascularization is then a significant source of new hemorrhages (Figure 10.2). Besides, retinal detachment can also occur.

Patients may complain of sudden blurring of vision in one eye – eventually, during the course of the disease 50–90% of patients presents bilateral involvement – decreased vision or floaters. Vision problems should prompt differential diagnosis with giant cell arteritis, a large vessel vasculitis that affects older patients. Focal neurological deficits can rarely occur, probably because of vasculitic involvement of cerebral arteries leading to clinical and subclinical strokes.[1] A high index of suspicion is required for diagnosis, in particular in cases of young males in which neurological deficits are associated with ocular symptoms (i.e., blurring of vision or vision loss) and possibly with a positive history of ocular and neurological disturbances (e.g., history of headache or previous episodes of transient ischemic attacks). Attention must be paid to distinguish hemianopsia, a typical symptom of stroke, from true vision loss in these patients.

In some cases seizure and migraine have also been reported in patients affected by Eales disease.[5]

Eales disease is considered as a diagnosis of exclusion and confirmed only after ruling out all possible infections and systemic etiologies. Systemic conditions – such as SLE, sarcoidosis and even diabetes – and infectious diseases – such as herpes simplex virus, syphilis or tuberculosis – should be ruled out, especially if the patient is immunocompromised. Complete blood tests – including an autoimmunity panel, and cultures and serological tests for infections, as appropriate – should be performed, together with an adequate neuroimaging evaluation.

If stroke is suspected, then a CT brain scan and CT angiogram of intracranial vessels should be ordered in the acute setting. Brain MRI may show acute infarction within multiple vascular territories with restricted diffusion and brain swelling. Multiple infarctions may be present at different stages of healing. MRI may also show white matter T2-hyperintensities involving both hemispheres, indicative of leukoencephalopathy. Brain MRI or CT angiography is crucial because it may show multiple and irregular stenosis involving both anterior and vertebrobasilar circulation. In some cases, vessel-wall MRI may be useful to distinguish atherosclerotic stenosis from vasculitis.

Cerebrospinal fluid (CSF) examination is not routinely performed, but it may show a slight increase in protein level and lymphocytic pleocytosis. Some authors also report the presence of oligoclonal bands in CSF.[5,6]

However, the diagnosis of Eales disease is primarily clinical and requires fundus oculi examination and a fluorescein angiogram, which reveals retinal vascular leakage. Optical coherence tomography (OCT) may also be useful.

## Treatment

The treatment of Eales disease depends on the stage of the disease and is not well established. In the acute inflammatory stage, oral corticosteroids are the mainstay of therapy (prednisolone 1–2 mg/kg body weight). In some cases, posterior sub-Tenon steroid injection can be considered. As with other autoimmune disorders, immunosuppressive therapy, such as cyclosporine, methotrexate and azathioprine, may be employed with the aim of preventing relapses.

A pathophysiological association with mycobacterium tuberculosis has been suggested, probably through immunological hypersensitivity mechanisms, but never demonstrated. Thus, antitubercular treatment should be reserved only for patients who have positive test for TB (either skin or blood test).

In order to prevent complete vision loss, in the ischemic phase, retinal laser photocoagulation to ischemic zones is beneficial in reducing neovascularization and vitreous hemorrhages. In the proliferative phase, intravitreal injection of vascular endothelial growth factor inhibitors (anti-VEGF agents) will stop neovascularization, but can cause tractional retinal detachment.[4,7]

## References

1. Azad SV, Takkar B, Venkatesh P. Eye and Vasculitis. *J Vasc.* 2016;**2**: 108.

2. Crawford CM. Primary Retinal Vasculitis Vs Eales' Disease. *Int J Open Access Opthalmology.* 2016;**1**(3): 1–8.

3. Rosenbaum JT, Sibley CH, Lin P. Retinal Vasculitis. *Curr Opin Rheumatol.* 2016;**28**(3): 228–235.

4. Das T, Pathengay A, Hussain N, Biswas J. Eales' disease: diagnosis and management. *Eye (Lond).* 2010;**24**(3): 472–482.

5. Biswas J, Raghavendran R, Pinakin G, Arjundas D. Presumed Eales' disease with neurologic involvement: Report of three cases. *Retina.* 2001;**21**(2): 141–145.

6. Gordon MF, Coyle PK, Golub B. Eales' disease presenting as stroke in the young adult. *Ann Neurol.* 1988;**24**(2): 264–266.

7. Biswas J, Ravi RK, Naryanasamy A, Kulandai LT, Madhavan HN. Eales' disease – current concepts in diagnosis and management. *J Ophthalmic Inflamm Infect.* 2013;**3**: 11.

# 1.2.d.4  Vasculitis with Prominent Eye Movement: Cogan Disease

Nikoloz Tsiskaridze, Alexander Tsiskaridze

## Case Presentation

A 28-year-old man was admitted to the emergency department with sudden left-sided weakness and sensory disturbance, and facial drop. In addition, he reported slowly progressive, but fluctuating, bilateral hearing loss, episodes of dizziness and vertigo, and periodic pain and irritation in both eyes for the last six months.

The patient had no history of hypertension, diabetes, heart disease or lipid profile abnormality. He reported no history of headaches or transient ischemic attacks before hospitalization. The patient rarely drank alcohol, was a non-smoker, and had not been using any illicit drugs. He had no family history of neurological disease.

The body temperature was 36.4°C, heart rate, 85 beats/min, blood pressure, 125/70 mmHg, respiratory rate, 20 breaths/min and oxygen saturation, 99% on ambient air.

Neurological examination revealed mild hearing loss on both sides, left central facial paresis, decreased muscle strength in the left extremities with positive Babinski sign and paraesthesia, together with a decrease in temperature and a pinprick sensation in the left side of the body.

Considering the patient's age and medical history, the following laboratory tests were made: total peripheral blood count, electrolytes, C-reactive protein (CRP), renal and liver function tests, thyroid function, serum lipids, extensive coagulation studies, complement level, rheumatoid factor (RF), antinuclear antibodies (ANA), antineutrophilic cytoplasmic antibody (ANCA), Coombs test, cryoglobulins, serum protein electrophoresis, lupus anticoagulant, antithrombin III, protein C, protein S, homocysteine, antiphospholipid antibodies, factor V Leiden mutation, prothrombin G202010A mutation and activated protein C resistance. All of those tests were normal except for elevated CRP (31 mg/l), erythrocyte sedimentation rate (ESR) (26 mm/h) and white blood cell count ($13.2 \times 10^9$/l). Tests for syphilis and Lyme disease were negative.

Urinalysis was normal. A lumbar puncture was performed. Cerebrospinal fluid (CSF) was acellular and the protein level was not elevated. Cultures of blood and CSF for bacteria, viruses and fungi were negative. Chest X-ray, electrocardiogram, 48-hour Holter cardiac monitoring, transthoracic and transoesophageal echocardiography with contrast were unremarkable. The initial brain CT performed on admission did not show any significant abnormalities. A repeat CT scan revealed lacunar infarction in the right posterolateral thalamus. Brain MRI showed increased signal intensity in T2-weighted images and decreased signal intensity in T1-weighted images in the right posterolateral thalamus adjacent to the posterior limb of the internal capsule, corresponding to the lacunar infarction, and dilated perivascular spaces. No enhancement with gadolinium was observed. MR

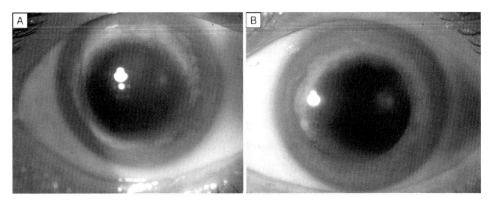

**Figure 1.2.18** Slit-lamp photographs showing corneal scarring secondary to interstitial keratitis in the patient's right (A) and left (B) eyes. Reprinted from Sevgi DD, Sobrin L, Papaliodis GN. Cogan syndrome with severe medium and large vessel vasculitis. *DJO.* 2016; 22(1): 32, (10.5693/djo.02.2015.09.002), copyright (2016), with permission of the Digital Journal of Ophthalmology.

angiography and duplex scanning did not reveal any abnormalities in the carotid and vertebral arteries; the intracranial vessels were normal as well. Ophthalmological examination showed non-suppurative inflammation in both eyes suggestive of interstitial keratitis (IK) (Figure 1.2.18).

Vestibulo-audiometric tests revealed bilateral signs of cochlear pathology with low-frequency sensorineural hearing loss. Based on the presence of ocular inflammation, audio-vestibular symptoms and alternative causes of inflammation or infection being ruled out, a diagnosis of Cogan syndrome (CS) was established. The patient started aspirin 100 mg/day and oral corticosteroid therapy. The focal neurological signs rapidly improved. At a three-month follow-up, the ophthalmological examination was normal, but hearing loss in both ears persisted.

# Diagnostic Algorithm

### Clinical suspicion of CS

- Age – 20–30 years, sex – no known predominance, race – mostly Caucasian, type of onset – mostly subacute. Clinical manifestations: (a) inflammatory ocular disease; (b) sensorineural hearing loss; (c) alternative causes of inflammation or infection excluded; (d) interval between the onset of ocular and audio-vestibular manifestations <2 years; (e) neurological manifestation – stroke of unknown etiology

### Clinical manifestations

- Ocular manifestations – interstitial keratitis (72–100%) (see figure), iritis or uveitis (37%), scleritis or episcleritis (23%), cataract (15%), conjunctivitis (10%), glaucoma (3%), retinal vasculitis, papillitis, vasculitic optic neuropathy, papilledema, subconjunctival hemorrhage, exophthalmos, orbital pseudotumor, central vein occlusion, central retinal artery occlusion, xerophthalmia and amaurosis. Slit-lamp examination – patchy, deep, granular corneal infiltrate

  - Audio-vestibular manifestations – progressive, usually bilateral hearing loss (>90%), vertigo/dizziness (90%), tinnitus (80%), nausea, ataxia, nystagmus, instability, vomiting, oscillopsia, cochlear hydrops. Caloric testing – absent vestibular function. Audiometry – sensorineural

(cont.)

## Clinical suspicion of CS

hearing loss at all frequencies, but mostly at the extremes. Auditory evoked potentials – reduced or absent. Cranial CT – intralabyrinthine calcific or soft-tissue attenuation. Cranial MRI – soft-tissue obliteration or narrowing of the membranous labyrinth

- Gastrointestinal manifestations (33%) – abdominal pain, diarrhoea, rectal bleeding, melena, hepatomegaly, hepatitis, esophagitis, liver steatosis
- Neurological manifestations (29%) – ischemic events/stroke, cerebral venous sinus thrombosis, encephalopathy, meningoencephalitis, seizures, cranial neuropathy, peripheral neuropathy, mononeuritis multiplex, trigeminal neuralgia, autonomic neuropathy, myopathy
- Cardiac manifestations (25%) – aortic dilatation, aortic valvular insufficiency, congestive heart failure, pericarditis, cardiomegaly, arrhythmia, silent coronary artery disease
- Genitourinary manifestations (20%) – hematuria, proteinuria, testicular pain
- Systemic vasculitis (10–15%) – retinal vasculitis, aortitis (coronary, carotid, subclavian, iliac, femoral and mesenteric arteries may be involved), multivessel involvement
- Mucocutaneous manifestations (5–10%) – erythematous or urticarial rash, vascular purpura, nodules or ulcerations of the limbs, genital organs and/or oral cavity
- Lymphatic manifestations (3–5%) – lymphadenopathy, splenomegaly
- Respiratory manifestations (3–5%) – pleuritis, dyspnea, cough, hemoptysis, pleuritic chest pain
- Constitutional/systemic manifestations – headache (19–40%), arthralgia (31–35%), arthritis (16–23%), fever (25–27%), myalgia (22%), weight loss (16%), rash (9–10%)

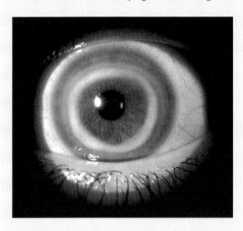

Interstitial keratitis (source: *N Engl J Med* 2018; 378: 852).

## Laboratory tests

- Peripheral blood count (elevated ESR, leukocytosis, anemia, thrombocytosis), CRP (elevated), antiheat shock protein 70 (Hsp 70), anticochlear antibodies, rheumatoid factor (RF), serology for various microorganisms, e.g., *Treponema pallidum*, chlamydia, *Borellia burgdoferi*. Immunological work-up: ANA, ANCA, circulating anticoagulant antibody, anticochlear antibodies, anticardiolipin antibodies, lupus anticoagulant, antibodies to smooth muscle, mitochondria, perinuclear

(cont.)

### Clinical suspicion of CS

constituents, phospholipids, factor VII and neutrophilic cytoplasm, cryoglobulins, total complement and its C3 and C4 fractions

#### Differential diagnosis

- Inflammatory eye disease (chlamydial infection, Lyme disease, herpes simplex and varicella zoster infection, leprosy, mycobacterium tuberculosis infection), inner ear dysfunction (viral infection, Ménière disease, autoimmune hearing loss, cerebellopontine tumor, vascular insufficiency, perilymphatic fistulas, drug toxicity, demyelinating disease), both eyes and inner-ear diseases (sarcoidosis, congenital syphilis, Whipple's disease, Susac syndrome, Vogt–Koyangi–Harada syndrome, KID (keratitis, ichthyosis and deafness) syndrome, Sjögren's syndrome, rheumatoid arthritis, systemic lupus erythematosis, antiphospholipid antibody syndrome, polyarteritis nodosa, Wegener's granulomatosis, microscopic polyangiitis, Takayasu's arteritis, relapsing polychondritis, Behçet's disease, ulcerative colitis, Crohn's disease, central nervous system lymphoma/leukaemia, retinocochleocerebral vasculopathy)

#### Treatment
*Ocular disease*

- Anterior ocular inflammation: topical glucocorticoids (prednisolone acetate), mydriatics – decrease ocular inflammation and photophobia, prevent synechiae, relieve ocular discomfort. Additional treatment: episcleritis, scleritis – nonsteroidal anti-inflammatory drugs (NSAIDs), systemic glucocorticoids. Refractory uveitis – anti-TNF treatment.

- Posterior ocular inflammation: systemic glucocorticoids (prednisone). Additional treatment – methotrexate, cyclophosphamide, cyclosporine, TNF inhibitor

*Inner-ear disease*

- Compromised auditory acuity: systemic glucocorticoids (prednisone). Additional treatment – cyclophosphamide, methotrexate, azathioprine, tacrolimus, leflunomide, mycophenolate mofetil, infliximab, TNF inhibitors

- Cochlear hydrops: diuretic therapy (hydrochlorothiazide, furosemide). Refractory cases – Cochlear implants

- Vestibular dysfunction: antihistamines (meclizine hydrochloride), benzodiazepines (diazepam), bed rest. Recurrent vestibular dysfunction – glucocorticoids, glucocorticoid-sparing therapy

*Systemic vasculitis*

- Prednisone. Additional treatment – methotrexate, azathioprine, mycophenolate mofetil, cyclophosphamide, cyclosporine, TNF inhibitors, tocilizumab, rituximab

# Case Discussion

Cogan's syndrome (CS) is a rare multisystem inflammatory disease named after American ophthalmologist David G. Cogan, who described a series of four cases in 1945.[1] There are two types of Cogan's syndrome: typical and atypical. Typical CS is defined as: (a) inflammatory ocular manifestations, classically presenting as non-syphilitic interstitial keratitis (IK); (b) audio-vestibular symptoms similar to those of Ménière's disease with an interval between the onset of ocular and audio-vestibular manifestations of less than two years. Atypical CS is characterized by: (a) different ocular manifestations, with or without IK; (b) audio-vestibular symptoms with (most importantly) a delay of more than two years between the onset of ocular and audio-vestibular manifestations.[2] The onset is usually subacute, with the patient typically being a young (20–30 years) Caucasian, and there is no known sex predominance. Pediatric CS has also been described, with a median age of 11.4 years and systemic manifestations being present in almost half of patients.[2]

The etiology and pathogenesis of CS remain unknown. Although a vasculitic process involving vessels of all sizes has been described in some patients, its role in the pathogenesis of the disease is undetermined. An infectious hypothesis has also been described, with chlamydia infection reported in some of the patients.[3] Lately, numerous studies have suggested autoimmune pathogenesis of CS, with some patients displaying autoantibodies against corneal and inner-ear antigens. Recently, antibodies to Hsp-70 have been described in some patients with the typical form of the disease.[4]

The clinical signs and symptoms typically manifest as ocular (inflammatory non-syphilitic IK) and inner-ear disease (Meniere-like symptoms of sudden onset of tinnitus and vertigo, accompanied by gradual hearing loss.) Systemic manifestations occur in 30–50% of the cases, with headache, arthralgia, fever, arthritis and myalgia being the most common constitutional symptoms.[5] Vasculitis has been described in 10–15% of patients, affecting vessels of all sizes. Aortitis has been described in 10% of cases. Patients can also present with various cardiac, neurological, gastrointestinal, respiratory, genitourinary, mucocutaneous and lymphatic manifestations.

For neurological manifestations, the patients can present with central (strokes/ischemic events, cerebral venous sinus thrombosis, aneurysm, encephalitis, meningitis/meningismus, encephalopathy, pituitary abnormality, optic neuritis, brainstem dysfunction, myelopathy) and peripheral nervous system (peripheral neuropathy, mononeuritis multiplex, autonomic neuropathy, cranial neuropathy, ophthalmoplegia, third nerve palsy, trigeminal neuralgia, facial neuropathy, myopathy) manifestations.[6] The majority of reported cases of ischemic stroke were diagnosed on a clinical basis without definitive radiological confirmation. Because of the small number of confirmed stroke cases, an established association between ischemic stroke and CS is lacking. A possible proposed mechanism could be related to vasculitis.[6]

Diagnosis of CS is clinical. No laboratory or radiographic tests are specific to CS. The diagnosis relies upon the presence of characteristic inflammatory eye disease and vestibulo-auditory dysfunction, with alternative causes of infection or inflammation being excluded. The most common laboratory findings are elevated ESR, CRP, anemia and thrombocytosis. Autoantibodies against different antigens have been described. Slit-lamp examination, audiometry and caloric testing are usually abnormal. Cranial CT can occasionally reveal intralabyrinthine calcifications. Brain MRI scans with gadolinium can reveal calcification or narrowing, and soft tissue obliteration of the vestibular labyrinth and cochlea.[7] Spinal fluid analysis can occasionally reveal inflammatory changes.

The differential diagnosis includes sensorineural hearing loss, congenital syphilis, Takayasu's arteritis, polyarteritis nodosa, Wegener's granulomatosis, Vogt–Koyanagi–Harada syndrome and Susac syndrome.

Treatment of CS is based on the assumption of an autoimmune mechanism for the disease. For ocular disease, topical and systemic glucocorticoids can be used. Vestibulo-cochlear, systemic and neurological manifestations are treated with systemic glucocorticoids. Vestibular dysfunction can be treated with antihistamines or benzodiazepines. Cochlear implants can be used in patients with severe progressive hearing loss. For patients still displaying symptoms after treatment, immunosuppressants (methotrexate, cyclophosphamide, mycophenolate mofetil, and leflunomide) and intravenous immunoglobulin can be used.

The prognosis of CS is variable, with most patients experiencing multiple disease relapses. The prognosis for ocular manifestations is generally good, but if deafness occurs, it is usually permanent.[8]

# References

1. Cogan DG. Syndrome of nonsyphilitic interstitial keratitis and vestibuloauditory symptoms. *Arch Ophthalmol*. 1945;**33**: 144–149.

2. Pagnini I, Zannin ME, Vittadello F, et al. Clinical features and outcome of Cogan syndrome. *J Pediatr*. 2012;**160**: 303–307.

3. Haynes BF, Kaiser-Kupfer MI, Mason P, Fauci AS. Cogan syndrome: studies in thirteen patients, long-term follow-up, and a review of the literature. *Medicine (Baltimore)*. 1980;**59**: 426–441.

4. Bonaguri C, Orsoni J, Russo A, et al. Mora P Cogan's syndrome: Anti-Hsp70 antibodies are a serological marker in the typical form. *Isr Med Assoc J*. 2014;**16**: 285–288.

5. Gluth MB, Baratz KH, Matteson EL, Driscoll CL. Cogan syndrome: a retrospective review of 60 patients throughout a half-century. *Mayo Clin Proc.* 2006;**81**: 483–488.

6. Antonios N, Silliman S. Cogan syndrome: an analysis of reported neurological manifestations. *Neurologist*. 2012;**18**: 55–63.

7. Casselman JW, Majoor MH, Albers FW. MR of the inner ear in patients with Cogan syndrome. *Am J Neuroradiol*. 1994;**15**: 131–138.

8. Study Group for Cogan's Syndrome, Grasland A, Pouchot J, Hachulla E, et al. Typical and atypical Cogan's syndrome: 32 cases and review of the literature. *Rheumatology (Oxford)*. 2004;**438**: 1007–1015.

# Vasculitis Secondary to Systemic Disease
## 1.3.a Systemic Lupus Erythematosis

Vildan Yayla, Hacı Ali Erdoğan, İbrahim Acır

## Case Presentation

A 41-year-old Syrian woman with a diagnosis of systemic lupus erythematosus (SLE) and antiphospholipid antibody syndrome (APS) presented with new seizures and worsening of left hemiparesis sequelae and general health condition. Her convulsions were described as deviation of the eyes, and paresthesia and clonic contractions in the right upper extremity. Her medical history showed SLE attacks, several ischemic cerebrovascular accidents (CVA) and seizures (Table 1.3.1). Neurological examination revealed confusion, poor cooperation/orientation, left-sided hemiparesis (4/5) and positive Babinski sign on the left side. Her treatment was planned as ASA 1 × 300 mg, clopidogrel 1 × 75 mg, warfarin according to the INR (International Normalized Ratio), levetiracetam 2 × 1000 mg and IV pulse methylprednisolone (1000 mg/day for five days). The dosage of levetiracetam was increased to 2500 mg/day.

**Table 1.3.1** Medical history of the patient

| Year | Clinical signs | Treatment |
|---|---|---|
| 2005 SLE + APS | Hemolytic anemia, malar rash, alopecia, arthralgia and recurrent miscarriage | HCQ and oral prednisolone HCQ stopped due to adverse effects AZA added in 2008 |
| 2014 | LA+, anti-ds DNA (+), ANA (+) 1/1000, | Coronary artery bypass graft surgery |
| 2016 follow-up in our hospital | | AZA 2 × 50 mg, prednisolone 4 mg/day |
| 2017 CVA | Dysarthria and vertigo (bilateral MCA-PCA infarction) | ASA + CLP |
| 2018 CVA | Dysarthria and hypoesthesia | ASA + CLP |

**Table 1.3.1** (cont.)

| Year | Clinical signs | Treatment |
|---|---|---|
| 2018 symptomatic epilepsy + CVA | Partial seizure | Warfarin and IV pulse steroid (three days) |
| 2018 CVA | Left-sided hemiparesis and ineffective INR | ASA and warfarin |
| 2018 CVA | Dysarthria and left-sided hypoesthesia | ASA+ warfarin and LMWH, CP |
| 2018 | | Rituximab was started and stopped due to adverse effect MMF was started |
| 2018 CVA | Facial palsy (INR: 5) | IV pulse steroid (five days) and CP |
| 2019 CVA | Ataxia and memory loss | CP, ASA and warfarin |

HCQ: hydroxychloroquine, AZA: azathioprine, CP: cyclophosphamide, CLP: clopidogrel, LMWH: low-molecular-weight heparin, MMF: mycophenolate mofetil

Cranial MRI revealed acute infarcts with restricted diffusion in the right parietotemporal and left frontal areas on diffusion-weighted imaging (DWI) sequences (Figure 1.3.1). Occlusions of bilateral internal carotid (ICA), middle, anterior and posterior cerebral arteries (MCA, ACA and PCA) were detected on carotid and cranial MR angiography (MRA) (Figure 1.3.2).

Cerebral digital subtraction angiography (DSA) revealed narrowing of bilateral proximal ICA and MCA, left ACA and right PCA with decreased blood flow, and also occlusions in the supracavernous segment of the right ICA and the right ACA. DSA findings suggested vasculitis related to lupus. Electroencephalography (EEG) showed slow and poorly organized background activity. Echocardiography was normal. On laboratory examination, mild anemia (WBC $5 \times 10^3/mm^3$, RBC $4.6 \times 10^6/mm^3$, platelets $356 \times 10^3/mm^3$, hemoglobin: 11.1 g/dl) and increased acute-phase reactants (ESR: 22 mm/h and CRP: 8mg/l) were detected. Hepatic and renal functions were normal. The patient was diagnosed with pneumonia and piperasilin/tazobactam treatment was started. Because of agitation, aggression, visual hallucination and suicidal thoughts, the patient was evaluated by psychiatry and diagnosed with secondary psychosis related to steroid treatment. Quetiapine, clonazepam and halo-peridol treatment was recommended. Systemic findings worsened and prednisolone $1 \times 40$ mg/day orally and IVIG 30 g/day for five days was given. Since the focal seizures and agitation continued, the dosage of levetiracetam was reduced and valproic acid $2 \times 500$ mg/day was added.

The patient was diagnosed with vasculitis related to lupus, and cyclophosphamide 1 g IV and uromitexan were added to the treatment. Respiratory distress developed and the patient was referred to the intensive care unit.

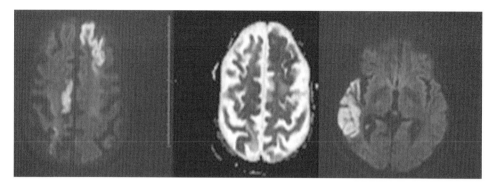

**Figure 1.3.1** DWI and ADC MR revealed acute infarcts with restricted diffusion in the right parietotemporal and left frontal area.

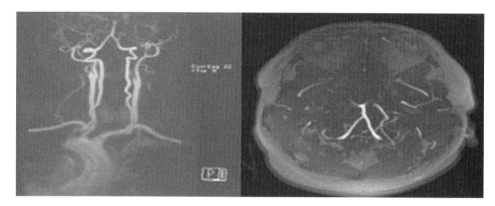

**Figure 1.3.2** Carotid and cranial MRA revealed bilateral ICA, MCA, ACA and PCA occlusion.

# Diagnostic Algorithm

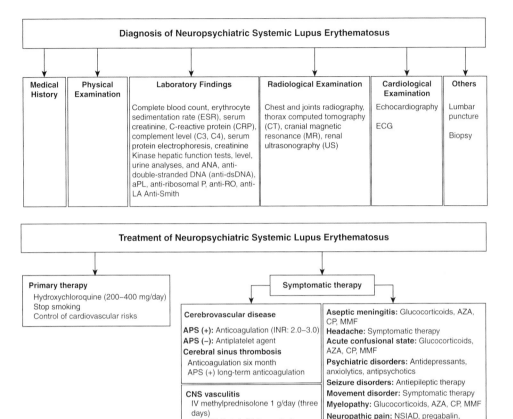

## Case Discussion

SLE is an autoimmune chronic progressive disease that involves many organs and systems. SLE may affect the central and peripheral nervous systems (CNS, PNS) and causes different neuropsychiatric symptoms, which range from subclinical conditions to life-threatening neurological and neuropsychiatric symptoms.[1] SLE is more common in women of childbearing age (15–40 years).[1] Neuropsychiatric syndromes of systemic lupus erythematosus (NPSLE) is observed in 10–80% of SLE patients. Neuropsychiatric findings can be primary or secondary to the complications and treatment of SLE.[2] Although the cause of the disease is unknown, different genetic, environmental, immunological, ethnic and hormonal factors are involved in the pathology of SLE.[3] Arthralgia-arthritis, nephrotic syndrome, progressive glomerulonephritis, pleuritis, interstitial lung disease, pneumonia, pulmonary hypertension and embolism are common manifestations of SLE. Nineteen NPLSE syndromes have been defined and diagnostic criteria have been developed by ACR.[4]

The pathogenesis of NPSLE is multifactorial. Vascular and neuronal damage caused by inflammatory cytokines, autoantibodies and immune complexes are involved in the pathogenesis. Secondary factors such as infections associated with chronic immunosuppressive treatment, other organ failure, metabolic complications, hypertension and the toxic effects of treatment also play a role in the pathogenesis.[5]

## Stroke and CNS Vasculitis Related to SLE

Stroke and cerebrovascular disease are the most severe complications of SLE, and the incidence rate is approximately 3–20%, especially in the first five years of the disease.[6] In a meta-analysis, it was reported that SLE patients have a twofold higher risk of ischemic stroke, a threefold higher risk of intracerebral hemorrhage and an almost fourfold higher risk of subarachnoid hemorrhage (SAH) compared to the general population.[7] Many factors, such as a high level of antiphospholipid (aPL), hyperhomocysteinemia, lupus disease activity, cerebral vasculitis, emboli from Libman–Sacks endocarditis and accelerated atherosclerosis can cause stroke in SLE. Nearly 36% of APS patients have SLE, and the combination of these conditions can increase the risk of aPL-mediated stroke.[7] APS is an autoimmune disease that is associated with the persistent presence of aPL. It causes recurrent thrombotic events, miscarriages and thrombocytopenia. High levels of aCL, anti-β2GPI and phosphatidylserine/prothrombin antibodies are more strongly associated with cerebral infarction than an LA (+) alone.[7] Cerebral venous sinus thrombosis (CVST) is a rare complication of SLE and is responsible for 1% of all strokes.[8] Vasculitis is a rare manifestation, occurring in less than 7% of NPSLE.[9] Immune complex deposition in vascular endothelium, intrathecal immune complexes and other inflammatory mediators are involved in the pathogenesis of vasculopathy and vasculitis.

CNS vasculopathy usually affects small arterioles and capillaries leading to micro infarcts and hemorrhages. CNS vasculitis had an eight times greater mortality rate. Dissimilar to classical stroke symptoms, CNS vasculitis due to SLE may present with fever, severe headaches, confusional episodes and rapid progression to psychotic symptoms, seizures and coma. Brain biopsy is the gold standard for the diagnosis of CNS vasculitis, but it has high risk and limited sensitivity. Neuroimaging (cranial MRI, MRA and DSA) in combination with clinical features and laboratory studies are preferred for the diagnosis. Contrast enhancement and thickening of the vascular walls on cranial MRI, and segmental narrowing of small and medium vessels on DSA are highly suggestive of CNS vasculitis.[10]

## References

1. Daniel JW, Dafna DG. Clinical manifestations and diagnosis of systemic lupus erythematosus in adults. www.uptodate.com. Literature review current through: Mar 2020.Last updated: Dec.10,2019. (accessed January 2022).

2. Schur PH. Neurologic manifestation of systemic lupus erythematosus in adults. www.uptodate.com. Literature review current through: Mar 2020.Last updated: Feb 21, 2019. (accessed January 2022).

3. Cooper GS, Dooley MA, Treadwell EL, et al. Hormonal, environmental, and infectious risk factors for developing systemic lupus erythematosus. *Arthritis Rheum.* 1998;**41**(10): 1714–1724.

4. The American College of Rheumatology nomenclature and case definitions for neuropsychiatric lupus syndromes. *Arthritis Rheum.* 1999;**42**: 599.

5. Hanly JG, Kozora E, Beyea SD, Birnbaum J. Review: Nervous system disease in systemic lupus erythematosus. Current status and future directions. *Arthritis Rheumatol.* 2019;**71**: 33.

6. Saadatnia M, Sayed-Bonakdar Z, Mohammad-Sharifi G, Sarrami AH. The necessity of stroke prevention in patients with systemic lupus erythematosus. *J Res Med Sci.* 2012;**17**: 894–895.

7. Holmqvist M, Simard JF, Asplund K, Arkema EV. Stroke in systemic lupus erythematosus: A meta-analysis of population-based cohort studies. *RMD Open* 2015;**1**: e000168.

8. Duman T, Demirci S, Uluduz D et al. Cerebral venous sinus thrombosis as a rare complication of systemic lupus erythematosus: subgroup analysis of the VENOST study. *J Stroke Cerebrovasc Dis.* 2019;**28**(12): 104372.

9. Rowshani AT, Remans P, Rozemuller A, Tak PP. Cerebral vasculitis as a primary manifestation of systemic lupus erythematosus. *Ann Rheum Dis.* 2005;**64**: 784–786.

10. Pomper MG, Miller TJ, Stone JH, et al. CNS vasculitis in autoimmune disease: MR imaging findings and correlation with angiography. *Am J Neuroradiol.* 1999;**20**: 75–85.

# 1.3.b Behçet's Disease

Uğur Uygunoğlu, Aksel Siva

## Case Presentation

A 27-year-old man with a history of a new headache was referred to our center for a second opinion. He described his headache as throbbing, involving the entire head and being quite severe over the last several weeks. There was no nausea or sensitivity to light or sound. Cranial MRI revealed two lesions: one extended from the right thalamus to the mesencephalon with gadolinium enhancement and the second was on the posterior limb of the left internal capsule (Figure 1.3.3). He had been treated elsewhere with intravenous methylprednisolone (IVMP) 1 g daily × 10 days and he stated that his headache disappeared completely after this treatment. When he was evaluated in our outpatient clinic, he had no complaints and his neurological examination was unremarkable.

Given that the patient described recurrent oral aphthous ulcers, and the MRI features were highly suggestive of the neurological involvement of Behçet's syndrome (BS), the patient was evaluated for BS. However, no genital ulcers or uveitis were observed, and the pathergy test was negative. Thus, BS could not be diagnosed according to the International Study Group (ISG) criteria (Table 1.3.2). Although we still considered the diagnosis of BS, even though the patient did not meet ISG criteria, the patient was not put on immunosuppressive treatment, as the evidence for BS was too weak to start long-term immunosuppressive treatment. Other diagnoses are also needed to be considered in this patient (Table 1.3.3). In that context, we decided to perform a repeat MRI one month later, which is a general approach in the setting of undetermined inflammatory diseases.

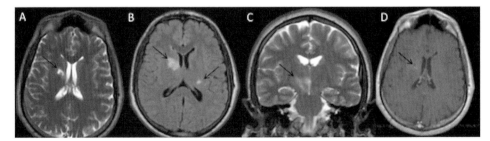

**Figure 1.3.3** Cranial magnetic resonance imaging of the patient during the headache episode. (A) Axial T2 W image shows right thalamic lesion. (B) Axial FLAIR image shows the lesions in the right thalamus and left internal capsule. (C) Coronal T2 W image reveals a lesion extending from the right thalamus to the mesencephalon. (D)Axial T1 W gd (+) image illustrates the contract enhancement pattern in parenchymal neuro-Behçet's syndrome (p-NBS).

**Table 1.3.2** International criteria for classification of Behçet's syndrome

Recurrent oral ulceration

Minor aphthous, major aphthous or herpetiform ulceration observed by a physician or reported reliably by patient

Recurrent at least three times in one 12-month period

*Plus 2 of:*

Recurrent genital ulceration

Recurrent genital aphthous ulceration or scarring, especially males, observed by physician or reliably reported by patient

Eye lesions

Anterior uveitis

Posterior uveitis

Cells in vitreous on slit-lamp examination

*or*

Retinal vasculitis observed by qualified physician (ophthalmologist)

Skin lesions

Erythema-nodosum-like lesions observed by physician or reliably reported by patient

Pseudo folliculitis

Papulopustular lesions

*or*

Acneiform nodules consistent with Behçet's disease – observed by a physician and in post-adolescent patients not receiving corticosteroids

Positive pathergy test

An erythematous papule, >2 mm, at the prick site after the application of a sterile needle, 20–22 gauge, which obliquely penetrated avascular skin to a depth of 5 mm; read by a physician at 48 hours

However, three weeks later, the patient presented with dysarthria and right-side weakness. MRI revealed a left thalamic lesion with contrast enhancement and a lesion on the anterior limb of the left internal capsule. The cerebrospinal fluid cell count and protein were normal and no oligoclonal bands were detected. He was treated with IVMP 1 g daily × 10 days and put on azathioprine 150 mg/d and an oral steroid since the MRI features were compatible with the neurological involvement of BS, and the patient had had frequent CNS involvement within a short period. He recovered fully from this relapse after IVMP. The oral steroid was tapered and stopped within six months. The patient has remained stable since then.

**Table 1.3.3** The differential diagnosis of Neuro-Behçet's syndrome

The differential diagnosis of neuro-Behçet's syndrome

Neurologic diseases
- Multiple sclerosis
- Stroke in young adults
- Primary CNS vasculitis
- Primary CNS lymphoma
- Brainstem glioma
- Amyloid-beta related angiitis

Systemic diseases with neurologic involvement
- Sarcoidosis
- Systemic vasculitis
- Wegener granulomatosis
- Metastatic disease

Systemic infections with neurologic involvement
- Tuberculosis
- Whipple disease
- Cat scratch disease
- Syphilis

## Diagnostic Algorithm

## When Should We Suspect Neurological Involvement of BS?

The onset of a subacute brainstem syndrome in a young man, especially of Mediterranean, Middle Eastern or Oriental origin that includes cranial nerve findings, dysarthria, unilateral or bilateral corticospinal tract signs, with or without weakness, ataxia and mild confusion should raise the possibility of Neuro-Behçet's Syndrome (NBS). Given that dysarthria, ataxia and hemiparesis are the major clinical features of NBS accompanying a headache in almost all cases, MRI and cerebrospinal fluid might help clinicians to differentiate a headache occurring in Neuro-Behçet's syndrome from a non-structural headache in BS.

The patient or his family should be interviewed, regarding the presence of systemic findings of BS. In BS, there is likely a history of oral aphthous ulcers and other systemic manifestations of the disease. Many patients may have never consulted a physician because of the mild nature of their systemic symptoms, or may be missed because they do not develop a full-blown picture of the disease.

Table 1.3.4 illustrates how to approach a patient with suspected Neuro-Behçet's Syndrome.

## Case Discussion

Behçet's syndrome, originally described in 1937 by the Turkish dermatologist Hulusi Behçet, a distinct disease with oro-genital ulceration and uveitis known as the "triple-symptom complex," is an idiopathic chronic relapsing multisystem vascular-inflammatory disease of

**Table 1.3.4** The diagnostic flow chart for NBS

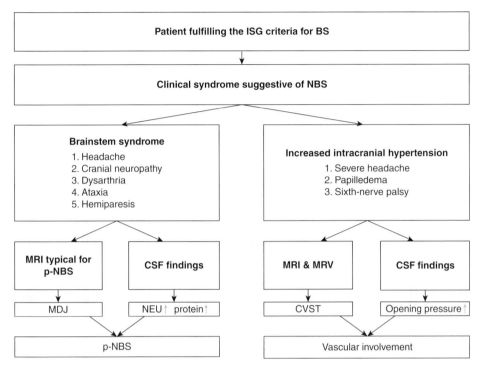

BS = Behçet's syndrome; CSF = Cerebrospinal fluid; CVST = Cerebral venous sinus thrombosis; ISG = International Study Group; MDJ = mesodiencephalic junction; NBS = neuro-Behçet's Syndrome; MRI = Magnetic resonance imaging; MRV = Magnetic resonance venography; NEU = Neutrophil; p-NBS = parenchymal neuro-Behçet's syndrome

unknown origin. The disease affects many organs and systems, causing mucocutaneous lesions, eye inflammation, musculoskeletal problems and also involves major vessels. There may be cardiac, pulmonary and gastrointestinal as well as nervous system involvement.[1]

Neurologic involvement in BS is an important cause of morbidity, and approximately 50% of patients are moderately to severely disabled after 10 years of disease. The Cerrahpaşa diagnostic criteria for NBS are "the occurrence of neurological symptoms in a patient that fulfills the International Diagnostic Criteria for BS, but are not otherwise explained by any other known systemic or neurological disease or treatment, and in whom objective abnormalities consistent with NBS are detected either on neurological examination, neuroimaging studies (magnetic resonance imaging-MRI) and/or abnormal cerebrospinal fluid (CSF) examination."

Patients with BS may present with different neurological problems, related either directly (primary) or indirectly (secondary) to the disease. Direct neurological involvement of BS may be classified into two forms: (1) parenchymal (p-NBS) or (2) vascular involvement.[2]

## Parenchymal NBS

Parenchymal NBS, with an incidence of 75% in the neurological involvement of BS, usually presents with an acute-subacute brainstem syndrome characterized by headache, cranial neuropathy, dysarthria, ataxia and hemiparesis as the most prominent symptoms.[3] While the headache is also the cardinal symptom of vascular involvement, differentiation of the neurologic type should be done cautiously together with the MRI features, as the long-term treatment differs between these two types of neurologic involvement.[4]

MRI patterns are of the utmost importance of distinguishing p-NBS from the other disorders mimicking p-NBS. The most common areas affected in p-NBS are the mesodiencephalic junction (MDJ), pons and medulla oblongata. MDJ lesions tend to extend upward to involve the diencephalic structures, and downward to involve the pontobulbar region, which is the most common radiological finding observed in p-NBS. Outside the brainstem, spinal cord involvement is also observed in p-NBS. Long-segment myelopathy occurs in most cases, which mimics neuromyelitis optica spectrum disorder (NMOSD) and myelin oligodendrocyte glycoprotein (MOG) antibody-associated disorders (MOGAD).[5] However, the recently described "Bagel Sign" pattern of spinal cord involvement in BS may be helpful for differentiating NMOSD and MOGAD from p-NBS as this pattern has not been observed in these disorders so far. The "Bagel Sign" is characterized by a central lesion with a hypo-intense core and a hyper-intense rim, with or without contrast enhancement.

Headache is the most common neurologic symptom seen in BS and can have various causes. It may be the presenting symptom of either forms of NBS, it can be seen as a symptom of ocular inflammation or may be independent of the disease, simply being a primary headache of the migraine or tension type. Up to 20% of people with BS may report a bilateral, frontal, moderately severe paroxysmal migraine-like throbbing pain, which is not true migraine and not uncommonly accompanies exacerbations of systemic findings of BS such as oral ulcerations or skin lesions. A headache that is not related to either p-NBS or cerebral venous sinus thrombosis is likely to be a toxic-vascular headache triggered by the immune-mediated disease activity in susceptible individuals. However, BS patients who report a severe headache of recent onset in the absence of any neurologic deficit and not consistent with any primary headache should be evaluated carefully to rule out the onset of NBS.

## Vascular Involvement

The main type of vascular involvement is cerebral venous sinus thrombosis (CVST) associated with a better prognosis than p-NBS. The clinical manifestations vary by the site and extent of venous thrombosis. Major vascular involvement other than CVST includes aneurysm and/or dissection. The sites of involvement include the common carotid, internal carotid, middle cerebral, superior cerebellar, anterior cerebral, anterior communicating and vertebral arteries.

CVST occurs in up to 20% of BS patients with neurological involvement. In such patients, the principal clinical features (severe headache, papilledema and sixth-nerve palsy on neurological examination) are compatible with intracranial hypertension. Most studies show that BS-associated CVST has a good prognosis in contrast to other etiologies causing CVST. The systemic features of BS in CVST patients, especially those living in endemic regions, should be looked for. CVST is usually subacute or chronic; only about 25% of cases exhibit clinical features for more than one month. Hemiparesis, impaired consciousness and epileptic seizures are uncommon in CVST patients with NBS. This may be explained by the extremely low probability of seeing hemorrhagic venous infarcts associated with NBS-CVST. Cranial MRI and magnetic resonance venography (MRV) will show that the most commonly involved dural venous sinuses are the superior and transverse sinuses, followed by the sigmoid and straight sinuses. Single-sinus occlusion is more frequent than multiple occlusions. However, if treatment is delayed because of misdiagnosis, multiple sites may be affected in the later stages of BS-CVST and in a few may compromise the optic nerves, resulting in blindness. Additionally, clinicians should be aware that cranial MRI and MRV scans may not show sinus thrombosis, even if the clinical findings strongly suggest its presence. In such situations, MRV of the thoracic and cervical venous structures should be evaluated. Irrespective of whether the neuroimaging data are abnormal or normal, we generally perform a spinal tap to study CSF pressure and contents in the suspected cases. Two case series found that CVST was more common in younger patients, supporting the idea that age is important in terms of NBS presentation. Interestingly, despite the observation of an elevated opening pressure, the CSF is free of inflammatory changes in BS-CVST patients.

### CSF Findings

During the acute phase of p-NBS, the CSF shows inflammatory changes in most cases of p-NBS with an increased number of cells, up to 100 and sometimes more per ml, neutrophils being the predominant cells, and modestly elevated protein levels. However, early lymphocytic pleocytosis should not be excluded. When neutrophilic pleocytosis is the case, they is later replaced by lymphocytes. The oligoclonal band positivity rate is low, at a rate of 20% or less.

## Prognosis

Brainstem or spinal-cord involvement, frequent relapses, early disease progression and high CSF pleocytosis are poor prognostic features for NBS, as indicated by International Consensus Recommendation (ICR). [6,7] Initiation with severe disability, primary or secondary progressive course, fever at onset, relapse during steroid tapering, meningeal signs and bladder involvement can be associated with poor outcome.

## Treatment

Due to multisystemic involvement of BS, long-term treatments should be decided by a multidisciplinary team. The first goal of the treatment in NBS is to suppress the acute episode in order to shorten the recovery time with minimal disability, and the second goal is to prevent further attacks. However, as there have been no controlled trials for the management of neurologic involvement, long-term treatments depend on clinical experience. In this regard, prognostic factors should be taken into account in choosing the appropriate treatment, together with the patient's age, gender and preferences.

High-dose intravenous methylprednisolone (IVMP) pulses for 5–10 days, followed by a slow oral tapering is the first choice for treating acute episodes. The dose and duration of steroid treatment vary amongst centers. Colchicine, azathioprine, cyclosporine, cyclophosphamide, methotrexate, chlorambucil, thalidomide, interferon alpha, anti-TNF agents and IL-6 blockers are among the drugs used for preventive treatment of the systemic features of BS, and have been tried for CNS involvement as well.

Currently, the only drug that has been shown to be effective based on Class IV evidence is infliximab for the treatment of p-NBS.[8] Although the efficacy of azathioprine isn't clear in NBS, there are a few reports suggesting that it may be effective. In many centers, azathioprine is the first-line drug to initiate once patients develop p-NBS, as also suggested by the 2018 updated European League Against Rheumatism (EULAR) recommendations. We tend to start infliximab in patients in whom azathioprine fails and sometimes as a first-line therapy in patients who present with a severe acute attack of p-NBS and who have poor prognostic factors. Given that cyclosporine-A is associated with increased risk of neurologic involvement, it should be avoided in patients with NBS and immediately stopped in patients developing NBS whilst taking cyclosporine-A.

Since the recurrence of CVST is very rare, the duration of azathioprine treatment in CVST controversial. In our practice, we usually use azathioprine at least five years, and before cessation of azathioprine we consult a rheumatologist and neuro- ophthalmologist on whether azathioprine is required for systemic features of BS other than CVST.

The addition of anticoagulant medication to steroids is controversial, as BS patients with CVST are more likely to have systemic large-vessel disease, including pulmonary and peripheral aneurysms that carry a high risk of bleeding. The complication rate with warfarin should be considered. Results of anticoagulation treatment for BS are controversial in CVST.

## References

1. Kantarci O. Neuro-Behçet's syndrome. In: *Mayo Clinic Neurology Grand Rounds.* Rochester: Mayo Clinic; 2018.

2. Kocer N, Islak C, Siva A, et al. CNS involvement in Neuro-Behcet's syndrome: an MR study. *Am J Neuroradiol.* 1999;**20**: 1015–1024.

3. Siva A, Kantarci OH, Saip S, et al. Behçet's disease: diagnostic and prognostic aspects of neurological involvement. *J Neurol.* 2001;**248**: 95–103.

4. Siva A, Saip S. The spectrum of nervous system involvement in Behçet's syndrome and its differential diagnosis. *J Neurol.* 2009;**256**(4): 513–529.

5. Uygunoglu U, Zeydan B, Ozguler Y, et al. Myelopathy in Behçet's disease: the Bagel Sign. *Ann Neurol.* 2017;**82**(2): 288–298.

6. Uygunoğlu U, Siva A. Behçet's syndrome and nervous system involvement. *Curr Neurol Neurosci Rep.* 2018;**18**(7): 35.

7. Uygunoglu U, Siva A. Behçet syndrome and the nervous system. In: Yazici Y, Hatemi G, Seyahi E, Yazici H (Eds), *Behçet Syndrome.* Springer: Cham; 2020, 73–82.

8. Zeydan B, Uygunoglu U, Saip S, et al. Infliximab is a plausible alternative for neurologic complications of Behçet disease. *Neurol Neuroimmunol Neuroinflamm.* 2016;**3**(5): e258.

# 1.3.c Sjögren Syndrome

Marilena Mangiardi, Sabrina Anticoli

## Case Presentation

A 50-year-old woman with a history of transient ischemic attacks (TIA) and raised blood pressure grade 1, was admitted to the emergency room because of speaking difficulties and a loss of strength in the right arm for about two hours on observed physical examination. Temperature was 36.5 °C, heart rate, 80 beats/min, blood pressure, 150/85 mmHg and respiratory rate, 21 breaths/min with an oxygen saturation of 99% on room air.

Brain magnetic resonance imaging (MRI) in diffusion-weighted images, showed recent ischemic lesions in the left hemisphere and MR angiography showed multiple arterial stenoses (left middle cerebral artery (MCA), left anterior cerebral artery (ACA), right intracranial internal cerebral artery (ICA)). No aneurysm, arteriovenous malformation or sinus thrombosis were found (Figure 1.3.4). Patient was eligible for intravenous thrombolysis with rtPA and after treatment neurological motor and language deficit improved.

Since extensive laboratory, cardiological and systemic vasculitis screening were negative, a diagnosis of isolated arteritis of CNS was supposed. Antiplatelets and steroid therapy was started. A few weeks later, the patient complained of a new transient episode of aphasic speech disorder; MRI showed more recent ischemic lesions (Figure 1.3.5) and arterial steno-occlusion features worsened, based on angiographic study. A second laboratory screening tested the

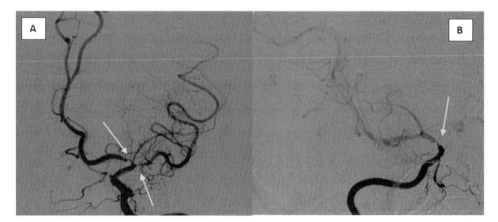

**Figure 1.3.4** (A) Angiography. Left internal carotid artery (ICA), oblique projection. Top ICA stenosis engaging the origin of the anterior cerebral artery (ACA) and the ipsilateral middle cerebral artery (ACM), with reduced representation of the downstream circle. (B) Angiography. Right internal carotid artery (ICA), oblique projection. Subocclusive stenosis of the ICA downstream of the emergence of the ophthalmic artery (yellow arrow) and reduced visualization of the downstream circle.

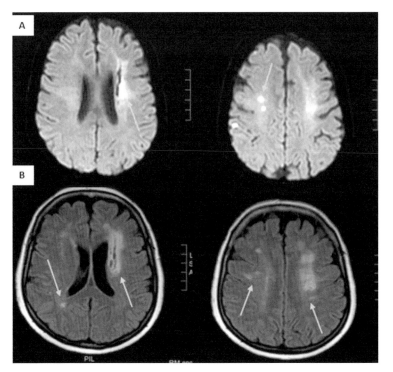

**Figure 1.3.5** (A) Brain MRI: DWI sequences. Multiple recent ischemic lesions appear in the right semi-oval center, left hemisphere and right subcortical frontal region with diffusion restriction. (B) Brain MRI: FLAIR sequences. Multiple bilateral cortico-subcortical hyperintense areas.

presence in the serum of Ro/SS-A, La/SS-B antibodies and raised PCR levels (28 mg/dl). Diagnostic suspicion of primary Sjögren syndrome (PSS)-associated cerebral vasculitis with stroke was raised, based on laboratory results and a positive Schirmer's test.

Salivary gland dynamic tracer emission CT with 99mTc-sodium pertechnetate showed decreased uptake in the parotid and submandibular glands. Immunosuppressive therapy with both IV cyclophosphamide and oral prednisone was started with clinical response and symptom control over a period of six months.

Following a clinical relapse related to a worsening of the neuroradiological picture, the patient was treated with rituximab, but the severe cardio-pulmonary complications associated with widespread cerebral edema and generalized seizures led to the death of the patient.

## Diagnostic Algorithm

Age = 50 years; average age of 54 years for women and 58 years for men at the first diagnosis. Gender = F:M 9–10:1. Annual incidence = 3.9–6.0 per 100,000 population. Type of presentation = PSS (prevalence of 0.9–3.5%) or secondary Sjögren syndrome (SSS) (association with other autoimmune diseases, such as AR, scleroderma, LES, mixed connective tissue disease, primary biliary cirrhosis). Clinical manifestation = *glandular symptoms* (xerostomia, xerophthalmia, local infection of the salivary glands, periodontal disease); *extraglandular symptoms* (arthritis, Raynaud's phenomenon, vasculitis, lymphoma, recurrent pancreatitis, lung disease, renal tubular acidosis, CNS and PNS diseases). Spectrum of CNS involvement in PSS = *focal* (motor and/or sensory deficit; aphasia/dysarthria; seizure;

brainstem syndrome; cerebellar syndrome); *diffuse* (acute or subacute encephalopathy; aseptic meningitis; cognitive dysfunction/dementia; psychiatric abnormalities); *spinal cord* (transverse myelitis; chronic progressive myelitis; neurogenic bladder; lower motor neuron disease; Brown–Sequard syndrome); *other* (optic neuropathy; multiple sclerosis-like disease). Neuroimaging for PSS-related vasculitis = variable and non-specific, with multiple bilateral ischemic infarctions in the white matter; angiography shows focal or multifocal segmental narrowing of both small and medium-sized blood vessels; occlusion may also be present. Treatment = isolated sicca symptoms may be managed symptomatically; extraglandular involvement generally requires immunosuppressive therapy, including corticosteroids, azathioprine, cyclophosphamide, intravenous immunoglobulin (IVIG), plasma exchange, infliximab and/or rituximab.

American-European Consensus Group International Classification Criteria for Sjögren syndrome

**I. Ocular symptoms:** a positive response to at least one of the following questions:

1. Have you had daily, persistent, troublesome dry eyes for more than three months?

2. Do you have a recurrent sensation of sand or gravel in the eyes?

3. Do you use tear substitutes more than three times a day?

**II. Oral symptoms:** a positive response to at least one of the following questions:

1. Have you had a daily feeling of dry mouth for more than three months?

2. Have you had recurrently or persistently swollen salivary glands as an adult?

3. Do you frequently drink liquids to aid in swallowing dry food?

**III. Ocular signs:** objective evidence of ocular involvement defined as a positive result for at least one of the following two tests:

1. Schirmer's test, performed without anesthesia (<5 mm in 5 min)

2. Rose Bengal score or other ocular dye score (>4 according to van Bijsterveld's scoring system)

**IV. Histopathology**: in minor salivary glands (obtained through normal-appearing mucosa) focal lymphocytic sialadenitis, evaluated by an expert histopathologist, with a focus score >1, defined as a number of lymphocytic foci (which are adjacent to normal appearing mucous acini and contain more than 50 lymphocytes) per 4 mm$^2$ of glandular tissue

**V. Salivary gland involvement**: objective evidence of salivary gland involvement defined by a positive result for at least one of the following diagnostic tests:

1. Unstimulated whole salivary flow (<1.5 ml in 15 min)

2. Parotid sialography showing the presence of diffuse sialectasis (punctate, cavitary or destructive pattern), without evidence of obstruction in the major ducts

3. Salivary scintigraphy showing delayed uptake, reduced concentration and/or delayed excretion of tracer

**VI. Autoantibodies:** presence in the serum of the following autoantibodies: 1. Antibodies to Ro (SSA) or La (SSB) antigens, or both

PSS: four of the six criteria in this table (including IV or VI), or three of the four objective criteria (III–IV–V–VI). In patients with an associated disease (e.g., another defined connective tissue pathology), the presence of point I or II, plus at least two of points III, IV and V, is suggestive of SSS.

PSS: primary Sjögren syndrome; SSS: secondary Sjögren syndrome; RA (rheumatoid arthritis); SLE: systemic lupus erythematosus; xerostomia: subjective feeling of mouth dryness; xerophthalmia: subjective feeling of eye dryness; CNS: central nervous system; PNS: peripheral nervous system

# Case Discussion

Sjögren syndrome is an autoimmune disease that predominantly affects women (female-to-male ratio of 9–10:1), with an average age of 54 years at the first diagnosis. The annual incidence has been estimated at 3.9–6.0 per 100,000 population. Sjögren syndrome can present as primary Sjögren syndrome (PSS) if it is isolated syndrome, or as secondary Sjögren syndrome (SSS) if associated with other connective tissue diseases (most commonly rheumatoid arthritis or systemic lupus erythematosus). The pathological features are lymphocytic infiltrations in the exocrine glands that determine xerostomia and dryness of the eye, and hyperactivity of B lymphocytes that induces the appearance of numerous circulating autoantibodies (Ro/SS-A, La/SS-B). Anti-SSA occurs in 33–74% of patients with Sjögren syndrome, anti-SSB (La) in 23–52%, and antinuclear antibodies in 59–85%.[1] Extra-glandular organs are involved in about a third of patients. These include: thyroid, lungs, kidneys, gastrointestinal tract, liver, central or peripheral nervous system, cardiovascular system and hematological involvement (malignant lymphoma).

Sjögren syndrome affects the nervous system in approximately 20% of cases and, of these, only 2–5% present CNS involvement. Neurological symptoms may precede the onset of sicca syndrome in a variable percentage of patients (25–92%). The most common neurological manifestations in Sjögren syndrome are sensory ganglionopathy (also known as sensory neuronopathy or sensory ataxic neuropathy), painful small-fiber neuropathy, longitudinally extensive transverse myelitis (LETM) and neuromyelitis optica (NMO). Nevertheless, there have been a few reported cases of ischemic and/or hemorrhagic stroke associated with Sjögren syndrome as the first symptomatic manifestation of the disease. Some patients may develop neurological disorders, on average, 7 years (range 1–16 years) after PSS diagnosis.[2]

Cerebral artery vasculitis secondary to the disease is likely the pathogenic mechanism of the ischemic damage in patients with PSS.

Vasculitis of small- and medium-sized vessels (rarely large arteries), is one of the mechanisms underlying CNS involvement in PSS. Recent meta-analysis has shown that patients with PSS have a significant increase in arterial stiffness measured with pulse wave velocity and intima-media thickness.[3] A high level of cytokines, such as IL-1, IL-6 and TNF-a, and pro-inflammatory molecules probably represents the cause of subclinical atherosclerosis in PSS. It has been speculated that the underlying molecular mechanism is mediated by chemotaxis of dendritic cells, monocytes and T cells into the intima. These markers include soluble thrombomodulin, antiendothelial cell antibodies, VCAM-1, ICAM-1 and asymmetric dimethylarginine.[4] Immunogenic studies have shown a higher frequency of HLA histocompatibility antigens in patients with Sjögren syndrome; in particular there is a high association with the HLA DQA1*0501 allele.

Neurological symptoms with acute onset in Sjögren-syndrome-affected patients may be different at the beginning, but these are mainly focal symptoms (aphasia, dysarthria, epileptic seizure), cerebellar or brainstem syndrome. Transient ischemic attack (TIA) with recurrent course and complete functional recovery between two consecutive events, seem to be the most common ischemic manifestations in patients with PSS and CNS involvement. In the few cases described, TIA correlated with stenosis of a cerebral artery, most frequently the middle cerebral artery. However, in some cases, the disease can have a recurring course, with several clinical bouts that remit after treatment with symptomatic drugs (anticonvulsants in patients with epilepsy) or oral anticoagulation (in a patient with recurrent ischemic episodes).

Neuroimaging findings for PSS-related vasculitis are usually variable and non-specific, with multiple bilateral ischemic infarctions in the white matter being the most common lesions. Meningeal enhancement and intracranial hemorrhage can also be seen. Angiography shows focal or multifocal segmental narrowing of both small and medium-sized blood vessels; occlusion may also be present. The same findings can be demonstrated in both CTA and MRA. Vessel wall MRI (VW-MRI) allowing differential diagnosis between vasculitis, where there is contrast enhancement of the involved arterial wall, and other causes of vascular narrowing (intracranial atherosclerotic plaque, reversible cerebral vaso-constriction syndrome, moyamoya disease, etc.).

The diagnosis of PSS requires four of the six criteria shown in the Diagnostic Algorithm section (including IV or VI), or three of the four objective criteria (III-IV–V-VI). In patients with an associated disease (e.g., another defined connective tissue pathology), the presence of point I or II, plus at least two of points III, IV and V, is suggestive of SSS. Lip minor salivary gland biopsy may be required to rule out other conditions that can cause dry eye, oral dryness or salivary gland hypertrophy.[5]

In the last three decades, therapeutic approaches in primary Sjögren syndrome have been based on the use of surrogate agents for sicca features and glucocorticoids and immunosuppressive agents for extraglandular involvement. While isolated sicca symptoms of Sjögren syndrome may be managed symptomatically, extraglandular involvement generally requires immunosuppressive therapy, including corticosteroids, azathioprine, cyclophosphamide, intravenous immunoglobulin (IVIG), plasma exchange, infliximab and rituximab.[6] Emerging immunosuppressant drugs and biologic therapies have increased the therapeutic spectrum available in the most severe situations, but their use is limited by the lack of specific licensing. There is even less scientific evidence on the treatment of patients who do not respond to first-line therapies. B-cell targeted agents seem to be the most promising future therapy, especially rituximab, which has shown improvement in vasculitis related to Sjögren syndrome.[7] The agents that block BAFF (B cell–activating factor of the tumor necrosis factor family) may also be a promising therapy.[8]

Advances in knowledge of the molecular mechanisms involved in the etiopathogenesis of primary Sjögren syndrome may allow the development of more effective, highly selective therapies without the adverse effects often associated with standard, less-selective drugs.

# References

1. Bournia VK, Vlachoyiannopoulos PG. Subgroups of Sjögren syndrome patients according to serological profiles. *J Autoimmun.* 2012;**39**: 15–26.

2. Berkowitz AL, Samuels MA. The neurology of Sjögren's syndrome and the rheumatology of peripheral neuropathy and myelitis. *Pract Neurol.* 2014;**14**(1): 14–22.

3. Yong WC, Sanguankeo A, Upala S, et al. Association between primary Sjögren's syndrome, arterial stiffness, and subclinical atherosclerosis: a systematic review and meta-analysis. *Clin Rheumatol.* 2019;**38**: 447–455.

4. Valim V, Gerdts E, Jonsson R, et al. Atherosclerosis in Sjögren's syndrome: evidence, possible mechanisms and

knowledge gaps. *Clin Exp Rheumatol.* 2016;**34**(1): 133–142.

5. Vitali C, Bombardieri S, Jonsson R, et al. Classification criteria for Sjögren's syndrome: a revised version of the European criteria proposed by the American-European Consensus Group. *Ann Rheum Dis.* 2002;**61**: 554–558.

6. Ramos-Casals M, Tzioufas AG, Stone JH, Sisó A, Bosch X. Treatment of primary Sjögren syndrome a systematic review. *J Am Med Assoc.* 2010;**304**: 452–460.

7. Seror R, Sordet C, Guillevin L, et al. Tolerance and efficacy of rituximab and changes in serum B cell biomarkers in patients with systemic complications of primary Sjögren's syndrome. *Ann Rheum Dis.* 2007;**66**(3): 351–357.

8. Pers JO, Devauchelle V, Daridon C, et al. BAFF-modulated repopulation of B lymphocytes in the blood and salivary glands of rituximab-treated patients with Sjögren's syndrome. *Arthritis Rheum.* 2007;**56**(5): 1464–1477.

# 1.3.d  Sarcoidosis

Dilcan Kotan, Aslı Aksoy Gündoğdu

## Case Presentation

A 49-year-old female patient was admitted to the emergency room with a complaint of sudden numbness in the left arm and left leg. Her history showed that she had been experiencing intermittent cough, extreme weakness, and general body pain for the past year and there was a diagnosis of autoimmune thyroiditis. There were no relevant diagnoses in her family history. Upon examination, the liver and spleen could not be palpated, there was no lymphadenopathy, the lung examination was normal, the heart sounds were rhythmic, and murmurs and additional sounds were not noted. In the neurological examination, there was left-sided frust hemiparesis, hemihypoesthesia and a positive Babinski sign. Cranial computerized tomography (CT) was isodense, and cranial diffusion magnetic resonance imaging (MRI) showed areas compatible with a hyperintense, apparent diffusion coefficient (ADC) hypointense acute infarct in B1000 sections in the posterior part of the right occipital lobe. Routine blood tests showed the following: HDL: 52 mg/dl, LDL: 180 mg/dl, and total cholesterol: 240 mg/dl. On carotid vertebral Doppler ultrasound, calcified atheroma plaques were present in the bilateral carotid bulb. No significant risk factor for stroke etiology was identified in the patient except for atherosclerosis and hyperlipidemia. Chest X-ray showed bilateral hilar fullness. Mediastinal lymphadenopathy and micronodular parenchymal infiltrations in the parenchyma of both lungs, thickening of the bilateral major fissure and multiple thin linear reticulonodular patterns with diffuse density were observed on high-resolution CT (HRCT). Respiratory function tests were normal. Advanced laboratory tests showed the following: a sedimentation rate of 44 mm/h; negativity for serum antineutrophilic antibody (ANA) and ANA profile, high rheumatoid factor (RF) at the border (18.9), high TSH (9.4); high anti-TPO (68 IU/ml <5.6); positivity for SS-A, SS-B and Ro-52 recombinant AMA-M2 (+++), positivity for direct Coombs IgG, positivity for anti-β-2 glycoprotein 1 IgG and a serum ACE (angiotensin-converting enzyme) level of 80 µg/l (N <40 µg/l ). Thyroid ultrasonography (USG) was compatible with thyroiditis. Salivary gland biopsy showed no inflammation or plasma cells.

In our patient, fluorodeoxyglucose (FDG)-positron emission tomography (PET)/CT showed pathological uptake in the mediastinal and abdominal lymphadenopathy areas, ground-glass opacity infiltration areas located in the bilateral lungs and intramedullary bone uptake, all of which are consistent with sarcoidosis. Pathologic investigation of the bone marrow biopsy material revealed non-caseating granulomas consisting of different dimensions of epithelioid histiocytes that stained positive for CD68 in light hypocellular

(a)                                         (b)

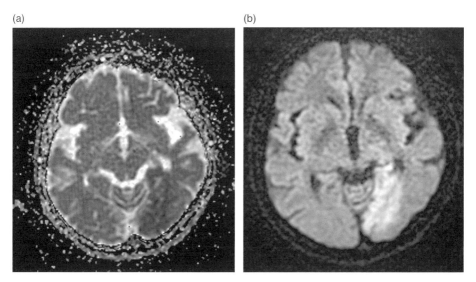

**Figure 1.3.6** Diffusion-weighted MRI showing hyperintensity (A) with decreased (B) ADC sections in the posterior part of the left occipital lobe.

regions. The presence of an "asteroid body," which is observed in the foci of granuloma structures, led to the diagnosis of sarcoidosis.

Based on the diagnosis of neurosarcoidosis (NS), oral corticosteroid and azathioprine treatment was suggested and followed.

# Diagnostic Algorithm

| Clinical suspicious of NS | |
|---|---|
| Age = 25-50 years;<br>Gender = Female ratio: 55-63%;<br>Type of onset = Acute, subacute, or chronic<br>Clinical manifestations: a) Focal neurological deficit; b)<br>Non-specific complaints (fatigue and general weakness) | Non specific<br>neurological<br>manifestations |

**Cranial CT =** Isodense,
**Diffusion MRI =** Hyperintensity with decreased ADC sections in the posterior part of the left occipital lobe compatible with acute ischemic stroke

| Differential Diagnosis | | | |
|---|---|---|---|
| **Infectious:**<br>Cryptococcosis,<br>Histoplasmosis,<br>Coccidioidomycosis,<br>Tuberculosis,<br>Syphilis,<br>Lyme disease,<br>HIV | **Inflammatory:**<br>Vasculitis,<br>Behçet's disease,<br>SLE,<br>MS,<br>ADEM,<br>Cerebral amyloid<br>angiopathy,<br>Acute inflammatory<br>demyelinating<br>polyradiculoneuropat<br>hy. | **Malignancies:**<br>Leptomeningeal<br>carcinomatosis,<br>Primary CNS<br>lymphoma,<br>Metastatic disease,<br>Gliomatosis cerebri,<br>Paraneoplastic<br>neuropathy | **Toxins:**<br>Alcohol,<br>Drugs,<br>Berylliosis |

| Diagnostic Studies |
|---|

**Blood Tests**
- CBC may show normochromic normocytic anaemia, lymphopaenia, megaloblastic changes or basophilic stippling.
- ESR, CK and aldolase may be elevated.
- Hypercalcaemia may occur in systemic involvement.
- Fasting glucose, glycosylated haemoglobin, and vitamin B-12 level
- BUN and creatinine to check renal functions
- ALT, AST, bilirubin, ALP and GGT to check liver functions
- Endocrine studies (thyroid function tests, sex hormones, growth hormone, insulin-like growth factor) should be performed to detect damage of the pituitary-hypothalamic axis
- C-ANCA to differentiate from Wegener granulomatosis
- Serum ACE levels are elevated but may be unreliable in isolated CNS sarcoidosis
- Protein immune electrophoresis

**CSF analysis**
- Findings are in normal limits in 30% of cases; therefore, serial CSF analyses may be performed.
- CSF pressure is frequently normal.
- May be xanthochromic and shows a white cell count of >50 mm3, elevated protein levels of >100 mg/dL, high CD4/CD8 ratio, elevated IgG index, or oligoclonal bands.
- In more than half of patients, ACE, lysozyme and beta2-microglobulin levels may be elevated.

**Tuberculin skin test**
- This test reveals anergy in systemic or pulmonary sarcoidosis. Nevertheless, in isolated NS, skin test has no diagnostic value.

**HRCT**
- Search for hilar adenopathy or granulomas

**FDG-PET**
- Useful to show the extent of inflammatory activity and to identify occult and reversible granulomas.
- May be performed to decide biopsy area

| Treatment of NS | | | | |
|---|---|---|---|---|
| **First-Line Treatment:** Corticosteroids<br><br>Intravenous pulsed methylprednisolone in doses of 500-1,000 mg for 3-5 days followed by daily doses of 1 mg/kg oral prednisone (tapering doses) | **Second-line Treatment Options:** Cyclophospha mide, Methotrexate, Azathioprine, Mycophenolate mofetil, Cyclosporine, Hydroxychloro quine, Infliximab Anti TNF-α | Antiaggregants for ischaemic stroke, Anticoagulants for cerebral venous sinus thrombosis | Intravenous immunoglobulins for peripheral nervous system involvement | Antiepileptics for epileptic seizures |

NS: Neurosarcoidosis; CT: Computerized tomography; MRI: Magnetic resonance imaging; DWI: Difusion weighted imaging; ADC: Apparent diffusion coefficient; CSF: Cerebrospinal fluid; HRCT: High-resolution computerized tomography; SLE: Systemic lupus erythaematosus; MS: multiple sclerosis; ADEM: Acute disseminated encephalomyelitis; CNS: Central nervous system; CBC: Complete blood count; ESR: erythrocyte sedimentation rate; CK: Creatine kinase; CRP: C-reactive protein; BUN: Blood urea nitrogen; ALT: Alanine aminotransferase; AST: Aspartate aminotransferase; ALP: alkaline phosphatase; GGT: gamma-glutamyl transpeptidase; ANCA: Antineutrophil cytoplasmic antibodies; ACE: angiotension-converting enzyme; Fluorodeoxyglucose (FDG)-Positron emission tomography (PET); TNF: tumor necrosis factor

# Case Discussion

Sarcoidosis is a chronic, idiopathic, inflammatory and granulomatous disease with multi-system involvement and an unknown etiology. Non-caseating epithelioid granulomas in the lungs, uvea, lymph nodes and skin are the characteristic findings of the disease. Granulomas have a central core of epithelioid and CD4 lymphocytes and a peripheral circle of CD8 lymphocytes, B cells and fibroblasts. The pathogenesis of the disease is still unclear. A genetic predisposition has been proposed; however, no single gene defect has been detected thus far.[1]

Sarcoid granulomas produce angiotensin-converting enzyme (ACE) and cause high cytokine levels. Serum ACE levels are elevated in more than half of sarcoidosis patients. Granulomas also produce high levels of cytokines and cause perivascular inflammation in the blood vessel walls and Virchow–Robin spaces. Sarcoid vasculitis is a very unusual clinical condition that mostly affects vessels of various sizes, including the abdominal aorta, and organs, such as the lungs, kidneys and skin. NS is a rare and important cause of cerebral vasculitis that can result in increased morbidity and mortality.[1,2]

A patient with a diagnosis of sarcoidosis may develop new neurological symptoms, or the presenting symptom of a patient with no prior diagnosis of sarcoidosis may be typical for NS. NS frequently occurs in patients with active disease and systemic involvement. Overall, 10–17% of patients have isolated NS. The disease commonly occurs in young adults aged 25–50 years, and a slight female predominance (55–63%) has been reported. NS has an incidence of 0.04–64/100,000, affects 5–16% of patients and involves the brain, spinal cord, optic nerves, peripheral nerves and muscles. The clinical signs and symptoms of NS depend on the affected part of the nervous system. Multiple cranial nerve palsies, optic neuritis, meningitis, encephalopathy, cerebrovascular events, seizures, hydrocephalus, myelopathy, dementia, peripheral neuropathy, myopathy and intraparenchymal tumors have been reported. Patients also suffer from non-specific complaints, such as fatigue and general weakness.[2,3]

Very rare presentations of NS are cerebrovascular events, such as ischemic stroke, transient ischemic attacks (TIAs), intracranial hemorrhage or venous thrombosis. At least half of the patients experience cerebrovascular events without a prior diagnosis of sarcoidosis. The possible mechanisms underlying NS-associated cerebrovascular events are cardiogenic embolism, artery-to-artery embolism, atherothrombosis, leptomeningeal inflammation, vasculitis, infectious angiitis, hypertension due to glomerulonephritis and intracranial arterial compression due to the mass effect of the granulomas. Sarcoidosis patients have an increased risk of other atherosclerotic diseases, such as myocardial infarction and peripheral arterial diseases.[2,3]

Clinically silent granulomatous vascular infiltrations are commonly discovered in postmortem studies. Small arterial perforators are most commonly affected in NS, whereas large vessels are rarely involved. Therefore, large-vessel and recurrent infarcts may occur, but small infarcts in the basal ganglia, thalamus or brainstem are more frequently observed. Hemorrhagic stroke in NS is often microhemorrhagic and occurs in the intraparenchymal and supratentorial regions. Granulomatous meningeal involvement has been proposed as a pathology underlying NS-associated cerebral venous sinus thrombosis. The superior sagittal sinus is the most commonly affected part, and patients usually present with symptoms of elevated intracranial pressure.[2–4]

There is no specific test for the diagnosis of NS. The Neurosarcoidosis Consortium Consensus Group has established diagnostic criteria indicating possible, probable or definite NS. In possible NS, typical clinical findings and diagnostic tests suggesting NS and no evidence of other causes should be provided. In probable NS, in addition to the previous criteria, there is a pathological confirmation of systemic granulomatous disease. Definite NS meets all of the above criteria, and the nervous system abnormality is consistent with NS and is one of two subtypes. While type A is characterized by evident extraneural sarcoidosis, type B is consistent with isolated NS.[2,3]

The first-line treatment for NS is corticosteroids. Spontaneous remission is very rare, whereas relapses occur in most cases. Therefore, long-term treatment is often required, especially in patients with severe CNS damage. To the best of our knowledge, there have been no controlled studies for NS to determine the dose and duration of treatment. In periods of exacerbation of the clinical symptoms, patients may be treated with intravenous pulsed methylprednisolone in doses of 500–1000 mg for three to five days followed by daily doses of 1 mg/kg oral prednisone (tapering doses) for months.[2,3,5]

Steroids cannot be used in cases of any contraindications, such as hypersensitivity or allergy. In patients with hypertension, diabetes or gastroduodenal ulcers, steroids should be used with caution. Chronic treatment with daily steroids may lead to aseptic necrosis of the femur or shoulder, osteoporosis, adrenal insufficiency or opportunistic infections. Trimethoprim-sulfamethoxazole should be given for the chemoprophylaxis of *Pneumocystis carinii* infection. Bisphosphonate, H2 blockers or proton-pump inhibitors should be given to avoid steroid complications. A low-carbohydrate and salt-restricted diet is recommended. Annual bone densitometry should be performed to monitor the development of osteoporosis.[2,3,5]

Second-line treatments, such as cyclophosphamide, methotrexate, azathioprine, mycophenolate mofetil, cyclosporine, hydroxychloroquine and infliximab, may be used in patients who are unresponsive to steroids or have a contraindication to steroids. Antitumour necrosis factor alpha (TNF-α) may be considered in refractory disease. In addition to immunosuppressant agents, antiaggregants should be added to treatment for ischemic stroke due to large-vessel vasculitis, and anticoagulants should be added for cerebral venous sinus thrombosis due to CNS vasculitis. Intravenous immunoglobulins may be administered for peripheral nervous system involvement. Myelopathy in sarcoidosis may be associated with bowel and bladder dysfunction. Antiepileptic drugs are needed in the case of seizures. Syndromes involving inappropriate antidiuretic hormone secretion and diabetes insipidus may result in an electrolyte imbalance, which needs to be corrected. Relapses are frequently observed in NS despite the effective use of first- and second-line treatments.[1-3,5]

In the follow-up period, gadolinium-enhanced MRI of the brain and spinal cord may be useful, while serum ACE levels are not used to evaluate the effectiveness of treatment. The most valuable parameters are the resolution of symptoms and a good clinical response of the patient. In NS, mortality mainly occurs as a result of hydrocephalus, sepsis and immunosuppressant-related side effects rather than cerebrovascular events.[2,3,5] NS should be considered in patients, especially young patients, experiencing recurrent TIAs, ischemic or hemorrhagic strokes, and having MRI findings suggestive of NS. The most important step for a clinician is to consider the possibility of NS in a stroke patient, which will aid in the early diagnosis, treatment and proper management of the disease.

## References

1. Iannuzzi MC, Fontana JR. Sarcoidosis: Clinical presentation, immunopathogenesis, and therapeutics. *J Am Med Assoc.* 2011;**305**(4): 391–399.

2. Degardin A, Devos P, Vermersch P, de Seze J. Cerebrovascular symptomatic involvement in sarcoidosis. *Acta Neurol Belg.* 2010;**110**(4): 349–352.

3. Ungprasert P, Matteson EL. Neurosarcoidosis. *Rheum Dis Clin North Am.* 2017;**43**(4): 593–606.

4. Bathla G, Watal P, Gupta S, et al. Cerebrovascular manifestations of neurosarcoidosis: an underrecognized aspect of the imaging spectrum. *Am J Neuroradiol.* 2018;**39**(7): 1194–1200.

5. Voortman M, Drent M, Baughman RP. Management of neurosarcoidosis: a clinical challenge. *Curr Opin Neurol.* 2019;**32**(3): 475–483.

# 1.3.e Inflammatory Bowel Disease

Gökhan Kabaçam, Merhmet Arhan, Murat Törüner

## Case Presentation

A 25-year-old female patient had been given a diagnosis of left-sided ulcerative colitis (UC) in 2010 and had a steroid-dependent clinical picture. Due to azathioprine intolerance, infliximab (IFX) therapy was started in 2014. In the third month of treatment she was hospitalized with a flare-up in UC. Following intense abdominal pain, abdominal Doppler ultrasonography (US) was performed. Due to suspicion of stenosis in the aorta, magnetic resonance (MR) angiography was performed, which revealed narrowing throughout the entire abdominal aorta. After these evaluations, a diagnosis of Takayasu arteritis (TAK) was made and methotrexate treatment was initiated which then caused an allergic reaction, and was therefore discontinued.

In May of 2016, the patient developed hypertension (HT) requiring multiple anti-HT agents. In her control MR angiography, she had 50% stenosis in the abdominal aorta, and 50–75 % stenosis in the proximal parts of the bilateral renal arteries. For the management of TAK with renal involvement, IFX was switched to rituximab. In August 2016, with another flare-up of UC accompanying TAK, she received 1000 mg pulse corticosteroid (CS) for three days followed by 0.5–1 mg/kg prednisolone for three months as maintenance treatment. Her UC entered remission, however she had uncontrolled HT despite multiple anti–HT agents, so a control angiography was performed which revealed stable narrowing in the abdominal aorta with progressive stenosis in proximal parts of the bilateral renal arteries of 95–100%. Renal scintigraphy showed atrophy in the right kidney. A stent was inserted into left renal artery and double antiaggregant therapy, including aspirin (ASA) + clopidogrel was initiated.

A month later, the patient had hematochezia and antiaggregant therapy was stopped. Cyclophosphamide was initiated for TAK. In July 2017, her UC was under remission but due to active vasculitis, adalimumab (ADA) therapy was initiated. Figures 1.3.7 and 1.3.8 show the narrowing in the abdominal aorta.

In October 2017, she was hospitalized again with a flare-up in UC under adalimumab treatment. Colonoscopy showed biopsy-proven disease activity (Rachmilewitz EIA = 8–10) of UC (Figure 1.3.9).

During this flare-up she was experiencing symptoms of bloody diarrhea, abdominal pain and weight loss (9 kg) over three months. C-reactive protein (CRP) was 82 mg/dl (N = 0–5), Hb = 10.3 g/dl, albumin 1.93 g/dl, without any signs of infection. Vedolizumab treatment was planned, however she refused to have any more medical treatments so total procto-colectomy with ilial pouch anal anastomosis was performed.

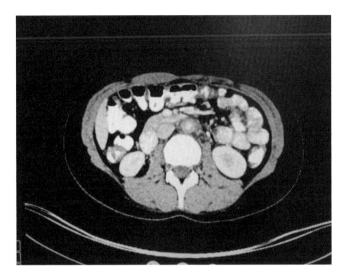

**Figure 1.3.7** CT scan showing narrowing in the abdominal aorta with normal intestinal walls (June 2017).

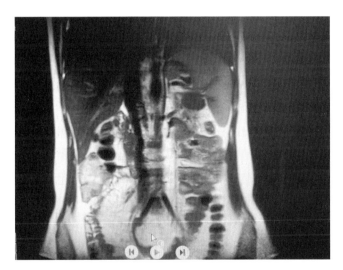

**Figure 1.3.8** MR angiography showing diffuse stenosis over the course of abdominal aorta (June 2017).

Pathological examination of colectomy specimen surprisingly showed non-necrotizing granulomas in the submucosa and subserosa, and segmental transmural inflammation (Figures 1.3.10 and 1.3.11). With that, her diagnosis was changed to Crohn's Disease (CD).

In the last visit she was asymptomatic without any medical treatment. CRP = 6 mg/dl (0–5 mg/dl), Hb =14 g/dl, albumin = 4.3 g/dl. Control MR angiography revealed irregular wall thickening in the aorta, and the orifices of the superior mesenteric artery and celiac arteries.

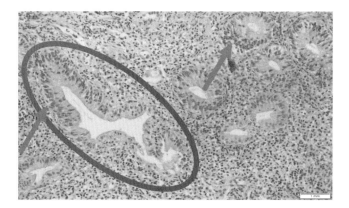

**Figure 1.3.9** Colonic pathology findings showing distortion, branching, regeneration (circle), and cryptitis (arrows) without any sign of granuloma.

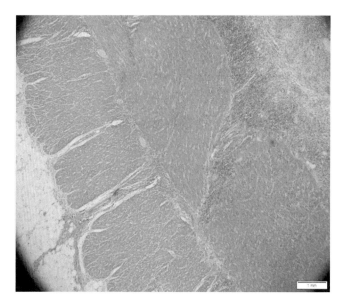

**Figure 1.3.10** Transmural inflammation.

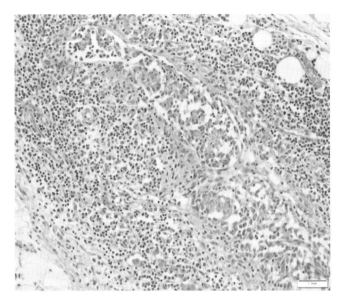

**Figure 1.3.11** Non-necrotizing granuloma in bowel wall.

# Diagnostic Algorithm

---

**Clinical Presentation of Vasculitis Secondary to Inflammatory Bowel Disease**

- Common type of vasculitides associated with IBD:
  - o Large-vessel vasculitis, mainly TAK
  - o Cutaneous vasculitis
  - o AAV, mostly GPA
  - o Central nervous system vasculitis
- Symptoms related to bowel ischemia due to mesenteric vessel involvement or gastrointestinal ulcers due to small vessel involvement.
- Most common form is CD + TAK
- Characterized by non-specific rise in acute phase reactants, constitutional symptoms (fever, abdominal pain, weight loss, rectal bleeding, nausea, diarrhea under immunosuppressive therapy) together with HT, difference in pulse/blood pressure between extremities, renal, neurological problems or rash in a patient with IBD
- IBD precedes TAK by median four years
- TAK presents 8–12 years early in cases with IBD
- There are some clues of genetic background and past tuberculosis history

---

**Laboratory Findings of Vasculitis Secondary to Inflammatory Bowel Disease**

- Elevation in acute phase reactants (CRP, ESR, calprotectin, etc.)
- ASCA, ANCA not helpful
- Doppler US, MR, CT, PET-CT to demonstrate narrowing or irregularity and enhancement in the affected vessel and organ
- Catheter based angiography is gold standard
- Endoscopic evaluation

---

**Etiological Investigations/Differential Diagnosis of Vasculitis Secondary to Inflammatory Bowel Disease**

- Microbiologic tests to exclude super-infections (stool microscopy, culture, entamoeba antigen testing, C. difficile toxin a&b, CMV – DNA, Tuberculosis, etc.)
- Renal function evaluation
- Endoscopy: focal (discontinuous) granular pattern over mild mucosal inflammation can be typical that may lead to difficulty in discriminating UC from CD at initial colonoscopy. Vasculitis-related ulcers are usually multiple, irregular and uneven based. Biopsy samples are hard to evaluate because superficial mucosal biopsies have a low diagnostic yield.

---

**Treatment of Vasculitis Secondary to Inflammatory Bowel Disease**

- Steroids (pulse steroid may be needed according to the severity of vasculitis)
- Biologic agents
- Cyclophosphamide
- Rituximab
- Angiographical treatment of major vascular abnormalities like stenoses
- Surgical treatment of significant stenoses, aneurysms or bleeding

# Case Discussion

Inflammatory bowel diseases (IBDs) are idiopathic, chronic inflammatory diseases of the intestinal system. However, vasculitides are also rare, chronic inflammatory disorders of the vascular system, some of which may present with involvement of the intestinal organs. These two different diseases are not only in the differential diagnosis for each other, depending on the clinical presentation, but they may also coexist at a rate not easily explainable by chance. There are several case reports and case series in the literature about this rare coexistance.[1,2] Common types of vasculitides that are associated with IBD are:

- Large vessel vasculitis, mainly Takayasu arteritis
- Cutaneous vasculitis
- Antineutrophil cytoplasmic antibody (ANCA)-associated vasculitides (AAV), mostly granulomatosis with polyangiitis (GPA)
- Central nervous system vasculitis.

Gastrointestinal manifestations may be seen in these and several other vasculitides due to involvement of the mesenteric vasculature leading to bowel ischemia. Granulomatous inflammation of the bowel is a characteristic sign of not only CD, but also small vessel vasculitides that affect arterioles and/or capillaries like AAV, including GPA, and large-vessel vasculitis like TAK. TAK or GPA are more commonly seen in CD patients.[2] Because our representative case has TAK, which is more commonly associated with IBD, we will discuss TAK here.

TAK is defined by granulomatous inflammation of the aorta and its branches. There is non-specific rise in acute-phase reactants without any specific laboratory marker. TAK is suspected in a case with constitutional symptoms with hypertension, differences in the pulse/blood pressure between extremities, and the diagnosis is made by Doppler US, MR or PET/CT showing inflammatory narrowing of the affected vessels on a clinical basis. It is rare, affecting 0.26–0.64 per 100,000 people and is more frequent in Asian populations.

The epidemiology of TAK in IBD is interesting. In a report of 44 TAK cases from France, 9% of the patients had CD, in North America out of 32 TAK cases, CD was found in 6% of the patients compared to the normal population prevalence of 0.2%. A Canadian study revealed 5% of the 160 TAK cases had IBD. In Japan, 9.2% of 142 TAK cases had IBD, whereas in Turkey 5.8% of the patients had IBD.[2] There is a female predominance in cases with concurrent disease.

The pathogenic mechanisms of this coexistence may be the genetic background. Among class I HLA molecules, HLA-A*24:02, -B*52:01 and -C*12:02 were expressed more in TAK+IBD than without IBD. According to the studies on HLA class II, HLA-DRB-1 *15:02, DQA-1*01:03, DQB-1*06:01, DPB-1*09:01 were more commonly presented in TAK and IBD.[3] IL12/IL23 pathway aberrations created tendencies toward UC, CD and TAK. A possible environmental risk factor for both TAK and IBD may be tuberculosis (TB) due to molecular mimicry of HSP-60 with HSP-65 of TB.

In the clinical course, commonly IBD precedes TAK by a median of 4 years (0.5–31 years), and in most cases IBD is already in remission at the onset of TAK,[4] which is 8–12 years earlier in cases with IBD. Anti-*Saccharomyces cerevisiae* antibody (ASCA) and ANCA testing may not be useful for predicting the association between TAK and IBD. If a patient with IBD develops constitutional symptoms like fever, abdominal pain, weight loss, rectal bleeding, nausea, diarrhea, hypertension or elevated acute-phase reactants under immuno-suppressive therapy, TAK may be the causative factor. If cross-sectional radiologic investigations reveal vasculopathy, catheter-based angiography is the gold standard for diagnosis and is required for therapeutic interventions. In the endoscopy, a focal (discontinuous) granular pattern over mild mucosal inflammation can be typical and may lead to difficulty in discriminating UC from CD at initial colonoscopy. Vasculitis-related ulcers are usually multiple, irregular and unevenly based.[3] Biopsy samples are hard to evaluate because superficial mucosal biopsies have a low diagnostic yield.

For the treatment of combined disease, most cases require steroids or biologic agents. There has been a good clinical response (55%) with biologics, that allowed tapering/discontinuation of steroids. In a literature search, four cases developed TAK during anti-TNF treatment, as in our case.[5] Pulse steroid, cyclophosphamide, rituximab or surgical treatment was necessary for management. Angiographic revascularization of the stenotic mesenteric vasculature may be necessary.

# References

1. Sy A, Khalidi N, Dehghan N, et al. Vasculitis in patients with inflammatory bowel diseases: A study of 32 patients and systematic review of the literature. *Semin Arthritis Rheum.* 2016;**45**(4): 475–482.

2. Kilic L, Kalyoncu U, Karadag O, et al. Inflammatory bowel diseases and Takayasu's arteritis: coincidence or association? *Int J Rheum Dis.* 2016;**19**(8): 814–818.

3. Akiyama S, Fujii T, Matsuoka K, et al. Endoscopic features and genetic background of inflammatory bowel disease complicated with Takayasu arteritis. *J Gastroenterol Hepatol.* 2017;**32**(5): 1011–1017.

4. Anderson E, Gakhar N, Stull C, Caplan L. Gastrointestinal and Hepatic Disease in Vasculitis. *Rheum Dis Clin North Am.* 2018;**44**(1): 1–14.

5. Hatemi I, Hatemi G, Çelik AF. Systemic vasculitis and the gut. *Curr Opin Rheumatol.* 2017;**29**(1): 33–38.

# 1.3.f  Cerebral Amyloid Angiopathy-Related Inflammation

Marialuisa Zedde, Rosario Pascarella, Jacopo C. De Francesco, Fabrizio Piazza

## Clinical Presentation

A 69-year-old male was admitted to the neurological ward because of the sudden onset of neurobehavioral symptoms (disorientation, agitation and confusion) and generalized seizures. His past medical history was completely unremarkable. Brain CT showed multiple bilateral hypodense areas with sulcal effacement and mass effect in the supratentorial compartment and a multifocal cerebral tumor was suspected. Electroencephalography showed bilateral theta slowdown of brain electrical activity.

The patient was treated using antiepileptic drugs and osmotic diuretics and the clinical course was characterized by persistence of spatial and temporal disorientation, psychomotor slowness, confusional status, dysarthria and right hemiparesis. The Mini-Mental State Examination (MMSE) score was 10/30.

Brain MRI showed bilateral asymmetrical T2 and fluid-attenuated inversion recovery (FLAIR) subcortical confluent hyperintensities encompassing several lobes (parieto-occipital lobes on both sides with precuneus involvement, Rolandic location with involvement of paracentral lobulus, bilateral frontal lobes) with corresponding sulcal effacement, mass effect and spontaneous leptomeningeal linear hyperintensities with contrast enhancement. Gradient echo (GRE) sequences showed multiple cortical and subcortical microbleeds. Blood tests were normal, including autoimmunity. Cerebrospinal fluid (CSF) examination showed mild hyperproteinorrachie (52 mg/dl, normal range, <45 mg/dl) with normal glucose content and cell count. CSF cultures and PCR for neurotropic viruses were normal. Molecular analysis of the apolipoprotein E gene revealed an apoE ε4/ε4 genotype. Based on clinical and neuroimaging findings a diagnosis of probable cerebral amyloid angiopathy-related inflammation (CAA-ri) was made, according to Auriel et al. criteria.[1] The patient was treated by IV administration of methyliprednisolone 1000 mg/day for five days with rapid clinical improvement up to regression of neurological changes; the MMSE score was 29/30 ten days after starting treatment and complete neuropsychological testing was normal at three months.

Brain MRI performed at three months showed complete regression of subcortical hyperintensities and leptomeningeal involvement on long TR sequences with persistence of chronic symmetrical leukoaraiosis and an increased number of cortical-subcortical microbleeds. Figure 1.3.12 shows the main neuroimaging findings.

(a)

(b)

(c)

(d)

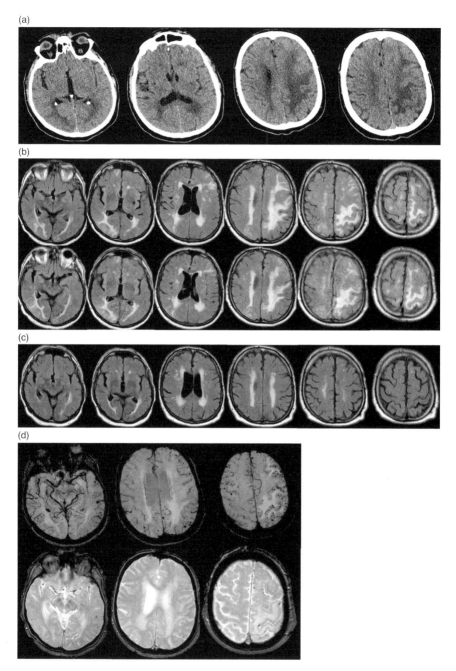

**Figure 1.3.12** Main neuroimaging findings of the proposed clinical case. (A) Unenhanced brain CT at hospital admission, showing multiple hypodense areas in subcortical white matter on both hemispheres without cortical involvement. (B) Brain MRI in the acute phase; axial FLAIR sequences before (first line) and after (second line) contrast administration, confirming the multiple areas of abnormal signal sparing the cerebral cortex with leptomeningeal contrast enhancement. (C) Brain MRI after three months. Unenhanced axial FLAIR sequences, showing the complete resolution of the previously identified signal abnormalities suggestive of vasogenic edema. (D) Brain MRI in the acute phase; SWI sequences (first line) and T2* sequences (second line) showing multiple hypointense dotted areas mainly in cortical and subcortical positions. In accordance with published diagnostic criteria, they are lobar microbleeds. It is easy to see the greater sensitivity of the SWI sequences compared to the T2* sequences in identification of the microbleeds.

The search for CSF anti-amyloid-$\beta$ (A$\beta$) autoantibodies turned out to be positive (at a concentration of 120.45 ng/ml).[17] In the acute phase, CSF levels of A$\beta$40 and A$\beta$42 examined using ELISA were, respectively, 5381 pg/ml and 337 pg/ml (normal >550 pg/ml) with total tau-protein levels 450 pg/ml [normal < 466] and phosphor tau-protein levels of 62 pg/ml [normal < 61]. These CSF biomarkers were persistently abnormal in the acute phase, remission phase and long-term follow-up.

After two years of follow-up, no clinical or neuroimaging recurrence of CAA-ri occurred and brain MRI was unchanged.

# Diagnostic Algorithm

| Grade of probability | Criteria |
|---|---|
| Possible CAA-RI | Age 40 years |
| | More than one of the following symptoms not directly attributable to an acute ICH: |
| | - Headache |
| | - impaired consciousness |
| | - behavioral change |
| | - focal neurological deficit |
| | - epileptic seizures |
| | MRI: proximate subcortical white matter with WMH |
| | More than one of the following cortico-subcortical hemorrhagic lesions: |
| | - cerebral macrobleeds |
| | - cerebral microbleeds |
| | - cortical superficial siderosis |
| | Absence of other infectious or neoplastic causes. |
| Probable CAA-RI | Age 40 years |
| | More than one of the following symptoms not directly attributable to an acute ICH: |
| | - headache |
| | - impaired consciousness |
| | - behavioral change |
| | - focal neurological deficit |
| | - epileptic seizures |
| | MRI: asymmetric, uni- or multifocal WMH-lesions in the proximate subcortical white matter. The asymmetry isn't a consequence of ICH. |
| | More than one of the following cortico-subcortical hemorrhagic lesions: |
| | - cerebral macrobleeds |
| | - cerebral microbleeds |
| | - cortical superficial siderosis |
| | Absence of other infectious or neoplastic causes |

CAA-ri diagnostic criteria from Auriel et al.[1]
CAA-RI: cerebral amyloid angiopathy-related inflammation, ICH: intracerebral hemorrhage, WMH: white matter hyperintensity

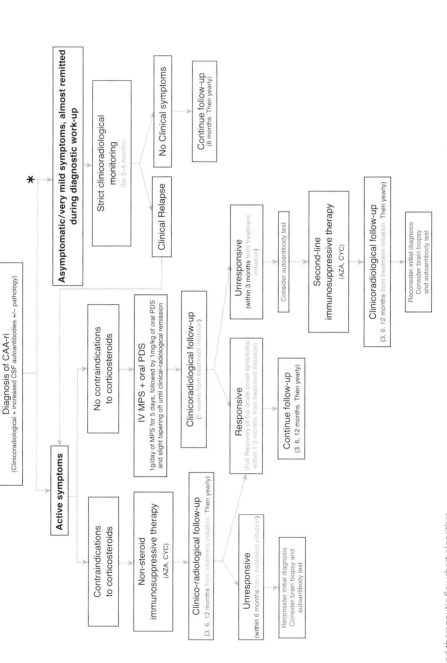

Diagnostic and therapeutic flowchart algorithm

Suggested flowchart for diagnostic and therapeutic decisions in the management of CAA-ri patients, inferred from current literature data and the last 7th years' experience in the iCAB International Network. Noticeably, this is a tentative algorithm that means to serve as a starting point in order to help in the difficult decision-making process, to monitor outcomes and to balance positive and negative effects of the different immunosuppressive drugs. The algorithm is currently a matter of validation through the iCAB International Network.

* The choice must be carefully weighted case-by-case, a closer clinical-radiological follow-up is mandatory.

# Case Discussion

The most common cerebral amyloid-related diseases are cerebral amyloid angiopathy (CAA) and Alzheimer's disease (AD). CAA is well known as a common cause of lobar intracerebral hemorrhage (ICH) in the elderly and AD is the most common cause of dementia and cognitive impairment. The first is characterized by deposition of Aβ in the walls of small- to medium-sized arteries, veins and capillaries of the leptomeninges and brain.[2]

Cerebral amyloid angiopathy-related inflammation (CAA-ri) is a rare and aggressive manifestation of both CAA and AD. It is probably underdiagnosed and not well known. CAA-ri represents a steroid-responsive type of dementia. Indeed, an early diagnosis has relevant treatment implications, being the unique treatable manifestation of CAA and AD.[3–6] CAA-ri is characterized by the acute/subacute onset of neurological symptoms, accompanied by MR evidence of cerebral vasogenic edema on FLAIR sequences, and cortical-subcortical microbleeds (MBs) and/or cortical superficial siderosis (CSS) on T2*-weighted gradient echo (T2*-GRE) or susceptibility-weighted imaging (SWI). The main differential diagnosis is represented by neoplastic, infectious, or other even more rare causes, such as posterior reversible encephalopathy syndrome (PRES).[5,7]

It has been very rarely described as spontaneous encephalitic-like manifestation in patients with AD (both sporadic and monogenic) and with greater frequency as an iatrogenic complication in immunotherapy trials in AD patients. It can occur spontaneously in patients with CAA, which probably represents a biological remnant of the coexistence of the two diseases in the brain, already known from histopathological studies.

It encompasses a wide range of clinical manifestations, including acute or subacute onset encephalopathy, subacute cognitive decline, changes of consciousness up to coma, focal neurological deficits, headache, confusion, epileptic seizures and focal neurological deficits.[8] Atypical forms of CAA-ri have also been reported, including radiologically isolated CAA-ri, minimally symptomatic CAA-ri, CAA-ri with isolated leptomeningitis and CAA-ri without MBs.[9–12]

The neuroradiological features are well described in both CAA and AD and have been coded in AD immunotherapy trials such as ARIA (amyloid-related imaging abnormalities) on MRI.[13–16] Some of these neuroradiological features are included in the new clinical-neuroimaging diagnostic criteria validated vs histopathology[1,17] after the first criteria by Chung et al.[7] The most striking neuroradiological features, according to the above-mentioned criteria, is the presence of mono or bilateral white matter hyperintensities extending to the immediately subcortical white matter in long TR sequences associated with cortico-subcortical micro- and macrobleeds.[17] Auriel et al.[1] reported a sensitivity of 82% and a specificity of 97% for their probable criteria in identifying biopsy-proven CAA-ri. The diagnostic criteria proposed by Auriel et al.[1] added to the previous ones proposed by Chung et al.[7] CSS as marker of CAA is included in the modified Boston criteria for CAA diagnosis.[18] Indeed, CSS is a neuroradiological sign highly specific of CAA[19] and it is associated with an even higher ICH risk than MBs.[20]

The gold standard for diagnosis remains histopathology; however, the existence of clinico-radiological criteria validated vs histopathology dramatically reduces the need for brain biopsy in clinical practice, both for diagnostic purposes and when proposing long-term immunosuppressive treatment. Indeed, the term CAA-ri includes two different histopathological pictures that cannot be differentiated on the basis of clinical presentation, neuroimaging and non-invasive tests: inflammatory CAA (ICAA) and amyloid-β-related angiitis (ABRA). The histopathology of ICAA is significant for perivascular inflammation;

conversely, ABRA is characterized by transmural and intramural inflammation, often with granuloma formation.[21] Without pathological data is not possible to make a differential diagnosis between ABRA and ICAA, but there are no significant differences in the treatment and in the response to it.[1] Moreover, both pathologic forms can co-occur, supporting the overlap between non-vasculitic and vasculitic forms of CAA-ri. The clinical and radiological findings of both variants are remarkably similar.

To date a systematic review has collected 213 distinct pathologically proven cases of CAA-ri/ABRA, from 104 publications.[8] To these must be added cases published without histopathological confirmation, based on the diagnostic criteria of Auriel et al.[1]

Although probably underdiagnosed, only a small proportion of CAA and AD patients develop CAA-ri and its cause remains unclear. Detectable anti-Aβ antibodies in the CSF can be considered an important clue to the pathophysiology of CAA-ri[17,22] and a useful diagnostic support. The prognostic role of the variations over time of the antibody titer in CSF is being defined to predict the response to therapy, the need for second-line immuno-suppressive therapy and the possibility of recurrence. In fact, although CAA-ri was initially described as a monophasic manifestation strongly responsive to steroid treatment, cases of short and long-term relapses are increasingly reported, as well as cases of prevalent leptomeningeal involvement. These are probably disease subtypes not yet fully character-ized from a biological and natural history point of view, which are the subject of ongoing research.[23]

What has been described currently[3,17] is that anti-Aβ antibody titers decrease upon immunosuppressive treatment from high levels in the acute phase to low levels in the clinical and/or neuroradiological remission phase. Otherwise, the CSF may be normal, but often shows a pleocytosis and/or mild raised protein (increased IgG). Amyloid bio-markers in CSF have a typical profile in CAA depending on the presence of CSS.[24]

Another support for the diagnosis is the determination of the APOE genotype, because is reported in the literature that the ε4 allele seems to be associated with an increased risk of developing CAA-ri,[5,25,26] but there are cases associated with the ε3 allele[4] and the ε2 allele.[27] One large neuropathological study found that either apo ε4 or ε2 could potentiate CAA pathology in both the parenchymal and meningeal vasculature.[28] The apoE gene is closely related to sporadic CAA and AD and there is evidence that apo ε4 facilitates amyloid deposition in patients with CAA or AD. The ε2 allele is less represented in AD patients, but is a known vascular risk factor and both ε2 and ε4 alleles are risk factors for CAA and CAA-related ICH.[29]

The first-line treatment is high-dose steroids, preferably by IV administration for a short time possibly followed by oral tapering-off. There is no consensus on the dose or on the overall duration of the treatment, as different therapeutic regimes are described in the literature; in fact, there are still no homogeneous prospective data with large numbers on the natural history of the disease and on the response to treatment. Second-line therapy is even less homogeneously characterized, but the greater number of reports considers oral azathioprine and/or IV cyclophosphamide.

In the literature it is reported that about half of patients with CAA-ri respond to first-line steroid therapy with partial-to-complete remission on a clinical and/or neuroradiological basis, but there are biases in the interpretation of case reports and case series, often retrospective and with incomplete data, as well as relating to cases that arrive at the diagnosis because they are more serious from the point of view of the clinical presentation. A retrospective series of 48 CAA-ri patients[23] supports the effectiveness of immunosuppressive treatment and suggest that early treatment may both improve the initial disease course and reduce the likelihood of recurrence. A prospective multicenter collaborative effort is therefore needed to define the natural history of treated and untreated CAA. This is one of the objectives of the Inflammatory Cerebral Amyloid Angiopathy and Alzheimer's Disease Biomarkers International Network (iCAβ). Furthermore, since CAA-ri is a possible manifestation of the two main cerebral amyloid-related diseases, CAA and AD, which can coexist in a not insignificant percentage of subjects, a further open question on the natural history of CAA-ri is that of the impact of the underlying disease and how CAA-ri affects the course of underlying CAA, AD or CAA+AD. Other open questions concern the effect of CAA-ri on the natural history of the underlying disease, as some data are present in the literature for patients with AD, even in the presymptomatic phase, on the iatrogenic form of CAA-ri in immunotherapy trials for AD.[13]

It is noteworthy that in some cases CAA-ri represents the first clinical manifestation of the underlying cerebral disease in patients who have no known prior history of CAA or AD. Therefore it is necessary to consider CAA-ri in the differential diagnosis in patients with rapid cognitive decline, acute and persistent alterations of consciousness and also epileptic status, in particular in the elderly, in order to reduce the diagnostic delay and promptly carry out treatment.

# References

1. Auriel E, Charidimou A, Gurol E. Validation of clinic-radiological criteria for the diagnosis of cerebral amyloid angiopathy-related inflammation. *JAMA Neurol.* 2016;**73**: 197.

2. Greenberg SM, Bacskai BJ, Hernandez-Guillamon M. Cerebral amyloid angiopathy and Alzheimer disease – one peptide, two pathways. *Nat Rev Neurol.* 2020;**16**: 30–42.

3. DiFrancesco JC, Brioschi M, Brighina L, Ruffmann C, Saracchi E. Anti-A autoantibodies in the CSF of a patient with CAA-related inflammation: A case report. *Neurology.* 2011;**76**: 842–844.

4. DiFrancesco C, Touat M, Caulo M, Gallucci M. Recurrence of cerebral amyloid angiopathy-related inflammation: A report of two cases from the ICAβ International Network. *J Alzheimers Dis.* 2015;**46**: 1071–1077.

5. Kinnecom C, Lev MH, Wendell L, Smith EE. Course of cerebral amyloid angiopathy-related inflammation. *Neurology.* 2004;**68**: 1411–1416.

6. Berkowitz AL, Baker JM, Miller JJ, Greenberg SM. Mystery case: Cerebral amyloid angiopathy-related inflammation. *Neurology.* 2014;**83**: 1678–1679.

7. Chung KK, Anderson NE, Hutchinson D. Cerebral amyloid angiopathy related inflammation: Three case reports and a review. *J Neurol Neurosurg Psychiatry.* 2011;**82**: 20–26.

8. Corovic A, Kelly S, Markus S. Cerebral amyloid angiopathy associated with inflammation: A systematic review of clinical and imaging features and outcome. *Int J Stroke* 2018;**13**(3): 257–267.

9. Kang P, Bucelli RC, Ferguson CJ. Teaching neuroimages: cerebral amyloid angiopathy-related inflammation presenting with isolated leptomeningitis. *Neurology.* 2017;**9**: e66–e67.

10. Liang JW, Zhang W, Sarlin J. Case of cerebral amyloid angiopathy-related inflammation – is the absence of cerebral microbleeds a good prognostic sign? *J Stroke Cerebrovasc Dis.* 2015;**4**: e319–e322.

11. Renard D, Wacongne A, Thouvenot E. Radiologically isolated cerebral amyloid angiopathy-related inflammation. *J Stroke Cerebrovasc Dis.* 2017;**6**: e218–e220.

12. Banerjee G, Alvares D, Bowen J. Minimally symptomatic cerebral amyloid angiopathy-related inflammation: three descriptive case reports. *J Neurol Neurosurg Psychiatr*. 2019;**90**: 113–115.

13. Sperling RA, Jack CR Jr, Black SE. Amyloid-related imaging abnormalities in amyloid-modifying therapeutic trials: Recommendations from the Alzheimer's Association Research Roundtable Workgroup. *Alzheimers Dement*. 2011;**7**: 367–85.

14. Ketter N, Brashear HR, Bogert J. Central review of amyloid-related imaging abnormalities in two phase iii clinical trials of bapineuzumab in mild-to-moderate Alzheimer's disease patients. *J Alzheimers Dis*. 2017;**57**(2): 557–573.

15. Barakos J, Sperling R, Salloway S, MR Imaging Features of Amyloid-Related Imaging Abnormalities. *Am J Neuroradiol*. 2013;**34**: 1958–1965.

16. Arrighi HM, Barakos J, Barkhof F, Tampieri D. Amyloid-related imaging abnormalities-haemosiderin (ARIA-H) in patients with Alzheimer's disease treated with bapineuzumab: a historical, prospective secondary analysis. *J Neurol Neurosurg Psychiatry*. 2016;**87**: 106–112.

17. Piazza F, Greenberg SM, Savoiardo M. Anti-amyloid β autoantibodies in cerebral amyloid angiopathy-related inflammation: implications for amyloid-modifying therapies. *Ann Neurol*. 2013;**73**: 449–458.

18. Linn J, Halpin A, Demaerel P, et al. Prevalence of superficial siderosis in patients with cerebral amyloid angiopathy. *Neurology*. 2010;**74**(17): 1346–1350.

19. Wollenweber FA, Baykara E, Zedde M, Gesierich B. Cortical superficial siderosis in different types of cerebral small vessel disease. *Stroke*. 2017;**48**(5): 1404–1407.

20. Wollenweber FA, Opherk C, Zedde M, Catak C. Prognostic relevance of cortical superficial siderosis in cerebral amyloid angiopathy. *Neurology*. 2019;**92**(8): e792–e801.

21. Salvarani C, Hunder GG, Morris JM. Aβ-related angiitis comparison with CAA without inflammation and primary CNS vasculitis. *Neurology*. 2013;**81**(18): 1596–1603.

22. DiFrancesco JC, Longoni M Piazza F. Anti-Aβ autoantibodies in amyloid related imaging abnormalities (ARIA): Candidate biomarker for immunotherapy in Alzheimer's disease and cerebral amyloid angiopathy. *Front Neurol*. **6**: 207.

23. Regenhardt RW, Thon JM, Das AS. Association between immunosuppressive treatment and outcomes of cerebral amyloid angiopathy-related inflammation. *JAMA Neurol*. 2020;**22**: e201782.

24. Catak C, Zedde M, Malik R, Janowitz D, Soric V. Decreased CSF levels of β-amyloid in patients with cortical superficial siderosis. *Front Neurol*. 2019;**10**: 439.

25. Piazza F, Winblad B. Amyloid-Related Imaging Abnormalities (ARIA) in immunotherapy trials for Alzheimer's disease: Need for prognostic biomarkers? *J Alzheimers Dis*. 2016;**52**(2): 417–420.

26. Carmona-Iragui M, Fernández-Arcos A, Alcolea D. Cerebrospinal fluid anti-amyloid-β autoantibodies and amyloid PET in cerebral amyloid angiopathy-related inflammation. *J Alzheimers Dis*. 2016;**50**(1): 1–7.

27. Xu YY, Chen S, Zhao JH, Chen XL. A case of cerebral amyloid angiopathy-related inflammation with the rare apolipoprotein +2/+2 genotype. *Front Neurol*. **10**: 547.

28. Nelson PT, Pious NM, Jicha GA, Wilcock DM. APOE-+2 and APOE-+4 correlate with increased amyloid accumulation in cerebral vasculature. *J Neuropathol Exp Neurol*. 2013;**2**: 708–715.

29. Marini S, Crawford K, Morotti A, Lee MJ. Association of apolipoprotein e with intracerebral hemorrhage risk by race/ethnicity: A meta-analysis. *JAMA Neurol*. 2019;**76**(4): 480–491.

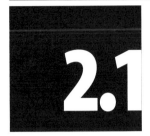

# Meningovascular Syphilis

Thierry Adoukonou

## Case Presentation

A 45-year-old, right-handed man was admitted to our hospital on December 23th, 2019 for generalized tonic-clonic seizures. With no context of fever or high blood pressure, he presented on the following day a right-side hemiparesis. No past history of venereal disease was noted. His temperature was 36.7 °C and blood pressure 135/81 mmHg. The brain CT scan showed an infarction in the left middle cerebral artery territory (Figure 2.1.1). Laboratory test results showed glycemia: 0.89 g/l, blood cell count normal. Neck vessels showed no abnormality and cardiac echography was normal. The *Treponema pallidum* hemagglutination (TPHA) test was negative, but the Venereal Disease Research Laboratory (VDRL) test was positive. The cerebrospinal fluid study revealed lymphocytotic pleiocytosis with 90 cells/μl and a positive test for VDRL. A diagnosis of meningovascular syphilis was made. The patient was given penicillin G intravenously at 20 million units per day for two weeks and physiotherapy. On discharge the patient could walk and recovered from his impairment. The prescribed treatment was aspirin 100 mg per day and phenobarbital 100 mg per day.

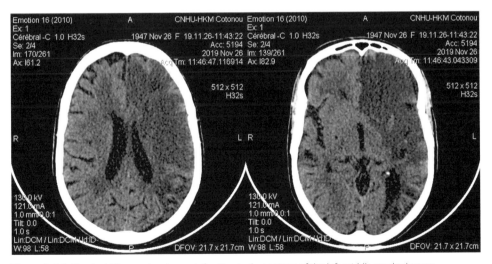

**Figure 2.1.1** Cerebral CT-scan showing an infarction in the territory of the left middle cerebral artery.

# Diagnostic Algorithm

---

**CLINICAL SUSPICION**

- Young people (20–50 years), suddenly neurological impairment

- No vascular risk factor, positive for HIV

- Past history of syphilitic chancre or sexual transmitted disease or high risk sexual behaviour

- Clinical vascular syndrome (middle cerebral artery)

---

⬇

---

**DIAGNOSIS**

- Brain CT scan or MRI: infarction in middle cerebral artery or multiple location with segmental arterial narrowing or dilatation
  or occlusion (vasculitis) in angiography or angio-CT or angio-MRI

- CSF: lymphocytic pleicytosis and elevated protein (>50 mg/dl), **VDRL (Venereal Disease Research Laboratory) positivity**

- Blood: systemic inflammation (elevated C-reactive protein: CRP), Reactive serum treponemal test (TPHA-VDRL), Rapid
  Plasma Reagin

- Absence of other cause of stroke (ECG, echocardiography, neck and intracranial artery Doppler, biology)

---

⬇

---

**TREATMENT**

- Intravenous injection of aqueous crystalline penicillin G at doses of 18–24 million units per day for 10–14 days, +/–
  probenecid 500 mg orally four times a day for 10–14 days or

- Procaine penicillin G, 2.4 million units intramuscularly (IM) once daily plus probenecid 500mg orally four times a day, both
  for 10 to 14 day, or;

- Ceftriaxon 2 g intravenously daily for 10–14 days.

- Alternative: benzathine penicillin G, 2.4 million units IM once per week for up to three weeks after completion of these NS
  treatment regimens to provide a comparable total duration of therapy

- Management of vascular risk factors

- Aspirin 100 mg/day?

---

# Case Discussion

Syphilis is one of the most prevalent infectious diseases, especially in developing countries. Its incidence is estimated at around 12 million new cases each year.[1] Due to the widespread use of antibiotics, the early stage of syphilis is rare. Indeed the tertiary stage is the most common and is characterized by cardiovascular syphilis and neurosyphilis. In Africa, a recent systematic review showed that neurosyphilis accounted for about 3% of all meningitis cases[2] and was not uncommon in patients with human immunodeficiency virus (HIV). About 46% of all neurosyphilis was recorded among HIV-infected patients. In a case–control study of stroke conducted in Tanzania, syphilis was more common in stroke patients (24.7%) than in age- and sex-matched controls (12.7%) with an odds ratio of 2.8 (95% CI: 1.6–4.6).[3] In another large hospital-based study the prevalence of meningovascular syphilis among stroke and transient ischemic attack (TIA) patients was 4%.[4] This incidence is frequently high among young patients with ischemic stroke.

Pathologically there are lesions which are fairly well correlated with the clinical manifestations. Thus inflammation of the leptomeninges and subarachnoid spaces is observed. The vessels crossing this space are the seat of inflammatory phenomena with lymphocytic cellular infiltration in the tunics of the arteries (media and adventitia) and also hyperplasia of the intima of the arteries, which can go as far as occlusion of the vessels. Varying lesions of endarteritis are commonly observed. These lesions relate to the cortical and leptomeningeal superficial vessels and can extend to the arteries of medium and large caliber, but rarely the small arteries. In addition, lesions of fibrosis are sometimes observed and more rarely lesions of syphilitic gum. The latter are made up of perivascular lymphocyte infiltrates of plasma cells and multi-nucleated giant cells or even of caseous necrosis.[5,6] In a few cases, hemorrhagic lesions have been described, probably due to rupture of vessels damaged by the pathological lesions described above.

The clinical presentation depends on the location of the stroke. It commonly involves the territory of the middle cerebral artery and multiple locations are not exceptional. It is most often encountered in young patients. A history of syphilitic chancre is found in almost half of the cases. However, the time between this chancre and the occurrence of stroke may range from a few months to several years. The onset is variable and is acute most of the time, but a quarter of patients present a progressive or subacute onset. Prodromes are often seen, including headache, dizziness, insomnia, and personality and psychiatric disorders. It is not uncommon for a stroke to follow subacute syphilitic meningitis. The classical vascular syndromes are observed, but in some cases unilateral parkinsonism and other extrapyramidal signs have been observed.[7] Spinal-cord infarction has also been reported.

Brain imaging (MRI or CT scan) shows the lesions (infarction or hemorrhage) and indicates the location (territory involved). However, arterial imaging (angiography, angio-MRI or angio-CT scan) is essential for the diagnosis. The typical finding is segmental arterial narrowing, dilatation or occlusion, the pattern of infectious vasculitis. This pattern can help to distinguish atherosclerotic lesions. Aneurysms have also been reported.

Study of the CSF helps in making the diagnosis of meningovascular syphilis. CSF VDRL test positivity is essential for the diagnosis. The CSF fluorescent treponemal antibody absorption (FTA-ABS or Nelson test) has a high sensitivity. CSF study shows elevated cells (>5 cells/μl, lymphocytic pleiocytosis) and elevated protein (>50 mg/dl and sometimes >100 mg/dl). Polymerase chain reaction (PCR), if available, can help in the diagnosis.

A rapid plasma regain (RPR) test on serum will be positive in most cases.

# Diagnosis

The diagnosis is based on a combination of the past history of the patient, clinical features, imaging abnormalities and the findings of CSF and serological tests.

✓ Young patient (under 45 years) without vascular risk factors, positive for HIV

✓ Past history of chancre
✓ Inflammatory systemic signs (elevated C-reactive protein (CRP))
✓ Stroke signs (infarction or rarely hemorrhage) on brain imaging and vasculitis signs in angiography, angio-CT scan or angio-MRI.
✓ Reactive serum treponemal test, CSF-VDRL test positivity, lymphocytic pleiocytosis or protein >50 mg/dl.
✓ Absence of another cause of stroke

## Treatment

The goal of the treatment is to ensure normalization of the CSF and to commence secondary prevention.

As with the treatment of the other forms of syphilis the gold standard is the intravenous injection of aqueous crystalline penicillin G at doses of 18–24 million units per day for 10–14 days. It is sometimes recommended to add probenecid 500 mg orally four times a day for 10–14 days. Alternative treatment is ceftriaxone 2 g intravenously daily for 10–14 days.

Care must be taken in the use of penicillin in case of a Jarissch–Herxheimer reaction. Patients who fulfill thrombolysis criteria for ischemic stroke can benefit from this treatment with a high level of safety.

Monitoring is very important for meningovascular syphilis. This monitoring includes serologic monitoring (efficacy of the treatment on the fourfold reduction of RPR titers) and eradication on the CSF examination. CSF must be checked every three months until normalized. Brain imaging needs to be redone and arterial abnormalities must also be checked. Sometimes the vasculopathy can persist despite successful the treatment (based on normalization of CSF and serological tests).

Secondary prevention includes hygienic measures (prevention of sexually transmitted diseases) and the use of aspirin.[7–9] Any vascular risk factors must also be managed.

## References

1. Hook EW 3rd, Peeling RW. Syphilis control – a continuing challenge. *N Engl J Med.* 2004;**351**: 122–124.

2. Marks M, Jarvis JN, Howlett W, Mabey DCW. Neurosyphilis in Africa: A systematic review. *PLoS Negl Trop Dis.* 2017;**11**(8): e0005880.

3. de Mast Q, Molhoek JE, van der Ven AJ, et al. antiphospholipid antibodies and the risk of stroke in urban and rural Tanzania: A community-based case-control study. *Stroke.* 2016;**47**: 2589–2595.

4. Cordato DJ, Djekic S, Taneja SR, et al. Prevalence of positive syphilis serology and meningovascular neurosyphilis in patients admitted with stroke and TIA from a culturally diverse population (2005–09). *J Clin Neurosc.* 2013;**20**: 943–947.

5. Holmes MD, Brant-Zawadzki MM, Simon RP. Clinical features of meningovascular syphilis. *Neurology.* 1984;**34**(04): 553–556.

6. Harriman D. Bacterial infections of the central nervous system. In: *Greenfield's*

*Neuropathology.* Chicago: Yearbook Medical Publishers; 1976. 238–238.

7. Ahbeddou N, El Alaoui Taoussi K, Ibrahimi A, et al. Stroke and syphilis: a retrospective study of 53 patients. *Rev Neurol (Paris).* 2018;**174**(05): 313–318.

8. Behrous R, Malek AR, Chichkova RI. Meningo-vascular syphilis: Revisiting an old adversary. *Pract Neurol.* 2011: 32–37.

9. Shulman JG, Cervantes-Arslanian AM. Infectious etiologies of stroke. *Semin Neurol.* 2019;**39**(4): 482–494.

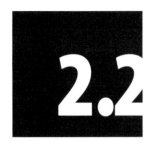

# Neuroborreliosis

Zeljko Zivanovic, Nikola Boban, Vladimir Galic

## Case Presentation

A 77-year-old patient was referred to a neurologist due to the recent onset of memory disturbances and signs of mild cognitive impairment. He did not have a significant past medical history and no other conventional risk factors for cardiovascular or neurological diseases, except hypertension. The patient was positive for a tick bite two years ago, followed by a classical erythema migrans. On a neurological examination, he did not have marked pyramidal deficit or a lesion of the cranial nerves, but presented with psychomotor impairment and short-term memory disturbance. A non-contrast brain CT scan showed several areas of chronic hypodensity in the corona radiata. Routine laboratory tests were unremarkable, except for a slightly elevated liver transaminase, while the extended coagulopathy work-up was within normal limits. The cerebrospinal fluid (CSF) analysis at admission showed lymphocytic pleocytosis (90 leukocyte cells/µl, 90% lymphocytes), elevated proteins (albumin 1.2 g/l), normal glucose level, *Borrelia burgdorferi* (Bb)-specific IgG antibodies detected by ELISA and confirmed by Western blotting. Serum analysis showed Bb-IgG antibodies, and the CSF/serum antibody index (AI) was positive. Further investigations did not reveal large-vessel disease or a cardiac source of ischemic stroke. Lipid profile and serum glycemia were normal, screening tests for neurotropic viruses and autoimmune disorders were negative. MRI of the brain showed diffuse, non-specific T2 W and FLAIR hyperintense, supratentorial white-matter lesions, without restricted diffusion, as well as signs of marked global brain atrophy (Figure 2.2.1.).

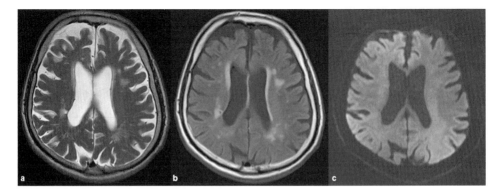

**Figure 2.2.1** Axial brain MRI: diffuse, non-specific T2 W (a) and FLAIR (b) hyperintense, white-matter lesions, without restricted diffusion (c). MRI signs of marked, global brain atrophy, without signs of contrast enhancement (not shown).

The diagnosis of late Lyme neuroborreliosis (LNB) with cerebrovascular complications was made, and therapy with intravenous ceftriaxone at a dose of 2 g daily was started for the next 21 days. In addition, the patient received antiaggregating therapy with acetylsalicylic acid (100 mg per day), with gastroprotection. The patient slowly improved and was discharged with a mild memory deficit. Serologic testing was reassessed four months after the antibiotic treatment and showed normalization of serum antibody titers and CSF parameters. At six-month follow-up, he did not have any new neurological or residual symptoms.

# Diagnostic Algorithm

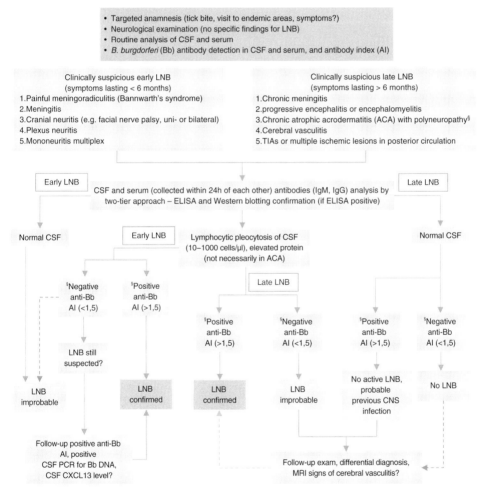

Diagnostic algorithm for adults with suspected early and late LNB, partially modified according to reference 9 ([§]in Europe)

**Table 2.2.1** Overview of antibiotic treatment for early and late LNB

| Antibiotics | Adult dose | Early LNB | Late LNB |
|---|---|---|---|
| | | Duration (days) | |
| Ceftriaxone | 2 g (i.v.) daily | 14 | 14–21 |
| Doxycycline | 200 mg (p.o.) daily | 14 | 14–21 |
| Penicillin G | 20 million IU (i.v.) daily | 14 | 14–21 |
| Cefotaxime | 6 g (i.v.) daily | 14 | 14–21 |

# Case Discussion

Lyme disease (LD) is one of the most prevalent arthropod-borne infectious diseases in endemic areas of the northern hemisphere, commonly reported in Europe and North America and sporadically in some parts of Asia.[1] Despite being known in Europe for a long time, as a dermatological and neurological disease, LD was named after the coastal town in Connecticut, USA, where it was first described in North America, having the original rheumatological presentation.[2] Lyme disease is a multisystemic, multistage disorder, caused by infection with spirochetes of the *Borrelia burgdorferi sensu lato* genospecies, and is transmitted by the bites of ticks belonging to *Ixodes ricinus* species complex.[3,4] Out of 20 different genospecies found so far,[1] three (*B. burgdorferi*, *B. afzelii*, and *B. garinii*) are responsible for human infections in different geographical regions.[5] *B. burgdorferi sensu stricto* is the most frequent cause of LD in North America, while *B. afzelii* and *B. garinii* are responsible for Lyme borreliosis in Europe.[6] LD generally affects the skin, manifesting as *erythema migrans*, yet it can involve joints, and the cardiovascular and nervous systems as well. The most frequent neurological manifestation of LD (collectively named Lyme neuroborreliosis) in Europe is Garin–Bujadoux–Bannwarth's syndrome,[7-8] which is characterized by painful radiculopathy, facial nerve palsy and meningitis with CSF lymphocytic pleocytosis.[9] Lyme neuroborreliosis, with either symptomatic meningitis or the involvement of cranial or spinal nerves, occurs in approximately 15% of LD patients in Europe.[10] Expansion of the disease to brain parenchyma is less common, while cerebrovascular progression, and especially stroke due to underlying LNB, appear to be unusual complications, affecting from 0.3% to 1% of patients in endemic areas.[11]

After being deposited in the skin, *B. Burgdorferi* migrates through the host tissues and into the blood or lymphatic system. As it spreads to distant sites within the human body, including the joints, and cardiovascular and nervous systems, the recruitment of inflammatory cells and release of cytokines continue. The spirochete is primarily a tissue-based organism and does not produce toxins or other degrading proteases. Thus, human manifestation of this infection at each stage is associated with a multifocal immune response.[12] Since research evidence shows that contact with this spirochete induces focal areas of inflammation in cells of the nervous system, the pathophysiology of a stroke in LNB is probably related to an inflammatory vasculopathy of intracranial vessels as well.[13]

The difference and heterogeneity among *B. burgdorferi senso lato* genospecies appear to be associated with the demographic differences and specific clinical manifestations of Lyme disease,[12] where *B. burgdorferi* is notably accountable for arthritogenic manifestations in North America. At the same time, *B. afzelii* causes infections of the skin and *B. garinii* is above all neurotropic and is represented in European cases of LNB.[6] The clinical course of LD is variable. It usually begins with a skin lesion, erythema migrans (stage 1), which is followed by early disseminated infection and neurological symptoms such are radicular pain, headache or cognitive dysfunction (stage 2, symptoms lasting less than six months) and finally, late disseminated infection manifesting as arthritis or acrodermatitis atrophicans (stage 3, with symptom duration between six months and several years). Neurological symptoms generally occur 4–6 weeks after the tick bite,[8] although only half of patients recall a tick bite, and approximately one-third of them report a local skin infection.[14] Pathophysiologically, Lyme neuroborreliosis can affect the peripheral nervous system, parenchymal central nervous system (CNS) and non-parenchymal CNS parts.[15] Besides this, in practice, a useful clinical distinction between early and late LNB is that meningitis, cranial neuritis, and radiculitis occur more in the former, while the latter may present as mild encephalopathy and peripheral neuropathy.[15] Generally, non-specific symptoms such as headache, meningismus, numbness and tingling, myalgia, fatigue and mild cognitive changes, without severe brain syndromes, are common findings among all patients.

## Early Lyme Neuroborreliosis

Peripheral nervous system involvement happens in 5–10% of patients with early LNB.[15] As stated before, the most common neurological display of early LNB in European endemic areas is painful, lymphocytic meningoradiculitis, known as Bannwarth's syndrome,[2] with preceding erythema migrans in only a few cases.[16] The distribution of peripheral nerve damage is variable, while the pain is often chronic, severe and lancinating, lasting for months after the infection and mostly worsening at night. In North America, LNB presents as subacute, lymphocytic meningitis with or without cranial nerve palsy, usually without painful radiculitis.[16] Other peripheral manifestations include plexus neuritis, mononeuritis multiplex and cranial neuropathy, particularly in the facial and optic nerves.[8] Encephalitis and myelitis are rare in this stage of LNB.

## Late Lyme Neuroborreliosis

Parenchymal involvement is rare, and patients may present with segmental myelitis or encephalitis, followed by clinical hallmarks like cerebellar ataxia, opsoclonus-myoclonus, apraxia or hemiparesis.[12] Other possible manifestations of late LNB include chronic meningitis, progressive encephalitis, encephalomyelitis and cerebral vasculitis.[9] When observing the less frequent manifestations of LNB, transient ischemic attack (TIA) or stroke is probably a secondary reflection of infection-induced cerebral endarteritis.[13] Stroke in patients with LNB has varying aspects. These patients may present with TIA or stroke,[17] subarachnoid hemorrhage,[18] intracerebral hemorrhage,[19] cerebral venous sinus thrombosis,[20] or aneurysm.[21] A recent meta-study analyzed 88 individual cases of LNB, and showed that multiple, ischemic brain lesions were present in over 60% of the patients, whereas intracranial and subdural hemorrhage and aneurysms were the least frequent cerebrovascular complications.[22] As presented in these results, LNB-induced vasculitis affected mainly large- and medium-sized arteries (middle cerebral, anterior cerebral and basilar).[22] However, one must be aware that small blood vessels may be involved, too, due to the low resolution of conventional angiography.

Lyme neuroborreliosis poses a clinical, diagnostic challenge for several reasons and fundamental limitations. Mostly, patients with LNB present to a neurologist from a few weeks up to a few months after a suspicious tick bite.[16] Thorough clinical examination and proper history-taking, asking the patient about tick bites and a subsequent, localized skin lesion can help in diagnosis. The diagnosis of LNB should be taken under consideration in areas endemic for *Ixodes* ticks. Neurologists in non-endemic areas need to acquire a travel history from patients who might have vacationed in an endemic region. Except for patients with erythema migrans, the diagnosis must rely on recognition of clinical signs and symptoms, along with routine CSF analysis and antibody studies of serum and CSF.[8] Direct detection and culturing the *B. burgdorferi senso lato* species are of low value for the diagnosis of LNB. After the spirochete disseminates, its count in a specimen of serum or CSF is meager and can hardly be multiplied, even by PCR,[13] especially in patients with chronic symptoms.[8] Therefore, the host's immune response is the most critical aspect of the assessment, which needs three to six weeks to develop, since serologic tests are often negative exceedingly early after infection.[10,15] Laboratory diagnosis of infection is made by the detection of antibodies by enzyme-linked immunosorbent assay (ELISA) and confirmed by Western blotting.[15] The IgM class of antibodies is highly cross-reactive; a positive result must be taken with caution in the absence of its IgG conversion.[15] Furthermore, to demonstrate CNS involvement, Bb-specific intrathecal antibody production must be detected (corrected for passive diffusion of anti-Bb antibodies through the blood–brain barrier), followed by estimation of CSF-to-serum antibody index, which remains the pillar of laboratory testing in Europe.[8,16] Studies of the C6 Lyme antibody and additional biomarkers (B lymphocyte chemoattractant chemokine CLCX13) are still ongoing and not conclusive enough to be used in everyday practice.[16] Knowledge of additional radiological features could support this diagnosis. LNB presents with a broad spectrum of neuroimaging findings, mostly dependent on the genospecies and the phase of the disease. Cranial neuritis is demonstrated with nerve enhancement on contrast-enhanced T1 W images and could be considered relatively specific. The facial nerve is most frequently affected (Figure 2.2.2), in up to 80% of patients with LNB, and it is bilateral in 25% of cases.[23]

The most frequently reported findings are chronic white-matter lesions, seen in approximately half of the patients with LNB. These present with multiple T2 W and FLAIR hyperintense lesions without restricted diffusion. However, these are considered non-specific and are seen late in the disease course. MRI can demonstrate lesions with restricted diffusion, typical for acute and subacute ischemic areas. Rarely, these lesions can also enhance, which is considered a sign of disturbed blood–brain barrier and could point to inflammation in vasculitis. A recent systematic review of the literature found that the average time from symptom onset of LD until the first cerebrovascular manifestations of LNB was 3.5 months.[22] Mostly, lesions were multiple and relatively equally distributed among vascular territories, with a small predilection for posterior circulation. The same authors reported that in patients with LNB, vascular neuroimaging suggested vasculitis in nearly 80% of cases (seen as irregularities of the vessel wall, occlusion, segmental narrowing or dilatation). Novel "black blood" techniques can improve sensitivity for vessel wall enhancement in LNB vasculitis.[24]

With enough time, the human immune system can reduce the number of *B. burgdorferi* on its own, albeit some might survive for several years, causing persistent symptoms.[12] All

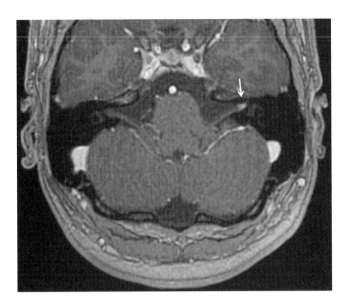

**Figure 2.2.2** Perineural enhancement (white arrow) of the left facial nerve.

manifestations, including LNB-induced vasculitis, when treated with the appropriate antibiotic regimens and on time, are highly responsive. However, some patients can have post-infectious, long-term sequelae. According to the current guidelines, adults with early LNB-induced CNS manifestations are treated with intravenous ceftriaxone (2 g daily) for 14 days, while those with late-onset LNB should receive the same therapy for 21 days.[8] Studies have shown that oral doxycycline has good blood–brain barrier penetration, reflecting sufficient CSF concentrations.[8] In addition, physical and occupational therapy, speech therapy, neuropsychological training, analgesics and non-steroidal anti-inflammatory drugs should be considered depending on various symptoms. Corticosteroids are not indicated since they interfere with immune-related killing of the spirochete. Prevention of LD relies primarily on wearing personal, protective measures and avoidance of endemic areas throughout the world.

In summary, previous case studies provided adequate data implying that late LNB can cause cerebral vasculitis. As a rare cause of TIA or stroke, neurologists should consider a diagnosis of LNB-induced vasculitis in patients with cryptogenic cerebrovascular events, without classical risk factors. Particularly in younger people, who present with a prominent headache or other LNB manifestations weeks or months before stroke onset, have any evidence of a vasculopathy on neuroimaging and come from endemic areas. Potential lack of awareness of this late LNB manifestation may lead to an unfavorable outcome. In these patients, cerebral angiography may reveal focal narrowing and dilatation of the affected arteries. A CSF examination is mandatory, as well as a careful differential diagnosis, especially since LNB-associated vasculitis may have a beneficial prognosis when appropriately treated.

# References

1. Mead PS. Epidemiology of Lyme disease. *Infect Dis Clin North Am*. 2015;**9**: 187–210.

2. Garcia-Monco JC, Benach JL. Lyme neuroborreliosis: clinical outcomes,

controversy, pathogenesis, and polymicrobial infections. *Ann Neurol.* 2019;**85**: 21–31.

3. Burgdorfer W, Barbour AG, Hayes SF, et al. Lyme disease – a tick-borne spirochetosis? *Science.* 1982;**216**: 1317–1319.

4. Piesman J, Gern L. Lyme borreliosis in Europe and North America. *Parasitology.* 2004;**129**: 191–220.

5. Baranton G, Assous M, Postic D. Three bacterial species associated with Lyme borreliosis: Clinical and diagnostic implications. *Bull Acad Natl Med.* 1992;**176**: 1075–1085.

6. Steere AC. Lyme disease. *N Engl J Med.* 2001;**345**: 115–125.

7. Kaiser R. Neuroborreliosis. *J Neurol.* 1998;**245**: 247–255.

8. Mygland A, Ljostad U, Fingerle V, et al. EFNS guidelines on the diagnosis and management of European Lyme neuroborreliosis. *Eur J Neurol.* 2010;**17**: 8–16.

9. Koedel U, Fingerle V, Pfister HW. Lyme neuroborreliosis-epidemiology, diagnosis and management. *Nature Rev Neurol.* 2015;**11**: 446–456.

10. Wittwer B, Pelletier S, Ducrocq X, et al. Cerebrovascular events in Lyme neuroborreliosis. *J Stroke and Cerebrov Dis.* 2015;**24**: 1671–1678.

11. Back T, Grunig S, Winter Y, et al. Neuroborreliosis-associated cerebral vasculitis: long-term outcome and health-related quality of life. *J Neurol.* 2013;**260**: 1569–1575.

12. Steere AC, Strle F, Wormser GP, et al. Lyme borreliosis. *Nat Rev Dis Primers.* 2017;**3**: 17062.

13. Halperin JJ. Strokes in patients with bacterial meningitis with a focus on pneumococcus and Lyme disease. In: Caplan L, Biller J. (Eds). Uncommon Causes of Stroke. Cambridge: Cambridge University Press; 2018. 26–38.

14. Ljostad U, Skogvoll E, Eikeland R, et al. Oral doxycycline versus intravenous ceftriaxone for European Lyme neuroborreliosis: a multicentre, non-inferiority, double-blind, randomized trial. *Lancet Neurol.* 2008;**7**: 690–695.

15. Halperin JJ. Neuroborreliosis. *J Neurol.* 2017;**264**: 1292–1297.

16. Pachner AR, Steiner I. Lyme neuroborreliosis: infection, immunity, and inflammation. *Lancet Neurol.* 2007;**6**: 544–552.

17. May EF, Jabbari B. Stroke in neuroborreliosis. *Stroke.* 1990;**21**: 1232–1235.

18. Chehrenama M, Zagardo MT, Koski CL. Subarachnoid hemorrhage in a patient with Lyme disease. *Neurology.* 1997;**48**: 520–523.

19. Martinez MS, Ibanez G, Herrero S, Garcia-Monco JC. Spontaneous brain hemorrhage associated with Lyme neuroborreliosis. *Neurologia.* 2001;**16**: 43–45.

20. Adamaszek M, Heinrich A, Rang A, Langer S, Khaw AV. Cerebral sinnuvenous thrombosis associated with Lyme neuroborreliosis. *J Neurol.* 2010;**257**: 481–483.

21. Polet JD, Weinstein HC. Lyme borreliosis and intracranial aneurysms. *J Neurol Neurosurg Psychiatry.* 1999;**66**: 806–807.

22. Garkowski A, Zajkowska I, Zajkowska A, et al. Cerebrovascular manifestations of Lyme neuroborreliosis – a systematic review of published cases. *Front Neurol.* 2017;**8**: 146.

23. Halperin JJ. Nervous system Lyme disease. *Infect Dis Clin North Am.* 2015;**29**: 241–253.

24. Smadi RN, Abdalla AH, Elmokadem AH, et al. Diagnostic accuracy of high-resolution black-blood MRI in the evaluation of intracranial large-vessel arterial occlusions. *Am J Neurorad.* 2019;**40**: 954–959.

# Tuberculosis Meningitis

## 2.3

Yared Z. Zewde, Seda Tadesse

## Case Presentation

A 28-year-old right-handed female patient presented to the emergency department with a complaint of sudden onset dizziness, postural imbalance, walking difficulty and falls of one day duration. She also had recent worsening of global headache, nausea without vomiting and visual obscuration on her right side with frequent collisions on the same side. She had a history of low-grade fever, mild global headache and lethargy for the past three weeks. A week before her presentation she visited a local clinic and was treated with paracetamol 1000 mg and unspecified parenteral antibiotics for 72 hours without improvement. Her family reported no prior history of diplopia, blurred vision, loss of consciousness, seizure, cough or contact with a chronic cougher. She worked as a secretary with no history of any drug use or similar illness in the past.

At the time of presentation, she was lethargic. Her temperature was 37.8 °C, blood pressure, 130/70 mm Hg, heart rate, 88 beats/minute and respiratory rate, 26 breaths/minutes with an oxygen saturation of 97% on room air. Physical examination of the head, neck, breast and lymph node, chest, cardiovascular, abdomen and musculoskeletal systems were not revealing. On neurologic examination, she was conscious and oriented to time, place and person. Visual acuity was 6/6 in both eyes using the Snellen chart, but a visual field test by confrontation found partial homonymous hemianopia on the right side. Fundoscopic, motor and sensory examinations were normal. She had dysmetria on the left upper limb, gait abnormality with a wide base and a tendency to fall to the left side. Neck stiffness was positive. Otherwise, she had no dysarthria, nystagmus or other signs of meningismus.

Considering the patient's presentation and epidemiology, brain magnetic resonance imaging (MRI) was done to exclude posterior circulation stroke complicating CNS infectious or inflammatory processes. The MRI showed left occipital-parietal and left cerebellar hemisphere T2 hyperintense lesions with diffusion restriction on diffusion-weighted imaging (DWI) (Figure 2.3.1).

Laboratory tests showed a raised erythrocyte sedimentation rate (ESR) at 82 mm/h, a white blood cell (WBC) count of 8200 cell/mm$^3$ with 67% neutrophils and hemoglobin of 9.8 mg/dl with mean corpuscular volume (MCV) of 77 femtoliters. Cerebrospinal fluid (CSF) analysis revealed a WBC count of 240/µl with 78% lymphocytes, a protein level of 330 mg/dl and a glucose level of 28 mg/dl. CSF Gene Xpert for Mycobacterium tuberculosis (MTB) was positive. Otherwise, Gram staining, Indian ink and Venereal Diseases Research Laboratory (VDRL) tests were negative. The chest X-ray was normal. Serology tests for HIV, HCV and HBV were non-reactive. The liver

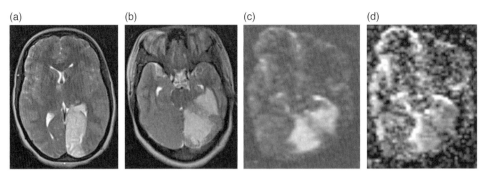

**Figure 2.3.1** (A, B) Axial T2 W MRI with left occipital and left cerebellar cortex hyperintensities with hyperintensities on DWI (C) and hypointensities on apparent diffusion coefficient (ADC) (D).

and kidney function tests were normal. Other causes of stroke were excluded after antinuclear antibodies (ANA), RF, electrocardiography (ECG), echocardiography and carotid Doppler ultrasound tests were normal.

She was diagnosed with left posterior circulation acute infarction due to post-infection vasculitis from tuberculosis meningitis (TBM) and started treatment with dexamethasone, anti-TB drugs and aspirin 100 mg daily. After four weeks of treatment, her clinical condition improved significantly and she was discharged with outpatient follow-up.

# Diagnostic Algorithm

| Clinical suspicion of TBM (infectious vasculitis)-associated stroke |
|---|
| *Age = children (< 4 years) and adults, TB endemic area*<br>**Clinical presentation**<br>*Prodromal phase (stage 1):* 1–3 weeks duration; insidious onset of fatigue, malaise, headache, low-grade fever, and loss of appetite; alert and oriented with no focal neurologic signs<br>*Meningitis phase (stage 2):* meningismus, protracted headache, vomiting, lethargy, confusion and mild focal neurology deficits (cranial neuropathies);<br>*Paralytic phase (stage 3):* rapid deterioration, seizure, multiple cranial nerve palsies, dense hemiplegia, delirium, stupor, coma and death if not treated<br>**Risk factors:** concomitant immunodeficiency state (malignancy, HIV infection, malnutrition, diabetes mellitus, alcohol abuse, chronic kidney disease), prolonged duration of pre-existing symptoms, the presence of hydrocephalus, high CSF neutrophil count, meningeal enhancement on initial brain imaging, the presence of stage II or III of meningitis, and the presence of tuberculomas |

| |
|---|
| **Brain CT:** obliteration of the basal cisterns by isodense or slightly hyperdense exudate, hydrocephalus, infarction due to arteritis<br>Brain CT with contrast: basal enhancing exudates, leptomeningeal enhancement, epididymitis<br>**Brain MRI:** infarction due to vasculitis in middle cerebral artery and its lenticulostriate branches, thalamoperforating branches from the posterior cerebral artery and basilar artery, and vasospasm in the middle cerebral artery, terminal carotid artery and posterior cerebral artery. Basal cisterns and leptomeningeal enhancement and parenchymal tuberculomas in T1-weighted (T1W) image with and without gadolinium contrast, T2-weighted (T2W) image, and T2 fluid-attenuated inversion recovery (T2 FLAIR) image; hyperintensity on the diffusion-weighted image (DWI) and hypointensity on apparent diffusion coefficient (ADC). |

| |
|---|
| **Brain MR angiography (MRA):** narrowed or occluded small- or medium-sized intracranial arteries with scant collaterals |

| Exclusion of mimickers of cerebral vasculitis | | | |
|---|---|---|---|
| **Systemic autoimmune disease**<br>Neurosarcoidosis<br>Neurolupus<br>Neuro-Behçet<br><br>**Large-vessel vasculitides**<br>Takayasu arteritis<br>Giant cell arteritis<br>**Medium-vessel vasculitides**<br>Polyarteritis nodosa (PAN)<br>Kawasaki disease | **Small-vessel vasculitides**<br>Immune complex-mediated (cryoglobulinemic, IgA associated, Henoch–Schönlein purpura)<br>ANCA-associated variants (microscopic polyangiitis, Wegener granulomatosis, Churg–Strauss disease)<br>Rheumatic syndromes (lupus, Sjögren syndrome, scleroderma) | **Non-infectious CNS vasculopathy**<br>**PACNS**<br>Fibromuscular dysplasia, neurofibromatosis, RCVS, CADASIL, MELAS, Sneddon's syndrome Divry–van Bogaert syndrome Osler's disease Moyamoya angiopathy **Metabolic disease** Fabry's disease | **Infectious CNS vasculitis**<br>Emboli from subacute bacterial endocarditis Basilar meningitis caused by tuberculosis or fungal infection Bacterial and viral infections (HIV, neurosyphilis, VZV) **Malignancy** Carcinomatous meningitis, Lymphomatoid granulomatosis |

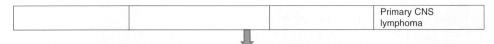

| | | | | Primary CNS lymphoma |

↓

| Investigating the causes of vasculitis infarction |
| --- |
| **Autoimmune disease:** acute-phase proteins (ESR, C reactive protein (CRP)), antinuclear antibodies (ANA), antineutrophil cytoplasmic antibodies (ANCA) titers, Complete blood count, complement level<br>**Systemic vasculitides:** Carotid Doppler ultrasound, cerebral arteries duplex ultrasound, transthoracic echocardiography,<br>**Prothrombotic state:** lupus anticoagulant, antiphospholipid antibodies, factor V leiden mutation, protein S, protein C, antithrombin III deficiency, hyperhomocysteinemia, ECG<br>**Infections:** CSF pleocytosis, HIV serology, VDRL/Treponema pallidum hemagglutination (TPHA), TB PCR, chest X-ray for pulmonary tuberculosis (PTB), varicella zoster virus (VZV) PCR<br>**CNS arteritis:** Brain MRI, MRA and cerebral angiography (intracranial arterial beading, diffuse microangiopathies, ischemia)<br>**Biopsy of the cerebral vessels and brain tissue:** Definitive diagnosis |

↓

| Treatment of cerebral infarction due to infectious vasculitis | |
| --- | --- |
| **Antituberculosis regimen:** isoniazid 300 mg day, ethambutol 1200 mg day, pyrazinamide 1500 mg day and rifampicin 150 mg day<br>**Antibiotics:** ceftriazone 2 gm day and vancomycin 1 gm day<br>**Anti-platelet:** aspirin 100 mg day<br>**Systemic steroid:** dexamethasone 12 mg day | **Hyponatremia** (49%): fluid replacement cerebral salt wasting (CSW) and free-water restriction syndrome of inappropriate antidiuretic hormone secretion (SIADH)<br>**Hydrocephalus** (42%): ventriculoperitoneal shunts and endoscopic third ventriculostomy<br>**Vasculitis and stroke** (15–57%): aspirin<br>**Epileptic seizure** (28%): antiepileptic in the first seizure<br>**Tuberculoma** (3%): Anti-TB for a long duration |

# Case Discussion

Tuberculosis is the leading public health problem with a huge morbidity and mortality burden worldwide. Tuberculous meningitis (TBM) occurs in 10% of patients with tuberculosis (TB) and stroke complicating the course of TBM in about 13–57% of patients. The mortality is about three times higher in TBM patients with stroke compared to those without infarction.[1] The risk factors for stroke in TBM include younger age, prolonged duration and advanced stage of TBM, presence of hydrocephalus, tuberculoma, basal meningeal enhancement and raised CSF white blood cell count.[2]

In TBM, stroke might develop insidiously and it can be a symptomatic or silent infarct (25%). Symptomatic infarct presents with focal neurologic deficits. The most common (49%) brain region that is vulnerable to the development of infarction is referred to as the "tubercular zone," which includes the basal ganglia, thalamus and internal capsule.[2] A different mechanism for the development of cerebral infarction in TBM has been hypothesized. The main pathologic culprit is the basal exudate, which induces inflammatory infiltration of the vessel wall with panarteritis. It is followed by proliferative reaction and fibrinoid necrosis of the large cerebral vessels, which results in vasculitis, thrombosis and vasospasm of large vessels with ischemia and infarction. Another mechanism, such as hypercoagulable state-induced venous sinus thrombosis or aneurysmal dilations, may increase the risk of infarction.

The focal neurologic deficits of TBM-associated cerebral infarction is often preceded by prodromal symptoms of fever, headache, fatigue and malaise.[3] A stroke usually occurs at stages 2 or 3 of TBM and it has a poor clinical outcome with high mortality. The clinical manifestation varies widely based on the location of the infarction. The most common symptoms, such as motor weakness, sensory impairment, movement disorders, seizure, apraxia and hypothalamic disorders might be associated with middle cerebral artery involvement in the anterior circulation. While ataxia, cranial nerve palsy, and altered consciousness might be attributed to posterior circulation involvement, which is identified in 20% of TBM-related stroke patients.

The diagnosis of stroke in TBM is based on clinical and neuroimaging evaluation. TBM patients who develop sudden deterioration with focal neurologic deficit warrant immediate evaluation with a brain CT scan. This detects infarction in 15–57% of TBM patients, where 75% of the lesions are located in the tubercular zone. Brain MRI is superior to CT in detecting acute infarct with high sensitivity, using DWI and ADC.

Brain MRI protocols such as T1-weighted (T1 W) imaging with and without gadolinium contrast, T2-weighted (T2 W) imaging and T2 fluid-attenuated inversion recovery (T2 FLAIR) imaging reveal intense basal meningeal enhancement, tuberculoma, cerebral infarction, hydrocephalus (communicating or non-communicating) or a combination. The diagnosis of acute stroke is confirmed by detecting hyperintensity on the diffusion-weighted image (DWI) and hypointensity on the apparent diffusion coefficient (ADC). CT/MR angiography may reveal brain vessel abnormalities (40%), such as narrowing of the terminal portion of the internal carotid artery and delayed circulation in the middle cerebral artery due to constriction of terminal carotid and middle cerebral arteries. Ventricular dilation might also cause a widely sweeping pericallosal artery or outward bowing of the thalamostriate vein.

After neuroimaging, lumbar puncture and CSF examination should be done. The opening pressure is usually moderately elevated with turbid CSF. The WBC count is between 100 and 500 cells/μl with lymphocytes prominent and there is increased protein concentration, usually between 100–500 mg/dl, and low CSF glucose concentration <45 mg/dl (<0.5 of serum glucose). CSF Gene Xpert assay diagnoses >90% of TBM including MDR-TB. AFB smear and culture of CSF might diagnose half of TBM cases.

There is no specific treatment for TBM-associated stroke.[4] The standard regimen of antituberculous drugs with dexamethasone will have a mortality benefit but doesn't change the long-term complications of TBM. The antiplatelet, antiaggregant, anti-inflammatory and antioxidant properties of aspirin reduce the risk of stroke by 19%.[5] The causes of other complications of TBM, including hyponatremia (49%) need to be identified. For cerebral salt-wasting syndrome, fluid and sodium replacement is the treatment of choice, while euvolemic hyponatremia in syndrome of inappropriate antidiuretic hormone (SIADH) should be treated with free-water restriction. CSF diversion surgeries such as ventriculoperitoneal shunts and endoscopic third ventriculostomy are indicated in patients with hydrocephalus (42%). Antiepileptic treatment is recommended after the first epileptic seizure (28%) is documented. Patients with tuberculoma (3%) might need to take anti-TB drugs for a long duration (18 months) or until the brain lesions are resolved.

Vasculitic stroke in TBM is associated with poor outcome, particularly infarction in the middle cerebral artery territory, and it also results in neurodevelopmental arrest in children.

## References

1. Tai MS, Viswanathan S, Rahmat K, et al. Cerebral infarction pattern in tuberculous meningitis. *Sci Rep*. 2016;**6**: 38802.

2. Misra UK, Kalita J, Maurya PK. Stroke in tuberculous meningitis. *J Neurol Sci*. 2011;**303**(1–2): 22–30.

3. Zhang L, Zhang X, Li H, et al. Acute ischemic stroke in young adults with tuberculous meningitis. *BMC Infect Dis*. 2019;**19**: 362.

4. Anuradha HK, Garg RK, Agarwal A, et al. Predictors of stroke in patients of tuberculous meningitis and its effect on the outcome. *QJM*. 2010;**103**: 671–678.

5. Misra UK, Kalita J, Sagar B, Bhoi SK. Does adjunctive corticosteroid and aspirin therapy improve the outcome of tuberculous meningitis? *Neurol India*. 2018;**66**(6): 1672–1677.

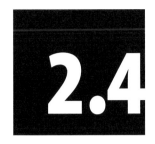

# Bacterial Meningitis

## 2.4

Marilena Mangiardi, Eytan Raz

## Case Presentation

A 76-year-old man with several vascular risk factors who had complained of fatigue, dizziness and headache for several days was admitted to the neurology department for sudden onset of left hemiparesis and slurred speech observed on physical examination.

Moreover, he had complained of fluctuating episodes of headache and gait disturbance over the last 10 days. There was no recent history of fever, travel, trauma or surgery.

Temperature was 37.5°C, heart rate, 85 beats/min, blood pressure, 130/70 mmHg and respiratory rate, 23 breaths/min, with an oxygen saturation of 99% on room air.

Brain magnetic resonance imaging (MRI) and magnetic resonance angiography (MRA) highlighted in both fluid-attenuated inversion recovery (FLAIR) and diffusion-weighted images a small acute ischemic infarct in the right temporal pole and an ipsilateral multifocal middle cerebral artery (MCA) irregularity (Figure 2.4.1).

The MRA showed an irregular appearance for both distal M1 and proximal M2, which was then confirmed on the cerebral angiogram (arrows on E and F). No aneurysm, arteriovenous malformation or sinus thrombosis were found. The patient was not eligible for intravenous thrombolysis with r-tPA due to prolonged timing from neurological symptom onset and no neuroimaging mismatch.

Primary stroke prevention therapy with acetylsalicylic acid 100 mg/day was started. After two weeks of hospitalization, the patient was discharged to home in fair general condition. Both mild balance disturbance and memory loss continued on neurological examination. Laboratory studies, including inflammatory panel and systemic vasculitis screening, were normal. No cardiological abnormality on either electrocardiogram or echocardiogram was found.

Two months later, because of change in gait with non-specific dizziness, a new subtle left hemiparesis and generalized epileptic seizures, the MRI was repeated. The images demonstrated a well-formed rounded lesion with diffusion restriction, peripheral and meningeal enhancement and diffuse surrounding vasogenic edema, consistent with a pyogenic abscess (Figure 2.4.2).

A lumbar puncture was performed, and the cerebrospinal fluid (CSF) results were normal except for a slight increase in protein (45 mg/dl). Inflammatory markers were normal. Human immunodeficiency virus (HIV) and hepatitis B and C serologies were negative. The combination of a third-generation cephalosporin (ceftriaxone) plus metronidazole was started empirically.

The patient underwent surgery that confirmed an abscess from *Staphylococcus aureus*.

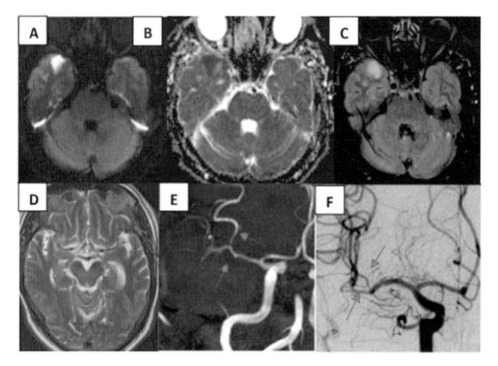

**Figure 2.4.1** (A) Diffusion-weighted image; (B) apparent diffusion coefficient (ADC) map; (C) FLAIR; (D) T2; (E) MRA; (F) digital subtraction angiography (DSA) image of right carotid injection frontal view, demonstrating a small acute ischemic infarct in temporal pole (red arrows on A-B-C). The MRA and cerebral angiogram show an irregular appearance for both distal M1 and proximal M2 (red arrows on E and F).

An antistaphylococcal penicillin (dicloxacillin) was used, based on antibiogram results, and antiepileptic therapy with levetiracetam 1500 mg/day was started.

Two years after surgery, follow-up MRI showed no evidence of the abscess with stable distal M1/M2 stenosis (Figure 2.4.3). The clinical and neurological picture gradually improved, until full recovery.

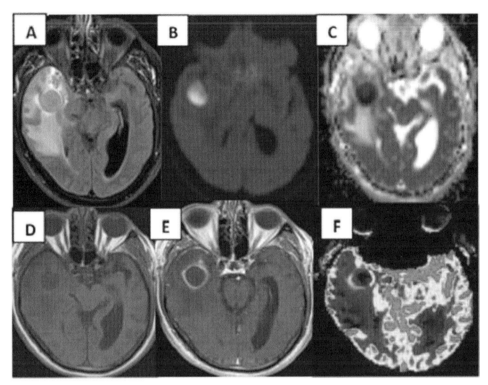

**Figure 2.4.2** Follow-up MRI after two months. (A) FLAIR, (B) diffusion-weighted image, (C) ADC map; T1 (D) before and (E) after gadolinium injection, (F) perfusion map. The images demonstrate a well-formed rounded lesion with diffusion restriction, peripheral enhancement and diffuse surrounding vasogenic edema, consistent with a pyogenic abscess.

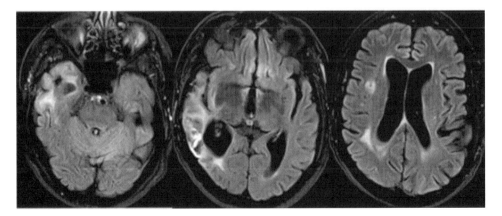

**Figure 2.4.3** Follow-up MRI after two years with FLAIR images demonstrating no evidence of the abscess.

---

**Bacterial meningitis with stroke**

---

**Age** = childhood and adults >65 years; **Gender** = F/M no difference; Annual incidence = 0.7–0.9 per 100,000 population (developed countries); 40 per 100,000 population (developing countries);
**Cumulative stroke incidence in bacterial meningitis** = 14%;
**Risk factors** = age; HIV/AIDS or other immunosuppressive conditions, cancer, diabetes mellitus and alcoholism;
**Risk factors for cerebrovascular events in ABM** = older age, female sex, otitis, sinusitis, immunosuppression, low GCS score and low leukocyte levels in CSF with higher serum erythrocyte sedimentation rates, classic triad at the onset; **Pathogenesis** = both septic emboli (as in case of endocarditis), and the inflammatory status induces plaque instability, narrowing of the vessel lumen and brain ischaemia (as in case of respiratory or urinary tract infections); **Clinical and neurological manifestation** = classic triad signs (fever, neck stiffness and behavioral changes); focal neurological deficit; seizures; gait disturbances; headache; dizziness; **Clinical examination signs and symptoms** = trending fever curves, looking for cardiac murmur, *Janeway lesions, **Roth spots, *Osler nodes, neck stiffness, Kernig and Brudzinski signs; **CSF analysis** = elevated cell counts and hyperprotein contents; CSF could be normal or reveal oligoclonal bands in some cases (e.g. meningovascular syphilis); **Angiographic studies** = arterial narrowing, vessel wall irregularities, focal dilatations, arterial occlusions, and thrombosis of the venous sinuses and/or cortical veins; **Transcranial Doppler** = increased cerebral blood flow velocity; **Bacterial meningitis- associatedstroke acute treatment** = Intravenous thrombolysis with r-tPA is ineffective and potentially dangerous due to high risk of bleeding; mechanical thrombectomy has a favorable outcome; high hemorrhagic risk when thrombectomy follows intravenous thrombolysis; **Anti-inflammatory drugs** = corticosteroids not certainly effective; use is recommended within the 4 h after antibiotic therapy administration.

---

r-tPA (recombinant tissue-type plasminogen activator), GCS (Glasgow coma scale); CSF (cerebrospinal fluid); Cbpa (curved DNA-binding protein); PilcC1 (pilin biogenesis protein); ICAM-1 (intercellular adhesion molecule-1); LFA-1 (lymphocyte function-associated antigen); TNF-α (tumor necrosis factor-α); NO synthetase (nitric oxide synthetase); BBB (blood–brain barrier); BCB (blood–cerebrospinal fluid barrier)

*Janeway lesions are rare, non-tender, small erythematous or hemorrhagic macular, papular or nodular lesions on the palms or soles only a few millimeters in diameter that are associated with infective endocarditis and often indistinguishable from Osler's node.

** Roth's spots, also known as Litten spots or the Litten sign are non-specific retinal red spots with white or pale centers, associated with infective endocarditis, but can occur in other conditions including hypertension, diabetes, collagen vascular disease, extreme hypoxia, leukemia and HIV.

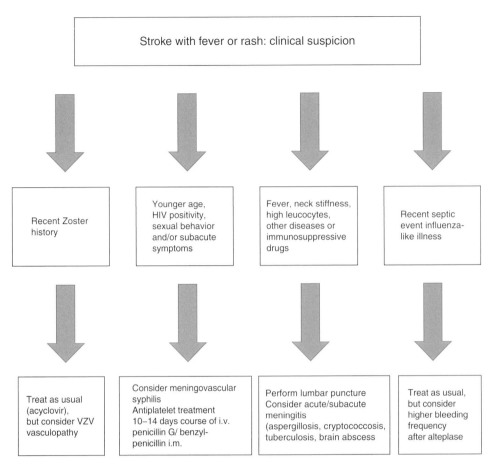

## Case Discussion

Acute bacterial meningitis (ABM) is frequently complicated with cerebrovascular events (CE). The annual incidence of ABM in developed countries has been estimated to be around 0.7–0.9 per 100,000 population, with a higher incidence rate in developing countries (40 per 100,000 population). The main risk factors for ABM are: age (childhood and adults >65 years), HIV/ AIDS or other immunosuppressive conditions, cancer, diabetes mellitus and alcoholism. Risk factors for cerebrovascular events in ABM include: otitis, sinusitis, immunosuppression, low GCS score and low leukocyte levels in CSF with higher serum erythrocyte sedimentation rates. The mortality and morbidity rate in patients with ABM-associated CE, varies between 46% and 62%; however, ABM was almost always fatal before the introduction antibiotic therapy.

Stroke has a cumulative incidence of 14% in patients with bacterial meningitis and, *Streptococcus pneumoniae* is the pathogen isolated with the highest frequency.[1] Clinical and experimental studies suggest that both bacterial and viral infections can be considered as stroke risk factors, regardless of age, owing to their role in triggering inflammation pathways that contribute to blood-vessel narrowing, causing brain infarction.[2] Indeed, stroke-related infections, can be due both to septic emboli (as in the case of endocarditis), and to the inflammatory status, which induces plaque instability, narrowing of the vessel lumen and brain ischemia (as with respiratory or urinary tract infections). All types of infection can trigger acute ischemic stroke, but a higher correlation rate has been observed with urinary tract infections, which are associated with a threefold greater risk of ischemic stroke within 30 days. A large prospective population-based cohort study showed that the stroke incidence is higher in the 14 days after infection for thrombotic stroke and during the subsequent period for cardioembolic stroke.[3]

The two primary mechanisms by which ABM causes CE are: inflammatory vasculopathy (including vasculitis and vasospasm), with greater involvement of the frontal lobe and the middle cerebral artery, and intravascular thrombosis.

Pathogens may use a variety of mechanisms to cross the subarachnoid space, inducing an inflammatory response from the brain's epithelial cells. After bacterial invasion, leukocytes migrate into the subarachnoid space. Virulence factors and adhesive proteins, such as CbpA and PilC1, interact with endothelial cells to promote bacterial adhesion and endocytosis. Endothelial cells express ICAM-1 which binds to LFA-1 on leukocytes to promote migration. These leukocytes also produce TNF-α and NO synthetase.

Leukocytes are then able to permeate into the CSF after bacteria infiltration that further damage the BBB and BCB. Pneumolysin, hemolysin/cytolysin, and $H_2O_2$ are bacterial toxins that stimulate apoptosis-inducing factor caspases, ultimately causing mitochondrial and neuronal death[4]

Finally, this inflammatory reaction induces perivascular smooth muscle contraction, (which causes vasospasm and vasculitis), coagulation-cascade activation, (causing intravascular thrombi) and the vascular basement membrane breakdown (resulting in cerebral edema).

CSF cytokines are inflammatory biomarkers associated with both a positive diagnosis and differentiation between ABM types, and they correlate with disease severity and prognosis.

Indeed, it has been shown that the CSF interferon-γ level is significantly higher in *pneumococcal meningitis* than in *meningococcal meningitis*.[5]

Moreover, in ABM-affected patients, CSF levels of soluble tissue factor, prothrombin and plasminogen activator inhibitor-1 are higher than in the healthy population or viral-encephalitis-affected patients.

When ABM-associated stroke is suspected, clinical examination is essential and should include the following: trending fever curves, looking for cardiac murmur, Janeway lesions, Roth spots, Osler nodes, neck stiffness, and Kernig and Brudzinski signs.

Laboratory and instrumental screening include peripheral blood test, blood cultures, transthoracic echocardiogram to screen for infective endocarditis (IE), lumbar puncture, and HIV/HCV blood test.

In about 40% of ABM patients, a focal deficit is observed on neurological examination. Since stroke or stroke-like symptoms can hide meningitis, the presence of at least one of the classic triad signs (fever, neck stiffness and behavioral changes), can suggest a ABM diagnosis. In 1–4% of ABM cases, patients will have good clinical recoveries initially, but after the first week will develop sudden changes in their level of consciousness or develop new focal neurological signs (delayed cerebral ischemia).

Several studies have highlighted that older age, female sex, otitis or sinusitis, immunocompromised state and the classic triad at the onset are most frequently associated with stroke.[6]

Angiographic studies can reveal arterial narrowing, vessel-wall irregularities, focal dilatations, arterial occlusions and thrombosis of the venous sinuses and/or cortical veins.

Increased cerebral blood flow velocity observed with transcranial Doppler, another marker of cerebral vasculopathy and arterial narrowing, is related to ABM-associated CE and poor outcomes.[7]

Intravenous thrombolysis with r-tPA is considered an ineffective and potentially dangerous treatment for stroke associated with bacterial meningitis (endocarditis embolism, tuberculous meningitis, meningovascular syphilis, brain abscess, etc.).

Literature data demonstrate that the risk of post-thrombolytic cerebral bleeding was higher than reported in stroke cases without endocarditis and that only a low percentage of cases could report a good outcome after r-tPA administration.

Instead, retrospective data indicate that a favorable outcome can be obtained after mechanical thrombectomy, but when thrombectomy follows intravenous thrombolysis, the hemorrhagic risk remains high.[8,9]

In patients with meningitis-associated stroke, dexamethasone use is recommended within four hours after antibiotic therapy administration (ESCMID guidelines).[10] Since the prothrombotic effect of high-dose dexamethasone treatment in bacterial meningitis is known, caution is needed in the use of steroids after the four-hour time window.

Although there is now a clear link between the neuroinflammatory response during ABM and the risk of CE, there are currently no experimental therapeutic protocols to test the efficacy and safety of using new anti-inflammatory drugs to target the components of the inflammatory cascade. The results on corticosteroids regarding their ability to reduce comorbidity in stroke are conflicting and inconsistent.

Future work will be needed that will test new anti-inflammatory drugs and genetic targets.

# References

1. Boldisen J, Dalager-Pedersen M, Schønheyder HC, Nielsen H. Stroke in community-acquired bacterial meningitis: a Danish population-based study. *Int J Infect Dis*. 2014;**20**: 18–22.

2. Sebastian S, Stein LK, Dhamoon MS. Infection as a stroke trigger. *Stroke*. 2019;**50**: 2216–2218.

3. Cowan LT, Alonso A, Pankow JS, et al. Hospitalized infection as a trigger for acute ischemic stroke: the atherosclerosis risk in communities study. *Stroke*. 2016;**47**: 1612–1617.

4. Siegel JL. Acute bacterial meningitis and stroke. *Neurol Neurochir Pol*. 2019;**53**(4): 242–250.

5. Coutinho LG, Grandgirard D, Leib SL, et al. Cerebrospinal-fluid cytokine and chemokine profile in patients with pneumococcal and meningococcal meningitis. *BMC Infect Dis*. 2013;**13**: 326.

6. Van de Beek D, de Gans J, Spanjaard L, et al. Clinical features and prognostic factors in adults with bacterial meningitis. *N Engl J Med*. 2005;**352**(9): 950.

7. Klein M, Koedel U, Pfefferkorn T, et al. Arterial cerebrovascular complications in 94 adults with acute bacterial meningitis. *Crit Care*. 2011;**15**(6): R281.

8. Marquardt RJ, Cho SM, Thatikunta P, et al. Acute ischemic stroke therapy in infective endocarditis: Case series and systematic review. *J Stroke Cerebrovasc Dis*. 2019;**28**: 2207–2212.

9. Engelen-Lee JY, Brouwer MC, Aronica E, van de Beek D. Pneumococcal meningitis: clinical-pathological correlations (MeninGene-Path). *Acta Neuropathol Commun*. 2016;**4**: 26.

10. Van de Beek D, Cabellos C, Dzupova O, et al. ESCMID guideline: diagnosis and treatment of acute bacterial meningitis. *Clin Microbiol Infect*. 2016;**22**: 37–62.

# Neurocysticercosis

**2.5**

Maria Cristina Bravi, Alfano Guido

## Case Presentation

A 34-year-old woman came to the emergency department with a progressively worsening headache over the last two weeks. She also reported a one-off episode of unexplained seizure in the previous three months. She did not report this to relatives or bring it to the attention of her general practitioner. She had lived in India in an overcrowded slum with three children and recently moved to Italy to live with her husband. At the time of admission to our department she was alert and did not show any focal neurological deficits, except for a slight ataxia of the left arm that she was unable to date. Her body temperature was 37.5 °C, heart rate 78 beats/min, blood pressure 120/78 mmHg, respiratory rate 24 breaths/min, with oxygen saturation 98 % on room air. On physical examination we found no other abnormalities. Her medical and family history were unremarkable and at the time she did not take any medications. The patient was initially given a CT brain scan that showed no abnormalities. Blood tests revealed only a slight peripheral eosinophilia (less than 9%).Three days after admission she experienced a second episode of seizure which started as partial, with rapid secondary generalization. We also performed a cranial MRI to rule out any other abnormalities not detected by cranial CT scan. We observed a subcentimetric focal oval lesion with peripheral enhancement in the right cerebellar hemisphere and a subcortical hypointense focal lesion, with peripheral intensity, in the left occipital lobe (Figures 2.5.1 and 2.5.2).

We promptly performed a CSF tap test. The fluid was clear, showing a mild increase in protein concentration (150 mg/dl),while the glucose concentration was in the normal range

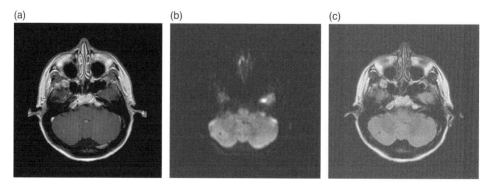

(a)          (b)          (c)

**Figure 2.5.1** (a) T1-weighted image after gadolinium administration: subcentimetric focal oval lesion with peripheral enhancement in the right cerebellar hemisphere. (b) DWI image: focal hypointense oval lesion in the right cerebellar hemisphere. (c) T2-FLAIR image: focal hypointense area with slight perilesional hyperintensity.

(a)

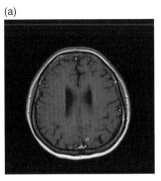

(b)

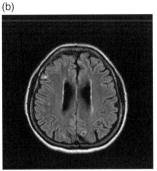

**Figure 2.5.2** (a) T2-weighted FLAIR image: subcortical hypointense focal lesion, with peripheral intensity, in the left occipital lobe. (b) T1-weighted image after gadolinium administration: subcortical focal lesion with peripheral enhancement, in the left occipital lobe.

(44 mg/dl). The tests for bacterial and fungal infection were negative, whereas the serological test enzyme-linked immune electrotransfer blot (EITB) was positive for antibodies to *Taenia solium*; we could therefore make a diagnosis of neurocysticercosis (NCC). The patient immediately started anti-inflammatory therapy with dexamethasone and levetiracetam 500 mg twice daily. After three days antiparasitic therapy with albendazole was added. She was discharged after full recovery. At one-year follow-up she was in good condition and free from seizure relapse.

# Diagnostic Algorithm

| Clinical suspicion of neurocysticercosis |
|---|
| Age = 2–95 years but peak incidence 20–50 years; gender = F:M 1:1; type of onset = acute (40%), subacute (30%), chronic (30%); clinical manifestation: seizures (60%), focal neurological deficits (16%), increased intracranial pressure (20%), cognitive decline (3%), involuntary movements (1%). History positive for immigration from endemic countries/local transmission in reported taeniasis cases |
| **Cranial CT** = CT sequences are more sensitive than MRI to detect calcified cysticerci. The lesions are visible as hyperdense nodules without peripheral edema (parenchymal calcification). Non-viable cysts <20 mm diameter (1–5 mm) |
| **Cranial MRI** = **Live cysts** (small, rounded with little or no edema or contrast enhancement). Cysts with tapeworm **scolex** visible as (hot-with-dot) internal asymmetric nodule in the cyst |
| **Degenerative cyst or colloid cyst** visible as a cyst < 2 cm in size with poorly defined borders, surrounded by edema and showing contrast enhancement |
| **Intraventricular** viable cysticerci in ventricles with loculated or obstructive hydrocephalus |
| **Racemose form and subarachnoid localization** large cysts, multilobed appearance localized within the CSF cisterns or within Sylvian fissures, often with arachnoiditis |
| Confirmed NCC etiological investigations |

| | |
|---|---|
| **Serologic testing**: use enzyme-linked immunoelectrotransfer blot (EITB) assay as a confirmatory test. EITB sensitivity is around | **Abnormalities in CFS** (mononuclear pleocytosis (<300 cells/ml), increased protein concentration (50–300 mg/dl), lower glucose |

| Confirmed NCC etiological investigations | |
|---|---|
| 98% in patients with two or more viable cysts or subarachnoid disease. Do not use enzyme-linked immunosorbent assays (ELISAs) because of poor sensitivity and specificity. Searching for alternative diagnoses if the serology is negative. **Peripheral eosinophilia** ($\leq$10%) | levels associated with poor prognosis. PCR assay for parasite DNA has been assessed with variable results |

| Treatment of NCC | | | |
|---|---|---|---|
| **Antiparasitic:** use in patients with viable parenchymal NCC<br><br>**1-2 cysts: albendazole\*** (15 mg/kg/d in two daily doses) with food for 10 d.<br><br>**> 2 cysts: albendazole** (15 mg/kg/d in two daily doses) combined with **praziquantel** (50 mg/kg/d in three daily doses) for 10 d | **Anti-inflammatory:** should be used whenever antiparasitic drugs are used or **dexamethasone** (0.1 mg/kg/d for 1-2 weeks followed by slow taper | **Antiepileptic:** first-line AEDs for at least two years after the last seizure. Poor adherence to AEDs therapy is the major factor for seizure recurrence Avoid phenobarbital due to high rates of drug interaction. Levetiracetam may be preferable. | **Surgery:** in addition to medical therapy the resection of lesions is indicated in patients with refractory epilepsy debulking or shunt placement in case of hydrocephalus from subarachnoid NCC |

\* Patients treated for more than 14 days should be monitored for leukopenia and hepatotoxicity. The main adverse effects are due to cysticidal activity of the antiparasitic therapy and treatment-induced inflammation, so during the early stage of the treatment there is a transient increase of seizures and headaches

# Case Discussion

NCC is the infection of the CNS by the larval stage of *Taenia solium,* a tapeworm that infests humans in endemic zones (Latin American countries, sub-Saharan Africa, China, India, southeast Asia) and who are the only definitive hosts of the adult parasite. Pigs and humans can be intermediate hosts that carry the larval form and both can ingest infective eggs present in human stools. Thus, pigs only represent intermediate hosts in the transmission of the disease to humans overall through ingestion of undercooked pork meat infected with cysts. Also, person-to-person transmission occurs via the fecal–oral route and this type of transmission seems to be more important.[1] More than 2000 cases of NCC are diagnosed in the USA every year as imported cases, while in some European countries there are about 45 cases per year (Portugal).[2] NCC has a wide range of clinical manifestations, but the most common are seizure and increased intracranial pressure. Focal neurological deficits are also possible due to edema around cysts or mass effects of cysticerci. Inflammatory reactions that occur because of cyst degradation might result in endarteritis, thrombosis with ischemic or hemorrhagic stroke. In particular some evidence suggests that 4–6% of NCC patients in an endemic area have a stroke. On the other hand, data from specialized centers show a prevalence of NCC in 2.5–7.3% of stroke patients. Patients with stroke and NCC that live in rural areas may be identified a long time after the acute event and this delay could be responsible for a spontaneous resolution of the lesion detectable through MRI.[3] Thus, routine corticosteroid administration is mandatory in patients with subarachnoid cysts, to avoid the risk of cerebral infarction. A careful history should be taken with particular attention to exposition as the latent period ranges from months to years between infection and clinical symptoms. Physical examination and radiological studies represent the key elements during the initial evaluation. The major determinant of the severity of the disease is the localization of the cysticerci and the intensity of the immune response by the host. Generally, *intraparenchymal NCC* (one or several cysts, degenerating lesions, calcified cysts only) presents with headaches and seizures that respond very well to antiepileptic drugs (AEDs). On the other hand, *extraparenchymal NCC* (basal subarachnoid NCC, NCC of the Sylvian fissures, intraventricular NCC, small cysts in subarachnoid space of the convexity) has a worse prognosis because of increased intracranial pressure and hydrocephalus, with high mortality when neurosurgery is not available. Children or young women with NCC may have a severe form of parenchymal NCC (*cysticercotic encephalitis*) with a high number of small, viable or degenerating cysts with an associated diffuse inflammatory reaction and cerebral edema. In this case, recurrent seizures, lack of consciousness and intracranial hypertension are the hallmarks of this condition. Other localizations, although rare, are represented by *spinal NCC* (localization of cysts in the subarachnoidal space or intramedullary with evidence of arachnoiditis, spinal dysfunction with paraparesis or incontinence) and *ocular NCC* (intraocular cysticerci in a small number of patients) so it is very useful to perform a fundoscopic examination to exclude retinal localization. Regarding to the diagnostic criteria for NCC, it is important to consider epidemiological factors such as those from living in an endemic region, frequent travel in endemic areas, or household contact with taeniasis. The detection of lesions highly suggestive of NCC on neuroimaging such as cystic lesions with a scolex area is a major diagnostic criterion for NCC. Positive serum antibodies on EITB, positive CSF antigen on ELISA, relief of symptoms after antiparasitic therapy, retinal cysticercosis on fundoscopic examination are also useful in the diagnosis of NCC. The differential diagnosis includes brain cancers, metastatic lesions, tuberculomas and overall toxoplasmosis for appearance of brain abscesses seen as ring-enhancing lesions on MRI and intracranial calcification. Before starting treatment, it is important to establish what type of brain involvement is present. Patients with viable cysts and diffuse cerebral edema should receive corticosteroids as first-line therapy. Patients with intraventricular or third ventricle localization require removal of the cysts by minimally invasive neuroendoscopy, while a standard surgical approach is required for cysts localized in the fourth ventricle. Patients with hydrocephalus should receive shunt surgery; those where the hydrocephalus is derived from subarachnoid NCC may benefit from surgical debulking. It is also recommended to treat all patients with corticosteroids to decrease brain edema in the perioperative period. Antiparasitic therapy is recommended after any surgical approach in the aforementioned patients. However, albendazole alone or in association with praziquantel should be given in the presence of one or two viable cysts or more than two viable cysts, respectively. AEDs should be given to all NCC patients who present with seizures and a poor adherence to AEDs is an important risk factor for seizure recurrence. The main factors for prognosis are the localization of the lesions (subarachnoid and intraventricular localizations have a worse prognosis), the number of viable or calcified cysts (one brain lesion has a better chance of good survival with no seizures), while cysticercotic encephalitis is often lethal.[4,5] As NCC continues to be one the most important cause of seizures in the world and in most developing countries is an important cause of hospital admission, in the future it is desirable that the burden of NCC be controlled through parasite control and eventually eradication.

# References

1. Del Butto OH. Neurocysticercosis: a review. *Scientific World Journal.* 2012: article ID 159821.

2. Gonzalez-Laranjo M, Devleesschauwer B, Trevisan C, et al. Epidemiology of teniosis/cysticercosis in Europe, a systematic review: Western Europe. *Parasit Vectors* 2017; **10**: 349.

3. Del Butto OH, Lama J. Short report: the importance of neurocysticercosis in stroke in rural areas of a developing Latin American Country. *Am J Trop Med Hyg.* 2013; **89**: 374–375.

4. Garcia HH, Nash TE, Del Butto OH. Clinical symptoms, diagnosis, and treatment of neurocysticercosis. *Lancet Neurol.* 2014; **13** (12): 1202–1215.

5. White AC, Jr, Coyle CM, Rajshekhar V, et al. Diagnosis and treatment of neurocysticercosis: 2017 Clinical Practice Guidelines by the Infectious Diseases Society of America (IDSA) and the American Society of Tropical Medicine and Hygiene (ASTMH). 2017 *IDSA/ASTMH Guidelines CID 2018*: **66**(8)e: 49–75.

# 2.6

# Varicella-Zoster Virus-Related: Cytomegalovirus (CMV) and Herpes Infections

Asma Akbar Ladak, Mohammad Wasay

## Case Presentation

A 36-year-old previously healthy male, with a recent exposure to chicken pox in the family, presented to a local hospital emergency room with new-onset seizures. He had a history of diffuse vesicular rash involving multiple dermatomes two weeks ago. During the illness he developed high-grade intermittent fever up to 38 8°C, along with severe diffuse headache. He was treated conservatively with antipyretics and discharged home. In the second week of his illness, he suffered three brief episodes of generalized tonic–clonic seizures. He was again taken to the emergency room, where he was given intravenous diazepam and loaded with levetiracetam. On neurological examination he was drowsy and disoriented with right hemiparesis. The cutaneous lesions diagnosed as "shingles" by our infectious disease expert were crusting. The laboratory investigations revealed a high total leukocyte count (20.8 × $10^9$). Liver function tests, hepatitis B and C serology and cerebrospinal fluid (CSF) analysis were all within normal limits. Polymerase chain reaction tests for *Mycobacterium tuberculosis* and herpes simplex virus (HSV), India ink stain, cryptococcal antigen and bacterial cultures of CSF were negative. CSF showed the presence of IgG varicella antibodies. Protein C and S levels were normal but serum homocysteine levels were elevated (32 µmol/l). Brain MRI showed bilateral superficial hemorrhagic infarcts and a MR venogram showed extensive cerebral venous sinus thrombosis (CVST) involving superior sagittal sinus, right transverse sinus and superficial veins. He was given intravenous acyclovir with adequate hydration and was started on oral levetiracetam. He was started on low-molecular-weight heparin (1 mg/kg SQ every 12 hours). His general condition improved gradually. He became afebrile and the cutaneous lesions continued to crust. No other skin lesion suggestive of purpura fulminans appeared. His headache disappeared and no seizure recurrence was observed. He became alert and oriented, while the hemiparesis improved. He was continued on anticoagulation for three months with an unremarkable course of recovery. A follow-up MRI showed recanalization of venous sinuses after four months with no lesions in the brain parenchyma.

## Diagnostic and Treatment Algorithm

Stroke and cerebral venous thrombosis (CVT) is a well-known complication of varicella-zoster virus (VZV). It must be suspected in all patients with typical skin lesions and neurological findings, especially focal neurological deficits. Brain imaging is a must, preferably contrast MRI and MR venography. Meningoencephalitis is not uncommon in patients with neurological involvement. A lumbar puncture should be done unless contraindicated in all patients. Cerebral VZV infection can be identified by IgG antibodies against VZV.

Many diagnostic kits (for example, Biofilm array) include VZV in their panel for meningo-encephalitis. If not included in the panel, it can be ordered separately. These antibodies are considered diagnostic for cerebral VZV infection.

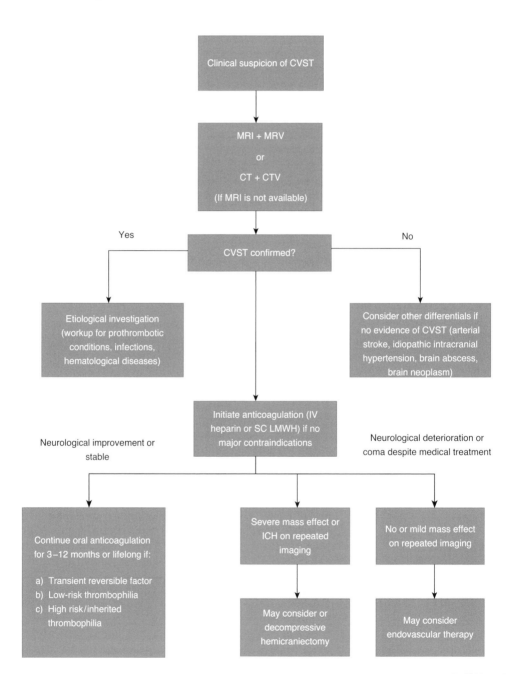

VZV infections are effectively treatable with acyclovir IV(10 mg/kg three times a day) for 10–14 days. CVT is treated with anticoagulation (low-molecular-weight heparin) for three to seven days followed by oral anticoagulation. Newer anticoagulants are currently the preferred choice for long-term anticoagulation rather than warfarin. In the absence of any hypercoagulable state, most patients require three to six months anticoagulation. Seizures are treated with antiepileptic drugs for six months or more. Most patients with acute CVT and seizures do not require long-term (more than two years) AEDs.

## Case Discussion

Varicella-zoster virus (VZV) is known to cause a benign self-limiting exanthem in children, rarely with any neurological manifestations. However, with increasing incidence of VZV in the adult population, severe neurological manifestations have been reported with cerebellar ataxia and encephalitis being the most common. VZV is also associated with cerebral vasculopathy, including cerebral artery stenosis, large artery disease, aneurysm, subarachnoid hemorrhage and cerebral venous sinus thrombosis (CVST).[1] Venous thrombosis secondary to VZV is rare and may occur during both primary infection and reactivation of virus. Patel et al. reported the case of a 25-year old male with a recent history of VZV infection presenting with severe throbbing headache and status epilepticus. CT revealed significant thrombosis in the left transverse, straight and sigmoid sinuses, confirming the diagnosis of CVST.[2] Headache and seizure history were also present in our case. Siddiqi et al. described two cases of CVST associated with VZV in protein C- and S-deficient patients.[3] Other cases of CVST associated with VZV have also been reported in the literature and one patient was reported to have both CVST and pulmonary embolism secondary to VZV due to widespread thrombosis.[4–6] VZV-associated CVST is attributed to blood vessels providing an anatomic pathway for the virus to spread, direct endothelial damage by the virus hence provoking thrombosis. There also has been a temporal link postulated between the development of skin lesions and thrombotic complications. The latency period of two to three weeks is the time during which endothelial damage occurs, leading to a widespread thrombotic process.[4] Patients with a procoagulant state like protein C- and S-deficiency and raised homocysteine levels have also shown a high occurrence of thrombosis.[3] VZV vasculopathy patients may not always have VZV DNA in the CSF, but diagnosis can be confirmed with anti-VZV antibodies.[2] Our patient not only had high homocysteine levels making him more susceptible to CVST, but also showed the presence of IgG varicella antibodies in the CSF. This report provides an insight into rare manifestations of varicella infection in adults. Studies investigating the possible mechanism of development of CVST would help improve management and therefore outcomes in these patients.

## References

1. Gilden D, Cohrs RJ, Mahalingam R, Nagel MA. Varicella zoster virus vasculopathies: diverse clinical manifestations, laboratory features, pathogenesis, and treatment. *Lancet Neurol.* 2009;**8**(8): 731–740.

2. Patel U, Ranjan R, Agrawal C, Patel N. Primary varicella zoster infection presented with cerebral venous sinus thrombosis in adult. *Int J Health Sci Res.* 2015;**5**: 568–572.

3. Siddiqi SA, Nishat S, Kanwar D, et al. Cerebral venous sinus thrombosis: Association with primary varicella zoster virus infection. *J Stroke Cerebrovasc Dis.* 2012;**21**(8): 917.e1–917.e4.

4. Khan R, Yasmeen A, Pandey AK, Al Saffar K, Narayanan SR. Cerebral venous thrombosis and acute pulmonary embolism following varicella infection. *Eur J Case Rep Intern Med.* 2019;**6**(10): 001171.

5. Gayathri K, Ramalingam P, Santhakumar R, et al. Cerebral sinus venous thrombosis as a rare complication of primary varicella zoster virus infection. *J Assoc Physicians India.* 2016;**64**(7): 74–76.

6. Sudhaker B, Dnyaneshwar MP, Jaidip CR, Rao SM. Cerebral venous sinus thrombosis (CVST) secondary to varicella induced hypercoagulable state in an adult. *Intern Med Inside.* 2014;**2**: 1.

# HIV Infection

Massimo Leone, Darlington Thole, Fausto Ciccacci, Maria Cristina Marazzi

## Case Presentation

Helen (invented name) came under our observation in 2015 when she was 11 years old. She suffered from severe stunting, her height being 123 cm, 3.56 Z-scores below the age-adjusted median value. Both parents were positive for human immunodeficiency virus (HIV+); she was therefore also HIV+, but could not start antiretroviral treatment (ARV) because stunting – a very common HIV-related phenomenon – was not considered to define acquired immune deficiency syndrome (AIDS) at the time. Months later, blood examinations showed a very low hemoglobin level of 5.4 g/dl. Common causes of anemia such as malaria, malnutrition, bleeding, and chronic conditions such as tuberculosis and leukemia were excluded and a diagnosis of *HIV-related severe anemia* was made; AIDS clinical stage 3 was fulfilled and ARV could be started. At that time the test and treat approach common in Western countries was not approved in Malawi or the rest of Africa.

One year after ARV, the viral load was persistently high (58.715 RNA copies/ml), poor adherence was hypothesized, home care and a repeat counseling program were started, but six months later the viral load was still high (78.162 RNA copies/ml).

Helen was a smart child, she lives in the bush about two hours walk from the HIV/AIDS health center in Balaka, a township in rural Malawi. She lived in a hut with two rooms shared by eight people, six of them younger then 14, no running water, no electricity and an outdoor toilet, a common condition in the country.

Helen was receiving a good support from her parents (both of them with undetectable viral load), good adherence could be ascertained and resistance to the first-line ARV was hypothesized. Second-line ARV was then started (abacavir 600 mg, lamivudina 300 mg, lopinavir 200 mg/ritonavir 50 mg).

After 18 days she developed acute difficulty in speaking, associated with right leg and arm weakness. No doctors or neurologists worked in the area. One day after onset she was brought to the HIV/AIDS health center, the Disease Relief through Excellent and Advanced Means (DREAM) health center in Balaka.

There she was visited by the senior clinical officer (DT). Since 2006 DT has shared a one-month period per year of work with an Italian neurologist (ML) at DREAM Balaka. He also took part in a number of teaching courses in neurology given to DREAM health workers by European neurologists. DT frequently discussed difficult cases with European neurologists online, thanks to a teleneurology system integrated into the DREAM center.

A general and neurological examination was performed. No fever was detected. Blood pressure, hearth rate, breathing, chest and heart auscultation were unremarkable, no murmurs on the neck, and radial and pedidial arterial pulses were symmetrical and normal.

The child could understand, but was not able to speak. There was no weight loss or malnutrition in her history. She could stand but was unable to walk alone. Strength was 4/5 on right leg and 3 ½/5 on the right harm and hand (she was right-handed). Muscle tone was moderately reduced on the right side, with no Babinski sign and normal pin prick sensation. There were no signs of cerebellar involvement.

Blood examination showed hemoglobin pf 10 g/dl, and platelets were increased to 883.000 $10^3/\mu l$, as they had been over the past two years. White blood cell count, glycemia, creatinine and transaminases were unremarkable. Investigations such as electrocardiogram, CT scan, echocardiography and blood clotting studies were not available in the area. No overt causes of stroke could be found (Table 2.7.1) and immune reconstitution inflammatory syndrome (IRIS) of the brain induced by the second-line ARV was hypothesized. A prednisolone oral course was started. She was taught some physiotherapy exercises to practice at home. Two weeks later her condition had much improved: she could walk alone, speak with only minor persisting difficulties, strength was 5–/5 on right leg and 4 ½/5 on the right arm and hand.

One and a half months after onset an electrocardiogram and a brain CT scan without contrast medium could be performed at the main national city hospital, six hours drive from the Balaka HIV center. The ECG was unremarkable, while the brain CT scan showed a left-sided hypodense cortical lesion in the motor area attributed to focal ischemia. No brain edema nor other brain lesions were found. Aspirin 100 mg/day was started.

Three months after starting the second-line ARV, the viral load was markedly reduced (<400 RNA copies/ml) and later on was permanently undetectable, platelets were normalized (149.000 $10^3/\mu l$) and stunting gradually resolved: height increased from 134 cm (more than three standard deviations below the median value) at initiation of the second-line ARV to 151.4 cm (between the median value and two standard deviations below the median value) on May 2020.

## Diagnostic Algorithm

In sub-Saharan Africa, 60% of the population live in rural areas far from health centers, below the poverty threshold (1.9 USD per day), making transportation to hospitals difficult

**Table 2.7.1** Classification of childhood arterial ischemic stroke. Acute CASCADE (Childhood Arterial Ischemic Stroke Standardized Classification and Diagnostic Evaluation) criteria

| Classification of childhood arterial ischemic stroke | |
| --- | --- |
| **Basic Subtypes** | **Expanded Subtypes** |
| Unilateral focal cerebral arteriopathy | *Anterior circulation with/without collaterals*<br>*Posterior circulation* |
| Bilateral cerebral arteriopathy of childhood | *With/without collaterals* |
| Aortic/cervical arteriopathy | *Dissection* |
| Cardio-embolic | |
| Other | |

Modified from Böhmer et al. *Stroke* 2019; 50: 83–87.

(there is no free service for this). In rural settings the clinical picture and some additional information guide the first-level differential diagnosis and approach.

**Attempting diagnosis of stroke in rural settings with no doctor/neurologist, imaging or health facilities**

Stroke includes focal or global disturbance of the cerebral function

Definite focal signs lasting more than 24 hours or leading to death

Signs must have developed of presumed vascular origin

- Unilateral or bilateral motor impairment (including uncoordination)
- Unilateral or bilateral sensory impairment
- Aphasia/dysphasia (non-fluent speech)
- Hemianopia (half-sided impairment of visual fields)
- Diplopia
- Forced gaze (conjugate deviation)
- Apraxia of acute onset
- Ataxia of acute onset
- Perception deficit of acute onset

A definite focal neurologic impairment must be present, or evidence of intracerebral ischemia or hemorrhage, or subarachnoid hemorrhage

Check for vital signs, blood pressure, heart rate, pathologic murmurs on heart and/or neck/cranial vessels, breathing, sweating, pupils, etc.

**Main differential diagnoses of stroke in rural settings**

| | |
|---|---|
| With fever | meningoencephalitis, malaria, infections, vasculitis, others |
| Without fever | Recent infections (ear, nose, lung, urinary or gastrointestinal tract etc.): brain abscess |
| | Epilepsy: brain mass such as tumor, abscess, vascular malformation, others |
| | HIV infection: immune reconstitution syndrome. Check for CD4, viral load, when last antiretroviral was started. Fever can occur |
| | Malnutrition: TB leading to brain damage/lesion |
| | Vasculitis |
| | Other causes |

# Case Discussion

Stroke has become the second most common cause of death worldwide and is the major (67.3%) contributor to the global burden of neurological disorders. In the last 20 years stroke has greatly increased in low- and middle-income countries (LMIC), while it has decreased in high income countries (HIC).[1] Stroke is among the first three main causes of death in 75% of countries in sub-Saharan Africa (SSA); the fast demographic and lifestyle changes contribute to the figure.[2] Causes of stroke and its risks factors may not be the same in SSA and Western countries; stroke is common in young people in SSA where HIV is the second main risk factor after hypertension and in a case control study conducted in Malawi, HIV was the main risk factor for stroke below 45 years.[3]

In SSA about 25 million people live with HIV; there are more than one million new infections per year and increased access to ARV, prolonging life expectancy, will further increase the burden of stroke in HIV+ patients.[4]

WHO reports that in SSA the percentage of adults who are hypertensive ranges from 16% to 40% (median 31%) and most hypertensive individuals are not aware of their condition.[5,6] The prevalence of diabetes is about 8%.[5] More than 60% of the SSA population live in rural settings where most hypertension and diabetes remain undetected, rarely treated and poorly controlled. And treatment gap for HIV remains high. All these factors heavily contribute to stroke in SSA.

Management of these and other modifiable risk factors for stroke at primary health care level needs to be improved. There is about one neurologist per million people in SSA so that task-shifting of neurology to local non-medical health workers is an unavoidable process[7]

Here we have presented the case of a young HIV+ patient living in a rural area of Malawi, an SSA country, who developed stroke.

The clinical history of this HIV+ child highlights the value of long-term partnership between neurologists from Western countries and local non-medical health workers to make task-shifts possible and effective.

## HIV and Stroke in sub-Saharan Africa and Malawi

A number of factors indicate that stroke in the SSA HIV+ population will continue to increase:

- HIV is the main risk factor for stroke in HIV patients below 45 years[1]
- 75% of the SSA population, including HIV patients, is younger than 45[2]
- severity of stroke, mortality and occurrence of stroke at younger ages are increased by socioeconomic disadvantages[8]
- about half of the SSA population live on 1.5 USD or less per day.

It is noteworthy that the risk of stroke further increases in very immunosuppressed patients starting antiretroviral therapy.

Stroke cases similar to Helen will probably be encountered more and more frequently.

Compared to stroke in Europe, cardiological factors, tobacco smoking, dyslipidemia and atherosclerosis are less frequent in SSA. Modifiable risk factors account for 82.7% of the risks for stroke in SSA[1]; more integrated prevention programs at primary-care level are necessary to treat these risk factors. HIV/AIDS centers have become a noticeable part of the primary health care system in SSA. Accordingly the United Nations indicated that management of HIV/AIDS and stroke (and other NCDs as well) should be unified at HIV/AIDS centers[9]; this approach could reduce the worrying increase in the double burden of HIV and stroke.

Helen lives in Malawi, an SSA country with a population of 18.5 million; 83% live in rural areas and 77% are younger than 45 years. HIV prevalence is 9.2% and hypertension affects about one-third of the adult population; stroke has become the fifth most common cause of death. The mortality rate (number of deaths per 100,000 general population) for stroke in Malawi is more than double that of Western countries. Malawi has very few (two to four) neurologists and there are 0.02 doctors per 1000 inhabitants (in Europe the mean is four doctors per 1000 inhabitants).[9,10] The vast majority of medical activities are performed by non-medical health workers; task-shifting neurology knowledge to local health workers is necessary.

In the last 20 years, many improvements in HIV/AIDS management have been recorded in Malawi and SSA.[11] Stroke could benefit from health-care models that have guided the improvement.

In 2005, Malawi had a high HIV prevalence (11.7–17.1%), health workers had very little knowledge about the condition and related diseases, cost of treatment per patient per year was high and only 3.1% of 2.6 million HIV+ patients could access antiretroviral treatment.

Continuous education and training of local health workers at HIV/AIDS centers have much increased and integrated their knowledge in medical fields, including virology, internal medicine, radiology, pediatrics, neurology, cardiology, pharmacology, management of other chronic conditions, etc. Nowadays, 84.1% of the HIV+ patients in the country receive ARV.

The DREAM health center where Helen was assisted introduced such a method.[12] DREAM is a public health program started in 2002 and now active in 11 SSA countries offering free health services at 49 HIV/AIDS health centers, 14 of which are in Malawi. The program follows more than 500,000 HIV+ patients and clinical activities are supported by 25 laboratories. All DREAM personnel are local. A key aspect of DREAM is regular teaching courses for local health personnel given by European specialists. Only 1.3% of patients per year are lost to follow-up. DREAM is scaling up health programs to manage chronic and non-communicable diseases (NCDs). A dedicated telemedicine service provides teleconsultations to support local activities remotely.[13] Thanks to the long-term partnership between European neurologists and local health workers, Helen could receive early diagnosis and successful treatment of her stroke.

One-third of the 25 million HIV+ patients in SSA and 40% of HIV+ children and adolescents in Malawi have no access to ARV; hopefully they will in the near future. After starting ARV, new strokes, such as IRIS of the brain are expected, particularly in the first six months and with low CD4 counts.[3] When starting ARV, HIV+ patients should be properly monitored and aspirin should be regularly given to prevent stroke. Long-lasting programs based on teaching and work-sharing with local non-medical health workers at HIV/AIDS centers is key to stroke prevention in SSA. Helen's story shows that many young HIV+ patients in rural areas will benefit from such approach – a practical way to bring neurology where there are no neurologists, doctors or tools to investigate the main causes of stroke.

# References

1. O'Donnell MJ, Chin SL, Rangarajan S, et al. Global and regional effects of potentially modifiable risk factors associated with acute stroke in 32 countries (INTERSTROKE): a case-control study. *Lancet*. 2016;**388**: 761–775.

2. www.worldlifeexpectancy.com/world-health-rankings (accessed January 2022)

3. Benjamin LA, Corbett EL, Connor MD, et al. HIV, antiretroviral treatment, hypertension, and stroke in Malawian adults: a case-control study. *Neurology*. 2016;**86**: 324–333.

4. www.who.int/hiv/data/en/ (accessed January 2022)

5. www.afro.who.int/publications/report-status-major-health-risk-factors-noncommunicable-diseases-who-african-region-0 (accessed January 2022)

6. Ataklte F, Erqou S, Kaptoge S, et al. Burden of undiagnosed hypertension in

sub-Saharan Africa: A systematic review and meta-analysis. *Hypertension*. 2015;**65** (2): 291–298.

7. Aslanyan S, Weir SJ, Lees KR, Reid JL, McInnes GT. Effect of area-based deprivation on the severity, subtype, and outcome of ischemic stroke. *Stroke*. 2003;**34**: 2623–2628.

8. Political Declaration of the High-level Meeting of the General Assembly United Nations. 2012. www.who.int/nmh/events/un_ncd_summit2011/political_declaration_en.pdf (accessed January 2022)

9. http://apps.who.int/gho/data/node.main.HWFGRP_0020?lang=en (accessed January 2022)

10. https://wfneurology.org/news-events/archived-news/2017-09-16-who-wfn-neurological-disorders-atlas (accessed February 2022).

11. Gupta N, Bukhman G. Leveraging the lessons learned from HIV/AIDS for coordinated chronic care delivery in resource-poor settings. *Healthcare*. 2015;**3**: 215–220.

12. https://dream.santegidio.org/?lang=en (accessed January 2022)

13. Leone M, Corsi FM, Ferrari F, et al. Teleneurology in sub-Saharan Africa: Experience from a long lasting HIV/AIDS health program (DREAM). *J Neurol Sci*. 2018;**391**: 109–111.

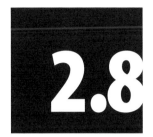

# Chagas Disease

## 2.8

Vinícius Viana Abreu Montanaro

## Case Presentation

A 40-year-old patient, with no known vascular risk factors, presented in the emergency room with sudden dizziness, incongruent speech and right hemiplegia with a duration of more than two hours. The patient was born and resided in the city of Cabeceiras in the Brazilian state of Goiás, a endemic region for Chagas disease (CD) in South America.

There was a delay in adequate medical treatment and correct diagnosis, which was made six hours after the event by neuroimaging (head computerized tomography). It was confirmed as ischemic stroke (IS); however, due to inadequate time of diagnosis and lack of health structure in his city he was not given intravenous thrombolysis.

Upon arrival, the patient was confused, aphasic and hemiplegic, with normal glycemic levels and no alterations in basic blood tests. Arterial pressure was 180/110 mmHg. No evident hepatosplenomegaly was detected on clinical examination. There was no previous history of an acute infection of Chagas disease and family members were also not aware of a family history of CD.

The patient evolved with a left middle cerebral artery infarct at the M2 level (Figure 2.8.1), on serological investigation CD positivity was discovered by two different

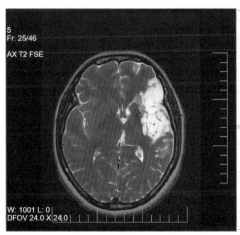
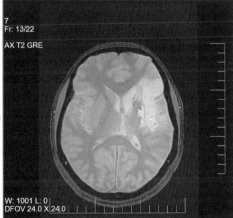

**Figure 2.8.1** T2-weighted and gradient echo (GRE) magnetic resonance imaging showing chronic middle cerebral artery (M2) infarction with minimal hemorrhagic transformation.

methods (ELISA and hemagglutination). The patient was unaware, until that moment, of the presence CD infection.

Transthoracic echocardiography showed systolic dysfunction (35% of ejection fraction), with cardiomegaly. Electrocardiography showed right bundle block. A cardioembolic etiology for the IS was made. There was no arterial cervical abnormalities on cervical Doppler. Later in the investigation no thrombophilia was found. The patient underwent rehabilitation at a specialized center; during follow-up in the neurovascular ambulatory room, difficulty in maintaining correct secondary prevention with anticoagulation was noted.

## Diagnostic Algorithm

> **Clinical suspicion of Chagas disease:**
> Young patient with IS (<50 years), embolic characteristics (large infarcts, hemorrhagic transformation, cortical strokes, more than one arterial territory) in neuroimaging, absence of classical vascular risk factors, presence of epidemiological data on CD (place of birth, vectorial transmission, etc.). It is common absence of history of an acute infection in the past

> Alteration in echocardiographym such as segmental dysfunction, apical aneurism, cardiomegaly; without other causes
> Eletrocardiography showing right bundle block

> Confirmation by two positive distinct serological tests (hemagglutination, ELISA, immunofluorescence)

> Decision on secondary prevention based on evidence of cardioembolism. The criteria are the same used for other cardioembolic etiologies so far, despite criticism. Acute management of IS does not change, as indication of intravenous or mechanical thrombolysis is the same as of any IS. There is a need for ambulatory follow-up by a neurologist and a cardiologist

## Case Discussion

Chagas disease is a vector-borne illness caused by the *Trypanosoma cruzi* parasite. It is the third most common parasitic infection worldwide and a major health problem in non-endemic regions.[1–3] The disease can initially manifest as an acute febrile illness characterized by fever, headache, facial edema and the classic *Romaña* sign, which can last between 6 and 12 weeks. A chronic form of infection can occur in approximately 40% of cases.[4] This form is characterized by cardiac involvement, including arrhythmias and cardiomyopathy.[5]

Over 16 million people are infected worldwide, with most cases in South America; however, cases involving immigrants have also been described, raising concerns about possible blood-borne transmission.[4] There is growing concern regarding Chagas disease prevalence, especially in the developed world, considering the changes in migration flows.[4]

The classical form of transmission of this infection is vector-borne, via *Triatoma infestans*.[5] It is important to notice that classical stercorarian transmission (through the feces of an infected vector) is relatively inefficient; generally, incidence of *T. cruzi* infections is estimated to be <1% per year. The highest estimated incidence of 4% per year is observed in the hyperendemic Bolivian Chaco.[5] There have also been concerns regarding other forms of contagion, such as consumption of contaminated açaí (a local fruit common in the north of Brazil) and through work-related illnesses of piassaba (a plant also common in the northern region) gatherers. Data also corroborates an increase in such alternative forms of infection.[5]

Besides cardiac and digestive system involvement, stroke, especially ischemic, has been related to Chagas disease. Although the correlation between Chagas disease and ischemic stroke (IS) has been described and studied, establishing a causal relationship may be difficult in some situations.[5,6] Data on the epidemiology of IS caused by or related to Chagas disease are scarce.

Most cases of IS in Chagas disease are of cardioembolic origin, since the chronic stage of the disease tends to affect the heart, and leads to the development of arrhythmias and cardiomyopathies. However, the cases of IS in patients without cardiac involvement have also been reported.[1] It is important to notice that most cases were not aware of CD infection before stroke.[4] Recently it has been found that the SSS/CCS TOAST classification to be superior in identifying the cardioembolic etiologies.[1] Individual factors such as the initial modified Rankin scale show a significant correlation with increased mortality and recurrence.[4] Also, recent recommendations of secondary prophylaxis have been questioned due to conflicting evidence, such as the embolic score IPEC\FIOCRUZ, which was proven not to be effective in adequately identifying patients at higher risk of recurrence of IS due to cardioembolism, which would warrant anticoagulation as secondary prophylaxis.[1]

Although acute treatment does not change due to this particular etiology, it is important for neurovascular physicians to recognize these neglected patients due to the need for improvement of management for secondary prevention (anticoagulation in all cardioembolic cases) and continuous cardiologic follow-up. Social and cultural difficulties that these patients suffer usually impairs adequate medical treatment, as shown in our case. The presence of epidemiological and clinical data suggestive of CD should always alert the possibility of the diagnosis. This usually happens in patients such as demonstrated in our case, with a reduced systolic function with no apparent cause in a patient from an endemic region. Other cardiac abnormalities, including arrhythmias (atrial fibrillation or flutter), segmentar hypokinesis, cardiac insufficiency syndrome with no known cause, etc. should also make the physician aware of the diagnosis. Unfortunately, so far no curative treatment for chronic CD has been approved.

The stroke physician should be aware of CD in these cases (epidemiological data, cardiac abnormalities, attention in vertical cases etc.), especially in a changing epidemiology scenario, with cases being reported outside the endemic regions. The correct secondary prevention can dramatically change the outcome of these patients.

# References

1. Montanaro VV, da Silva CM, de Viana Santos CV, et al. Ischemic stroke classification and risk of embolism in patients with Chagas disease. *J Neurol.* 2016;**263**: 2411–2415.

2. Carod-Artal FJ. Policy implications of the changing epidemiology of Chagas disease and stroke. *Stroke.* 2013;**44**: 2356–2360.

3. Mandell GL, Bennett JE, Dolin R. *Principles and Practice of Infectious*

*Disease, Edn 7*. 2010. Philadelphia, PA: Elsevier; 3481–3487.

4. Montanaro VVA, Hora TF, Silva CM, et al. Mortality and stroke recurrence in a rehabilitation cohort of patients with cerebral infarcts and Chagas disease. *Eur Neurol*. 2018;**79**: 177–184.

5. Montanaro VVA, Hora TF, Silva CM, et al. Epidemiology of concurrent Chagas disease and ischemic stroke in a population attending a multicenter quaternary rehabilitation network in Brazil. *Neurol Sci*. 2019;**40**(12): 2595–2601.

# 3.1

# Antiphospholipid Antibody Syndrome

Luana Gentile, Danilo Toni

## Case Presentation

In October 2015, a 43-year-old woman was admitted at 10.20 am to the emergency department (ED) with left brachial weakness on waking up (at about 4 am). She had a past medical history of arterial hypertension, migraine and a previous transient ischemic attack (TIA), and she was a current smoker. Neurological examination showed: left VII cranial nerve central palsy, left arm hemiplegia and mild-moderate sensory loss. Other cranial nerves were intact. NIH Stroke Scale (NIHSS) score was 7.

A brain computed tomography (CT) scan showed an area of focal hypodensity in the right parietal region, indicating a subacute ischemic lesion. Magnetic resonance imaging (MRI) detected ischemic fronto-parietal lesions with petechial hemorrhagic transformation and steno-occlusion of the proximal M1 segment of the right middle cerebral artery (MCA) (Figure 3.1.1).

Diagnostic angiography of the cerebral arteries (Figure 3.1.2) showed that the right MCA M1 segment was replaced by a tangle of vessels from which the lenticulostriate arteries stemmed, the right anterior cerebral artery (ACA) A1 segment was stenotic and the left internal carotid artery (ICA) siphon had severe stenosis.

She did not undergo revascularization treatment. Considering the patient's age and medical history, we performed the following diagnostic procedures: (a) transoesophageal echocardiogram, looking for patent foramen ovale, which was normal; (b) lab tests focusing on hypercoagulability and autoimmune diseases – C reactive protein levels (CRP) were normal;

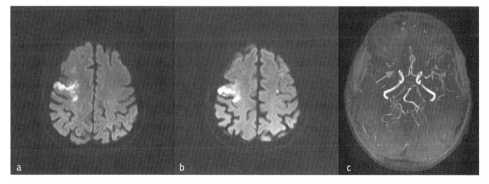

**Figure 3.1.1** (a, b) Diffusion-weighted imaging (DWI) shows acute ischemic fronto-parietal lesions with petechial hemorrhagic transformation; (c) Angio-MRI shows a steno-occlusion of the proximal M1 segment of the right MCA (arrow).

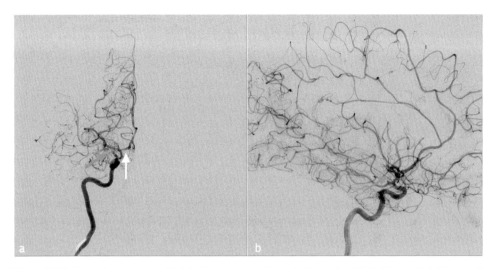

**Figure 3.1.2** Cerebral angiography: (a) right M1 segment occlusion (red arrow) and right A1 stenosis (white arrow); (b) right M1 segment replaced by a tangle of vessels (red arrow).

thrombophilia screening tests (homocysteine and cysteine levels, prothrombin gene mutation, protein S, protein C, and antithrombin III) showed only an heterozygosis mutation of MTHFR 677C>T and MTHFR 1298A>C; autoimmune screening panel (antineutrophil cytoplasm antibodies (ANCA), antinuclear antibodies (ANA), smooth muscle antibodies (SMA), anti-mitochondrial antibodies (AMA), lupus anticoagulant, anticardiolipin (aCL) and anti-β-2-glycoprotein I (b2GPI) antibodies, showed a level of aCL IgM of 21.10 MPL/ml (normal value <15.0) and b2GPI IgM of 23.6 UA/ml (normal value <20.0). During hospitalization, the clinical condition improved (NIHSS 3) and patient was discharged with antiplatelet and steroid treatment. About a month later, she returned to the ED with the sudden onset of slurred speech and right flattened nasolabial fold. An MRI + angioMRI showed new ischemic lesions in the left frontal lobe and both MCAs were filiform. We performed a lumbar puncture to exclude a primary angiitis of the central nervous system (PACNS); cerebrospinal fluid analysis showed no oligonal bands, no pleocytosis and the absence of neurotropic viruses. On the suspicion of antiphospholipid antibody syndrome (APS), we replaced antiplatelet therapy with anticoagulant treatment with vitamin K antagonist (VKA).

The patient did not visit at the outpatient clinic in the subsequent three years. In February 2018 she was again admitted to the ED for dysarthria, worsening in the last three days (NIHSS = 2). An MRI showed recent ischemic lesions in the right frontal cortex and in the left fronto-insular lobe. She reported two recent miscarriages: the first in 2016 and the second during the following year. Cerebrospinal fluid analysis was negative. Serological autoimmune screening confirmed high levels of aCL IgM (>50 MPL/ml) and of b2GPI IgM (>50 UA/ml) antibodies. The patient was discharged on therapy with acetylsalicylic acid (ASA) 100 mg and dabigatran 220 mg, in addition to steroid therapy. Follow-up lab tests four months later confirmed a high titer of aCL IgM (>50 MPL/ml) and b2GPI IgM antibodies (>50 UA/ml) and the diagnosis of APS. No recurrent events occurred within the next two-year follow-up (NIHSS = 2 and Modified Rankin Scale (mRS) score = 1).

# Diagnostic Algorithm

| SUSPICION OF ISCHEMIC STROKE RELATED TO ANTIPHOSHOLIPID ANTIBODY SYNDROME | |
|---|---|
| **Age** = 15–50 (85% of patients)<br>**Gender** = M:F 1:3.5 for primary APS, 1:7 for secondary APS | **History or evidence of non-neurological clinical manifestations:**<br>(1) venous thromboembolism: deep vein thrombosis, (2) pregnancy morbidity: early miscarriage (< 10 weeks of gestation), fetal loss (>10 weeks of gestation), pre-eclampsia, eclampsia, (3) other forms of arterial thrombosis: cardiac valve thickening or Libman–Sacks endocarditis, myocardial ischemia, ischemia of visceral organs, (4) hematological manifestations: thrombocytopenia, (5) dermatological manifestations: livedo reticularis, (6) renal diseases: thrombosis of renal arteries, acute or chronic renal failure. |

| NEUROIMAGING |
|---|
| no pathognomonic neuroimaging findings of APS |
| **Cranial CT:** can reveal the presence of single focal lesions or multiple areas of infarction and diffuse cortical atrophy, but the characteristics of these lesions are not distinguished from those of other etiologies<br>**Cranial MRI:** can show (a) isolated or multiple ischemic lesions, (b) diffuse and non-specific brain atrophy either isolated or in addition to parenchymal lesions, (c) multiple and diffuse white-matter hyperintense lesions (MS-like). Intracranial stenosis or occlusion is a frequent finding (> MCA territory)<br>**Cerebral angiography:** can reveal a vasculitis-like pattern with narrowing of multiple intracranial arteries |

| DIAGNOSTIC WORK-UP |
|---|
| Dosage of l.c. (aPLs)and exclusions of differential conditions associated with prothrombotic state or transient aPL positivity |

| Inherited Thrombophilia | Autoimmune or rheumatic disease | Infections |
|---|---|---|
| Factor VLeiden mutation<br>Prothrombin G20210A mutation<br>Protein S deficiency<br>Protein C deficiency<br>Antithrombin deficiency<br>MTHFR mutation | ESV/CRP<br>ANA, AMA, ANCA, SMA<br>Complement (C3-C4) levels<br>Direct Coombs test<br>Cryoglobulin | Bacterial: leptospirosis, syphilis, Lyme disease, [follow on]<br>tuberculosis,infective endocarditis, Streptococcus Klebsiella.<br><br>Viral: Hepatitis A, B, and C, HIV, HTLV-I, cytomegalovirus, varicella-zoster,EBV, rubeola, adenovirus, parvovirus |

| Acquired Prothrombotic Conditions | Other causes of stroke and/or prothrombotic state in the young |
|---|---|
| Malignancy<br>Medications (oral contraceptives) | PACNS (→cerebral angiography and lumbar puncture)<br>CADASIL (→MRI findings and NOTCH III gene mutation)<br>Fabry disease (→MRI findings and galactosidase alpha gene III mutation)<br>PFO (→transesophageal echocardiogram, transcranial Doppler ultrasound with saline bubble test) |

| | Revised Sapporo criteria for definite APS |
|---|---|
| aPL positivity<br>and<br>exclusion of alternative diagnosis to explain the clinical findings | At least one clinical criterion(avascular thrombosis or an adverse pregnancy outcome)<br>and<br>at least one laboratory criterion (presence of one or more specified aPLs <u>on two or more occasions at least 12 weeks apart)</u> |

| TREATMENT | |
|---|---|
| **Acute ischemic stroke (AIS)**<br>According to International Guidelines on AIS in non-APS patients: intravenous thrombolysis and/or thrombectomy<br>ATTENTION: aPLs can induce thrombocytopenia!<br>Primary endovascular thrombectomy may be considered as an alternative to intravenous thrombolysis in these patients | **Secondary prevention**<br>No consensus regarding optimal antithrombotic management<br>- VKAs (INR 2.0-3.0) are the treatment of choice<br>- In case of recurrence despite anticoagulation: increase INR target to 3.0–4.0 or add ASA<br>- Few data on DOACs |

# Case Discussion

Antiphospholipid antibody syndrome (APS) is an autoimmune disorder characterized by venous or arterial thrombosis and/or pregnancy morbidity in the presence of persistent antiphospholipid antibodies (aPLs).[1] It can occur as a primary condition or in the setting of a systemic autoimmune disease, particularly systemic lupus erythematosus (SLE). Clinical and laboratory features of the two forms often overlap, and many patients with primary APS may subsequently develop SLE. aPLs are a heterogeneous group of antibodies directed against phospholipid-binding plasma proteins, such as lupus anticoagulants (LA), anticardiolipin (aCL) and anti-β-2-glycoprotein I (b2GPI). APS has a prevalence of 1–5% in the general population and affects women more frequently than men with a ratio of 3.5:1 for primary APS and 1:7 for secondary APS (SLE related APS). The genesis of the prothrombotic state remains controversial. aPLs could induce thrombosis via several mechanisms: (1) interference with endogenous anticoagulant mechanisms, (2) platelet activation, (3) complement cascade activation, (4) expression of endothelial adhesion molecules. According to most recent theory the thrombosis is the consequence of a "two hit" model: the first hit (all conditions that increase oxidative stress such as smoking or infections) damages the endothelium integrity, while the second hit potentiates thrombus formation. Oxidation of b2GPI induces a conformational change which allows anti-b2GPI antibody binding.

According to the current classification criteria, clinical manifestations of APS include vascular thrombosis (thrombotic APS) and/or pregnancy morbidity (obstetric APS). There is also a rare form called catastrophic APS (CAPS) characterized by simultaneous thrombotic complications in multiple organs. Thrombotic APS is characterized by venous, arterial and small-vessel thrombosis: deep-vein thrombosis is the most frequent thrombotic manifestation of APS, but arterial events are the most life-threatening, and the central nervous system (CNS) is the most frequently involved site. Neurological involvement in APS is common and its occurrence increases morbidity and mortality. Recently APS neurological manifestations were classified as thrombotic and non-thrombotic.[2] CNS thrombotic manifestations include stroke, transient ischemic attack (TIA), and cerebral venous thrombosis (CVT). CNS non-thrombotic manifestations include cognitive dysfunction, migraine, seizure, MS-like syndrome, transverse myelitis, movement disorders and psychiatric symptoms. The Euro-Phospholipid Project, in a cohort of 1000 patients with APS, highlighted that the most common non-neurological manifestations in the APS was deep-vein thrombosis (38.9%), followed by arthralgia (38.7%), early fetal losses (35.4%) and thrombocytopenia (29.6%); among neurological manifestations, stroke occurred in 19.8% and TIA in 11.1% of cases. Ischemic stroke (IS) is the most common and severe arterial complication of APS in particular in young adults; considering all patients with cerebral ischemic events, the prevalence of aPLs in young adults < 50 years old has been reported to be 17.2%. The mechanisms of stroke in APS are both thrombotic and embolic, the latter due to cardiac involvement and valvular anomalies. Clinical manifestation of APS-associated IS depends on the location and size of the occluded vessel. Small arteries are frequently involved with lacunar subcortical IS, but about 50% of APS patients have intracranial stenosis or occlusion, classically in the MCA territory. A vasculitis-like pattern with narrowing of multiple intracranial arteries is also possible in APS. Occasionally, the extracranial carotid artery may be involved. Although not common, CVT can complicate APS or be the onset symptom.[3]

Diagnosis of stroke related to an underlying undiagnosed APS is not easy and is based on a combination of clinical features and laboratory findings. Diagnostic work-up must aim to investigate:[4]

– Medical history: the nature and frequency of thrombotic events, outcomes of pregnancies in female patients, other risk factors for thrombosis, such as contraceptive use.

– Physical examination: there are no pathognomonic physical findings of APS, but examination can show abnormal signs related to ischemia or infarction of the skin or viscera, or deep-vein thrombosis.

– Neuroimaging characteristics: there are no pathognomonic neuroimaging findings of APS, and lesions are often not distinguishable from those of other etiologies. The most common MRI abnormalities are: (a) isolated or multiple ischemic lesions in supratentorial regions or, less frequently, in the brainstem and cerebellum; (b) diffuse and non-specific brain atrophy isolated or in addition to parenchymal lesions; (c) multiple and diffuse white-matter hyperintense lesions (MS-like). Intracranial stenosis or occlusion is present in about half of patients, most frequently involving the MCA (31%). A vasculitis-like pattern with multiple sites of narrowing and dilation has also been described through angiography. Alterations of extracranial arteries are less frequent and three types have been described: (1) common carotid or internal carotid artery (ICA) stenosis or occlusion, (2) stenosis or occlusion of the origin of two or more large vessels (Takayasu-like pattern) and narrowing of the ICA in an atherosclerotic disease-like pattern.

– Laboratory testing for aPLs: aCL, IgG and IgM by enzyme-linked immunosorbent assay (ELISA), anti-b2-GPI antibodies, IgG and IgM, by ELISA, and LA testing detected by prolongation of a phospholipid-dependent clotting time. In contrast to IgG and IgM isotypes of aCL and anti-beta2-GPI, the association of the IgA isotypes with clinical thrombosis remains controversial.

According to the revised Sapporo classification criteria definite APS is considered a condition in which at least one of the two major clinical manifestations (thrombosis or pregnancy morbidity) is met, and one of three standardized laboratory assays demonstrate the persistence of aPLs for at least 12 weeks. Not every positive aPL test is clinically relevant: low-titer aPLs are common during infections, transient and not associated with clinical consequences. This is the reason why the confirmation of persistent medium- or high-titer aPLs on more than two occasions at least 12 weeks apart is required for the diagnosis of APS.[5]

In APS patients with angiographic anomalies, important differential diagnoses include PACNS and reversible cerebral vasoconstriction syndrome (RCVS). Both conditions are characterized by headache (recurrent thunderclap in RCVS, insidious and chronic in PACNS) and angiography anomalies ("Sausage on a string" sign in RCVS and irregular narrowing with ectasia in PACNS). RCVS is characterized by watershed cerebral ischemia, and subarachnoid hemorrhages (SAH) are also frequent. It is a non-inflammatory disease, usually treated with nimodipine and angiography pattern is reversible within 12 weeks. PACNS is characterized by a small and scattered cerebral ischemic pattern, lobar hemorrhage and SAH are very uncommon, cerebrospinal fluid classically shows abnormal findings (cell count >5 cells/μl or total protein concentration >45 mg/dl) in the majority of patients.

Prospective data on the therapeutic approach to stroke in patients with APS are scarce. In the acute phase, ischemic cerebrovascular events are managed according to international guidelines. For secondary prevention, long-term anticoagulation is the most common strategy and vitamin K antagonists are the treatment of choice, although there is no consensus regarding optimal antithrombotic management, due to lack of clinical trials. The thrombosis recurrence rate among APS patients remains high, despite adequate anticoagulation. If recurrence occurs with therapeutic INR (2.0–3.0), the target should be increased to 3.0–4.0 or aspirin should be added. Direct oral anticoagulants (DOACs) represent an interesting possible alternative to warfarin, but their use in APS patients is controversial. According to the 15th International Congress on Antiphospholipid Antibodies Task Force on Antiphospholipid Syndrome Treatment Trends in 2017, warfarin represents the only approved anticoagulant agent. Further studies on the use of DOACs are needed, particularly considering the young age of many patients, no need to monitor INR and the possible anti-inflammatory and antiangiogenic effect of DOACs.

# References

1. Linnemann B. Antiphospholipid syndrome: An update. *Vasa*. 2018;**47**(6): 451–464.

2. Ricarte IF, Dutra LA, Abrantes FF, et al. Neurologic manifestations of antiphospholipid syndrome. *Lupus*. 2018;**27** (9): 1404–1414.

3. Fleetwood T, Cantello R, Comi C. Antiphospholipid syndrome and the neurologist: from pathogenesis to therapy. *Front Neurol*. 2018;**9**: 1001.

4. Miyakis S, Lockshin MD, Atsumi T, et al. International consensus statement on an update of the classification criteria for definite antiphospholipid syndrome (APS). *J Thromb Haemost*. 2006;**4**(2): 295–306.

5. Cervera R, Piette JC, Font J, et al. Antiphospholipid syndrome: Clinical and immunologic manifestations and patterns of disease expression in a cohort of 1,000 patients. *Arthritis Rheum*. 2002;**46**(4): 1019–1027.

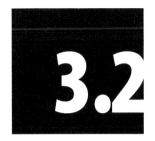

# Hyperhomocysteinemia

## 3.2

Maria Cristina Bravi, Sabrina Anticoli

## Case Presentation

A 16-year-old female presented to our emergency room complaining of headache and a single episode of a seizure during a beach volleyball match. She was alert but slightly confused, showing right facial paresis, a mild defect in motility in her upper right arm and slurred speech with NIHSS (National Institute of Health Stroke Scale) = 7. Temperature was 37.1 °C, heart rate 98 beats/min, blood pressure 139/87 mmHg, respiratory rate 25 breaths/min and $SpO_2$ 90% on room air. Her past medical history was unremarkable, while the family history was positive for deep venous thrombosis and myocardial infarction. Specifically, her paternal grandfather died aged 51 from a heart attack and her brother, aged 32, had dual episodes of deep venous thrombosis at 21 and 30 years, respectively. She was not taking any therapy. After a second episode of seizure that did not resolve with an intravenous dose of clonazepam, it transformed into status epilepticus with the appearance of respiratory insufficiency, so the patient underwent endotracheal intubation and stabilization of vital signs. After this, we performed a computed tomography (CT) brain scan that was negative for hemorrhagic or mass lesions. Then, a magnetic resonance study plus MRI venography were performed, which showed a wide area of ischemic lesion in the left frontal area and occlusion of the longitudinal superior venous sinus (Figures 3.2.1 and 3.2.2).

Thus, a diagnosis of stroke with cerebral venous thrombosis was made and she was promptly transferred to ICU for adequate treatment and management. Laboratory studies, including total peripheral blood count, biochemical screen, HbA1c, vitamin $B_{12}$, folic acid,

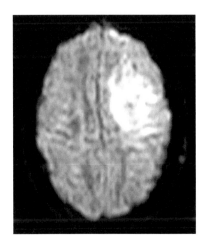

**Figure 3.2.1** DWI image: hyperintense lesion in the left frontal region.

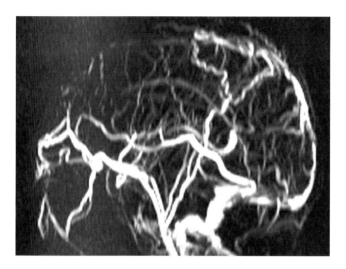

**Figure 3.2.2** Lateral MIP images of MR venography showing signal loss in the anterior half of superior sagittal sinus.

erythrocyte sedimentation rate (ESR), C reactive protein (CRP), thyroid, renal and hepatic functions were normal. Antinuclear antibodies (ANA), rheumatoid factor (RF), perinuclear antineutrophil cytoplasmic antibodies (P-ANCA), antineutrophil cytoplasmic antibodies (C-ANCA), lupus anticoagulant (LAC), antithrombin, protein S, protein C, Factor VIII levels, anticardiolipin antibodies, factor V Leiden mutation and activated protein C resistance were all in the normal range. However, plasma levels of homocysteine were increased (91 µmol/l with normal range from 5 to 12 µmol/l). She started an antiepileptic drug (levetiracetam 2 g/day) therapy, anticoagulation initially with LMWH and then with warfarin, maintaining an adequate INR range, and therapy with folic acid. After a few days her clinical condition consistently improved, her NIHSS was 3 because of the persistence of an alteration of the speech and a mild motor impairment of the right arm, so she was discharged from ICU and transferred to the stroke unit. She was then referred for genetic counselling and a mutation for the MTHFR (C677T) gene was found. A second MRI showed complete resolution of the cerebral venous occlusion, persistence of the ischemic area in the left frontal area and mild cerebral edema. She started a cycle of rehabilitation and after two weeks she was discharged with full recovery.

## Clinical presentation, diagnosis and management

Age = 15–70 years. Gender = F:M 1:3; type of onset = acute; race = Black people from southern Africa have lower HCY levels than white people

Clinical manifestation: focal neurological deficits, seizures, headaches, increased intracranial pressure

Past medical history positive for stroke/TIA at juvenile age and/or deep venous thrombosis

Causes: **Genetic defects** (deficiency of cystathionine β-synthase, mutation of $N^5$, $N^{10}$-methylenetetrahydrofolate reductase MTHFR C677T). **Nutritional deficiencies** (folate, vits $B_{12}$ and $B_6$). **Other causes:** chronic renal failure, hypothyroidism, pernicious anemia, cancer, drugs, smoking, increasing age (> 65), gastrointestinal malabsorption (celiac disease, Crohn's disease, giardiasis, diphyllobothriasis)

(cont.)

### Clinical presentation, diagnosis and management

**Cranial CT scan and angio CT scan** = Signs of brain infarction (parenchymal hypodense lesions in ischemic stroke, brain edema with midline shift or compression of ventricle, hyperdense lesions in cerebral hemorrhage), large-vessel occlusion or evidence of cerebral venous sinus thrombosis

**Cranial MRI** = Diffusion weighted imaging (DWI) hyperintensity with associated decreased apparent diffusion coefficient (ADC). FLAIR-weighted images areas of high signal intensity. Large arterial occlusion of the circle of Willis. Evidence of cerebral venous sinus thrombosis in MIP images of MR venography.

### Confirmed HHCY and etiological investigations

**Serologic testing**: HCY measured by immunoassay (normal HCY plasma concentrations in the fasting state range from 5 µmol/l to 15µmol/l), serum $B_{12}$ and folic acid measured by immunoassay

**Genetic counselling**: Evaluate the presence of MTHFR polymorphism particularly for a point mutation (C677T) on chromosome 1

Search for the presence of homozygous trait of cystathionine-β-synthase on chromosome 21

### Treatment of HHCY

**Vitamin supplementation:**

Vitamin $B_{12}$(5 µg/day)

Folic acid (400 µg/day)

Vit $B_6$ (3 mg/day)

**Additional measures:**

**Modification of lifestyle:**

Reduce alcohol and caffeine consumption, stop smoking, increase physical exercise, healthy diet with increasing consumption of fruit and vegetables, particularly green-leaf vegetables which contain folic acid.

Control renal function.

Control other cardiovascular risk factors, such as hypertension and dyslipidemia.

Peripheral blood count, iron, ferritin, urea and electrolytes, AST, ALT, ALP, GGT, creatinine, free T3, free T4, TSH, calcium, CRP, ESR, ANA, RF, C-ANCA, P-ANCA, LAC, anticardiolipin antibodies, APTT, fibrinogen, INR, antithrombin III, protein C, protein S, factor V Leiden, homocysteine, vitamin $B_{12}$, folic acid, vitamin $B_6$.

CT: computerized tomography; MRI: magnetic resonance imaging; DWI: diffusion-weighted imaging; ADC: apparent diffusion coefficient; CRP: C-reactive protein; ESR: erythrocyte sedimentation rate; ANA: antinuclear antibody; C- ANCA: antiproteinase-3 antibodies, P-ANCA: antimyeloperoxidase antibodies; LAC; lupus anti-coagulant; LMWH: low-molecular-weight heparin; INR: international normalized ratio

# Discussion

In 1969 McCully observed for the first time, during autoptic examination, that children affected by homocystinuria and hyperhomocysteinemia (HHCY) had evidence of wide-spread vascular thrombosis and atherosclerosis. Since then, many studies have established the relationship between HHCY and vascular disease. But what is homocysteine? Homocysteine (HCY) is a sulfur-containing amino acid derived from the metabolism of methionine, in which $B_{12}$ and $B_6$ vitamins are cofactors necessary to complete the metabolic pathway. Normal HCY plasma concentrations in the fasting state range from 5 µmol/L to 15 µmol/L. Genetic defects in HCY metabolism and nutritional deficiencies cause HHCY. Cystathionine β-synthase deficiency in the homozygous form (congenital homocystinuria) is the most common cause of severe HHCY (some patients show more than 400 µmol/l of HCY). This genetic defect is rare (1/200,000 births), and patients present mental retardation, ectopia lentis, skeletal deformities, severe atherosclerosis and thromboembolism, with a mortality of 20% in those untreated, while heterozygotes have plasma HCY in the range 20–40 µmol/l. Another genetic defect is represented by homozygous deficiency of $N^5$, $N^{10}$-methylenetetrahydrofolate reductase (MTHFR), an enzyme involved in the remethylation of HCY. A point mutation in MTHFR (C677T) has also been reported, but although it is quite common in the general population, it appears to be able to generate HHCY only in response to depletion of folic acid. HCY is also elevated in chronic renal failure, hypothyroidism and pernicious anemia, as well as in patients with several types of cancer, such as acute lymphoblastic leukemia and pancreatic, breast and ovarian cancers. Drugs, such as methotrexate and phenytoin can increase HCY levels by interfering with folate metabolism, while theophylline and hormone therapy increase HCY by reducing the synthesis of vitamin $B_6$. Cigarette smoking also acts in the same way. In fact, it has been observed that smokers have lower levels of vitamin $B_6$ than non-smokers, probably causing increased atherogenesis. Proton pump inhibitors can cause malabsorption through bacterial overgrowth in the small bowel and metformin can inhibit vitamin $B_{12}$ absorption, causing HHCY. The mechanism by which HHCY acts has been only postulated, but experimental evidence suggests that endothelial dysfunction generated by reactive oxygen species, platelet activation and thrombus formation play key roles in the pathophysiologic mechanisms of HHCY. Furthermore, HCY also affects the metabolism of endothelial-derived nitric-oxide-limiting nitric oxide production. Some authors have shown that HHCY is a risk factor for stroke/TIA, mainly in patients with other associated risk factors such as hypertension, dyslipidemia, smoking and carotid atherosclerosis.[1,2,3] It has also been demonstrated that HHCY can be an independent risk factor for venous thromboembolism and the association between HHCY and factor V Leiden further increases the risk of deep venous thrombosis.[4] It has also been reported that at age ≥80, 40% of patients referred for stroke prevention had HCY ≥14 µmol/l, and that metabolic $B_{12}$ deficiency was present in 10% of patients with stroke/TIA aged <50, 13% aged 50–70 and 30% above the age of 70. Furthermore, in the China Stroke Primary Prevention Trial (CSPPT) folic acid reduced ischemic stroke by 24% and a recent meta-analysis indicated that B vitamins combined with folic acid reduced the risk of stroke overall in patients with associated vascular risk factors.[5] Metabolic $B_{12}$, folic acid deficiency and HHCY remain common in patients with TIA or stroke.[6] Actually, according to recent American heart and Stroke Association Guidelines (AHA GL), routine analysis for HHCY among patients with a recent ischemic stroke or TIA is not indicated.[7] Even though HHCY is implicated in several vascular pathologies, such as stroke and cerebral venous thrombosis, it is far from being considered a biomarker of these conditions, but it might still be a good target for clinical interventions. In fact, patients with stroke and associated secondary cardiovascular risk factors could benefit from control of HCY, eventually adopting specific dietary plans. As HHCY is more frequent in young patients with stroke and this condition could have a serious impact on quality of life, serum $B_{12}$, folic acid and HCY should be measured and abnormalities treated.

# References

1. Welch GN, Loscalzo J. Homocysteine and atherothrombosis. *N Engl J Med*. 1998;**338**: 1042–1050.

2. Selhub J, Jaques PF, Bostom AG, et al, Association between plasma homocysteine concentrations and extracranial carotid-artery stenosis. *N Engl J Med*. 1995;**332**: 286–291.

3. Clarke R, Daly L, Robinson K, et al. Hyperhomocysteinemia: an independent risk factor for vascular disease. *N Engl J Med*. 1991;**324**: 1149–1155.

4. Den Heijer M, Kostor T, Blom HJ, et al. Hyperhomocysteinemia as a risk factor for deep-vein thrombosis. *N Engl J Med*. 1996;**334**: 759–762.

5. Quin X, Li J, Spence JD, et al. Folic acid therapy reduces the first stroke risk associated with hypercholesterolemia among hypertensive patients. *Stroke*. 2016;**47**: 2805–2812.

6. Ahmed S, Bogiatzi C, Hackam DG, et al. Vitamin $B_{12}$ deficiency and hyperhomocysteinaemia in outpatients with stroke or transient ischaemic attack: A cohort study at an academic medical centre. *BMJ Open*. 2019;**9**: e026564.

7. American Heart Association Stroke Council, Powers WJ, Rabinstein AA, Ackerson T et al. 2018 Guidelines for the Early Management of Patients With Acute Ischemic Stroke: A Guideline for Healthcare Professionals From the American Heart Association/American Stroke Association. *Stroke*. 2018;**49**: e46–e110.

# Hyperviscosity Syndrome

## 3.3

Francesca Romana Pezzella, Kateryna Antonenko, Larysa Sokolova

## Case Presentation

A 58-year-old male was admitted to the stroke unit with recurrent left hand weakness and dysarthria. Furthermore, the patient presented with non-specific clinical manifestations including weight loss, fatigue, blurred vision and intermittent nose bleeds for the past three months. In anamnesis vitae there was no history of stroke risk factors. On admission, his neurological examination revealed slightly decreased muscle strength in his left hand (grade 4/5), positive Babinski sign on the left side, diminished feeling of pain and warmth in the patient's left limbs (upper > lower limb) and mild dysarthria. In addition, no other nervous system abnormalities were detected.

Brain magnetic resonance imaging (MRI) revealed multiple areas of significant diffusion restriction in the cortico-subcortical level of the right temporal, frontal and parietal lobes – signs of recent ischemic lesions (Figures 3.3.1 and 3.3.2). Moreover, lacunar areas of gliosis were present in both hemispheres (Figure 3.3.2). MR-angiography did not show any pathology of the intracranial arteries.

To explore the etiology of the multiple acute and chronic ischemic cerebral infarctions, the stroke team performed carotid artery ultrasonography, echocardiogram, 24-hour Holter cardiac rhythm monitoring, standard thrombophilic screening (anticardiolipin antibodies, Protein C, Protein S, homocysteine, lupus anticoagulant) – all showed negative findings.

(a)     (b)     (c)

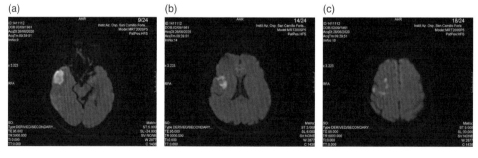

**Figure 3.3.1** Diffusion-weighted MR images, cortico-subcortical areas of significant diffuse restriction in the right temporal, frontal and parietal lobes. Neuroimages are courtesy of Professor Enrico Cotroneo, Director of the Neuroradiology Department, San Camillo Forlanini Hospital.

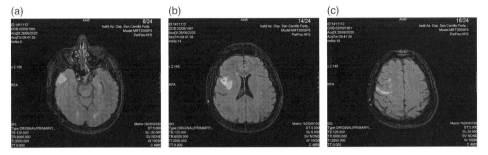

**Figure 3.3.2** FLAIR-weighted axial MR images, cortico-subcortical areas of high signal intensity in the right temporal, frontal and parietal lobes; lacunar areas of gliosis in both hemispheres. Neuroimages are courtesy of Professor Enrico Cotroneo, Director of the Neuroradiology Department, San Camillo Forlanini Hospital.

Laboratory studies detected anemia, hypoproteinemia and an abnormal albumin-globulin ratio. Further examinations were conducted and we revealed elevated serum monoclonal IgM (IgM – 5030 mg/dl, reference value: 46–304 mg/dl), and increased plasma viscosity (4.98 mPas reference value: 1.26–1.66mPas). Therefore, hematological disease was suspected, and the patient was ultimately diagnosed with Waldenström macroglobulinemia (WM) by bone marrow biopsy. We hypothesized that, in this patient, hyperviscosity syndrome caused by WM may have decreased blood flow and caused microcirculatory disorders, which consequently led to the development of cerebral infarction. In addition to secondary prevention for stroke (aspirin and atorvastatin), further treatment requiring chemotherapy was initiated at a local hospital after discharge. At the follow-up over one and a half years later, the patient had experienced no recurrence of stroke, and his serum IgM and plasma viscosity had decreased to almost normal values.

| Classic clinical triad of hyperviscosity disorders | | |
|---|---|---|
| **Mucosal hemorrhage** | **Visual disturbance** | **Neurologic** |
| Epistaxis bilateral<br>Gingival bleeding<br>Gastrointestinal bleeding<br>Retinal bleeding | Bilateral retinal hemorrhage<br>or thrombosis<br>Papilledema<br>Blurring<br>Diplopia | Headache<br>Dizziness and vertigo<br>Tinnitus and impaired hearing<br>Ataxia<br>Seizure<br>Ischemic stroke or cerebral<br>hemorrhage<br>Somnolence or coma |

| Major hematologic hyperviscosity syndromes | | |
|---|---|---|
| **Plasma abnormality** | **Increased cellularity** | **Decreased red cell deformability** |
| Waldenström macroglobulinemia<br>Myelomas<br>Polyclonal gammopathies | Polycythemia vera<br>Essential thrombocytopenia<br>Hyperleukocytic leukemias | Sickle-cell disease |

Peripheral blood count, blood protein, fibrinogen, D-dimer, blood urea nitrogen-to-creatinine ratio, lipid profiles, alpha-2 macroglobulins and immunoglobulins (in monoclonal and polyclonal immunoglobulinemias), routine tests of kidney and liver functions, measurement of plasma or serum viscosity by a viscosimeter

**Fundoscopy examination:** retinal vein dilatation with tortuous "sausage link" appearance on retinal veins, flame hemorrhages, papilledema, exudates, microaneurysms, central retinal vein occlusion
**Cranial MRI and CT:** multiple lacunar infarcts, Binswanger disease features, signs of cerebral venous thrombosis, intracerebral haemorrhages, large artery territorial infarctions
**Cranial MRA or CTA:** to exclude aneurisms, moyamoya syndrome, large artery occlusions

**Management of hyperviscosity syndromes:** supportive care, short-term treatment (emergency treatment), maintenance therapy to control underlying hematologic disorder

| Plasma abnormality syndromes | Increased cellularity syndromes | | | Decreased red cell deformability |
|---|---|---|---|---|
| | **Polycytemia vera** | **Essential thrombocytopenia** | **Hyperleukocytic leukemias** | **Sickle-cell disease** |
| • plasma exchange<br>• chemotherapy | • phlebotomy<br>• myelosuppressive treatment<br>• low-dose aspirin | • hydroxyurea<br>• low dose aspirin | • chemotherapy<br>• hydroxyurea<br>• leukapheresis | exchange transfusion |

# Discussion

Hematological disorders account for up to 8% of all ischemic strokes in different series. Hyperviscosity syndrome (HVS) refers to the clinical sequelae of increased blood viscosity. Blood viscosity is influenced by number of factors, including hematocrit, plasma protein and fibrinogen concentrations, cellular aggregation, red cell deformability and axial migration, vessel diameter and flow rate. Hematocrit, red cell deformability and plasma viscosity are the most important determinants of HVS.[1]

Increase in viscosity causes sluggish blood flow, relative decreased microvascular circulation and hypoperfusion of tissues. An increase in circulating proteins can also affect platelet aggregation and cause prolonged bleeding time. The severity of clinical symptoms is directly related to the increased levels of serum viscosity, with progressively more severe symptoms occurring as the individual patient's serum viscosity increases. The level of viscosity at which symptoms can initially present is variable from person to person depending on the underlying physiology.[2]

Whether elevated blood viscosity in subjects suffering acute stroke is causally related to the ischemic event or simply reflects the presence of secondary acute-phase reactants still remains controversial. Patients with acute and chronic cerebrovascular disease may have abnormalities involving blood viscosity, plasma viscosity, hematocrit, red cell deformability and fibrinogen.

Diseases that cause hyperviscosity can be divided into three main categories: plasma abnormalities, increased cellularity, and decreased red cell deformability. Each has a different rheological mechanism that leads to a hyperviscous state. Other conditions associated with hyperviscosity are: diabetes, inflammation, atherosclerosis and systemic low flow states/hemoconcentration in burn injury, inappropriate red cell transfusion, dehydration and circulatory shock.[1]

Plasma abnormalities due to increased production of high-molecular-weight globulins or macroglobulins are frequently found in patients with monoclonal and polyclonal immunoglobulinemias, most commonly in WM and myelomas, and less often in polyclonal gammopathies, attributable to various immune and infectious diseases, including Sjögren syndrome, rheumatoid arthritis, systemic lupus erythematosus, cryoglobulinemia, diabetes mellitus and HIV infection. Plasma hyperviscosity syndrome is a clinical entity that is characterized by mucous membrane bleeding, blurred vision, visual loss, lethargy, headache, dizziness, vertigo, tinnitus, paresthesia and, occasionally, seizures. There are sporadic cases and case series about the development of ischemic stroke in HVS with plasma abnormalities. Treatment with intravenous immunoglobulins is associated with a small risk of thromboembolic complications, as well as stroke, particularly in patients with underlying risk factors. The risk of thromboembolic events extends for days to weeks after intravenous immunoglobulin therapy.

Increased cellularity is observed in patients with polycytemia vera (PV), essential thrombocytopenia (ET) and hyperleukocytic leukemias. Patients with PV are at high risk for vaso-occlusive events, including cerebral ischemia. Although unusual, acute ischemic stroke may be an initial presentation of PV. The risk of events in the cerebral circulation is associated with older age and a prior history of thrombotic events. PV is characterized by overproduction of erythroid, myeloid and megakaryocytic cell lines, leading to elevated peripheral blood cell counts and an increased red cell mass, so the diagnosis of underlying pathology for stroke is often suspected based on laboratory findings. Ischemic strokes associated with ET are diagnosed in 0.25–0.5% of cases. A number of findings suggest that ET is an adjunctive risk factor for stroke in most cases, but is rarely the sole risk factor. The risk factors for thrombotic events in patients with ET include cardiovascular risk factors and the JAK2 V617F mutation, as well as patient age and history of thrombosis. Essential thrombocytopenia is suspected on the basis of elevated platelet count ($> 450,000/\mu l$) in the absence of any cause of reactive thrombocytosis. Very high white blood cell counts (e.g., >50,000 to >100,000/$\mu l$) in patients with leukemias are associated with hyperviscosity, that may result in microinfarcts and petechial hemorrhages.[1]

Sickle cell disease (SCD) is an autosomal recessive disorder of a gene mutation with sickle cell deoxygenated hemoglobin, which is poorly soluble and prone to polymerization and vessel occlusion. Furthermore, sickled hemoglobin distorts the cell membrane, causing ion imbalances, dehydrating red blood cells and making them stiff, and facilitating occlusion. Patients with SCD have chronic inflammation with high levels of interleukins, chemokines and cytokines. Increased expression of adhesion molecules enhances attachment of sickled red blood cells to the endothelium. The prevalence of stroke is 3.75% in patients with SCD. Recurrent cerebral infarction occurs in two-thirds of patients, usually within two to three years. Lesions on CT and MRI may be in deep and subcortical territories. Moyamoya syndrome is present in 20–30% of patients with SCD undergoing cerebral angiogram and predisposes to both ischemic stroke and intracranial hemorrhage.

It is well known that diabetes, inflammation and atherosclerosis are associated with rheologic manifestations. Hyperviscosity, hyperfibrinogenemia and altered rheologic factors may increase the risk of an ischemic stroke in certain conditions, including large-vessel stenoses, low flow and hypertensive small-vessel disease. However, a direct causative role for these rheologic factors in ischemic strokes remains speculative.[1]

The classic triad of hyperviscosity includes mucocutaneus bleeding, and visual and neurologic abnormalities. Neurologic manifestations can range from relatively mild headache and light-headedness to seizures and coma. Other manifestations may include heart failure, shortness of breath, hypoxia, fatigue and anorexia.[3,4]

The first assessment is a physical examination for signs of a tendency to bleed – bruises on the skin, or blood blisters in the mouth or the back of the eye. Epistaxis is a common presenting symptom, and if present in a patient with a possible paraproteinemia, should prompt additional evaluation for HVS, particularly fundoscopic examination, as evidence of ocular HVS can be present without visual symptoms and is a treatment indication. It is important to view the retina at the back of the eye using an ophthalmoscope. Fundoscopic examination is key because abnormalities are well-correlated with abnormal plasma viscosity. Classical changes include "sausage-shaped" blood vessels and small bleeds on the retina. The most severe ophthalmologic manifestation of HVS is central retinal vein occlusion, which can result in irreversible vision loss and has been reported for patients with IgM and non-IgM paraproteinemias. It is also important to assess the functioning of vital organs, primarily the heart and lungs.

Blood tests should be carried out to measure the complete blood count, full serum chemistries and coagulation profile, along with urinalysis. An elevated albumin-protein gap along with significant proteinuria on routine urinalysis suggest an underlying gammopathy. Measurement of plasma or serum viscosity by a viscosimeter assesses the diagnosis. Viscosity can be measured in absolute terms in centipoise (cP), or in relative terms compared to the viscosity of water (0.894 cP). A typical serum viscosity for a healthy patient is 1.5 cP, or 1.7 relative to water. The increased viscosity of serum relative to water relates primarily to its protein content. Typically, the higher the viscosity, the worse the symptoms.[4]

The general management of HVS involves supportive care, rapid therapies for symptomatic patients to reduce the causative substrate and measures to control the underlying hematologic disorder.

Plasma HVS is treated by plasmapheresis (plasma exchange) to remove the paraproteins and thereby reduce hyperviscosity and hypervolemia. Plasma exchange will decrease the plasma viscosity anywhere from 30–50% in a single session that exchanges one volume of the patient's plasma. Plasma exchange has been demonstrated to be effective for rapid symptomatic improvement, as well as reversal of retinopathy. Plasma exchange can be continued until there is symptomatic improvement in HVS, with concurrent initiation of chemotherapy. Chemotherapy selection is key in maintaining response and preventing HVS recurrence. Most data supports the use of a multidrug regimen in the setting of HVS.[4]

Phlebotomy is the mainstay for management of PV, with the goal of keeping the hematocrit below 45% in men and 42% in women. For patients at high risk of thromboses (i.e., age >60 years or prior thromboses), phlebotomy is often supplemented with adjunct myelosuppressive treatment. Adjunctive low-dose aspirin is reasonable for patients with PV and no history of major bleeding or aspirin intolerance.[1]

The treatment of essential thrombocythemia for symptomatic and high-risk patients (i.e., age >60 years or a prior thrombosis) involves hydroxyurea combined with low-dose aspirin.[1]

In addition to standard stroke care, patients with SCD and acute stroke should receive exchange transfusion with a goal of decreasing the HbS below 30%. Alternative therapies such as hydroxyurea or bone marrow transplant can be considered. The role of thrombolysis is unclear. In management of intracerebral hemorrhage in adults with SCD, neurosurgical expertise should be sought for aneurysms and surgical decompression if warranted.[5] During acute crises, oxygen and intravenous fluids are used to improve systemic and cerebral blood flow.

# References

1. Dashe JF. Hyperviscosity and strokes. In: Caplan LR, Biller J (Eds). *Uncommon Causes of Stroke.* Cambridge: Cambridge University Press; 2018. 408–417.

2. Perez Rogers A, Estes M. *Hyperviscosity Syndrome.* [Updated 2020 Apr 27]. Treasure Island (FL): StatPearls Publishing; 2020. www.ncbi.nlm.nih .gov/books/NBK518963/ (accessed February 2022).

3. Gertz MA. Acute hyperviscosity: Syndromes and management. *Blood.* 2018;**132**(13): 1379–1385.

4. Weaver A, Rubinstein S, Cornell RF. Hyperviscosity syndrome in paraprotein secreting conditions including Waldenstrom macroglobulinemia. *Front Oncol.* 2020;**10**: 815.

5. Talahma M, Strbian D, Sundararajan S. Sickle cell disease and stroke. *Stroke.* 2014;**45** (6): e98–e100.

# 3.4 Disseminated Intravascular Coagulation and Moschkowitz Syndrome

Kateryna Antonenko, Valeria Caso, Andrea Blass, Andrea Fiacca

## Case Presentation

A 68-year-old male was admitted to the stroke unit at the Santa Maria della Misericordia Hospital after complaining of what was later diagnosed as paraesthesia of his left hand and face that had lasted for about 10 min. The patient reported neither fever nor headache over the past three days.

On day two of admission, transient aphasia was diagnosed, therefore a plain brain CT was performed, which was normal. Laboratory findings revealed thrombocytopenia with a platelet (PLT) level of 23,000/µl. Hemolysis was found, due to microangiopathic hemolytic anemia: (hemoglobin level (Hb) 11.0 g/dl), presence of schistocytes (3%) in peripheral blood, increased level of lactate dehydrogenase (LDH) (max 1540 U/l) (normal 135–225 U/l). The creatinine level was 1.8 mg/dl. Based upon the above, the patient was diagnosed with thrombotic thrombocytopenic purpura (Moschkowitz syndrome) with recurrent TIAs. The hematological features deteriorated rapidly after 24 hours: PLT 6000/µl, Hb level 10.0g/dl, creatinine 1.5mg/dl, LDH 1077 U/l. Direct Coombs test was negative. Brain MRI revealed a small acute hyperdense area in the left cerebellum (Figures 3.4.1 and 3.4.2).

The patient was started on 100 mg aspirin after the MRI. A chest X-ray indicated aortosclerosis, while the lungs and heart were unremarkable. Abdomen ultrasound examination revealed splenomegaly (max diameter 13.5 cm), while the morphology and structure of the kidneys was normal. Urine and stool cultures investigated for *E. coli* 0157-H7 were negative. All of the investigated tumor markers (CEA, CA19-9, CA-125, CA 15–3, AFP, PSA) were negative. Anti-PLT, antinuclear (ANA) nuclear antigen (ENA), anticardiolipin (ACA), as well as anti-DNA antibodies, complements C3 and C4, circulating immune complexes (CIC, extractable) and lupus anticoagulant (LAC) were either normal or negative. ADAMTS-13 activity was less than 10%.

The patient was immediately started on a daily total plasma exchange (TPE) and corticosteroids. On the second day after treatment initiation, a transient speech disorder appeared and resolved without intervention. Five days later, the platelet count normalized to 100,000/µl.

At discharge, *after 8 TPEs over eleven days (once daily for the first five days and then again on days 7,9 and 11)* the following values were recorded: PLT: 328,000/µl, Hb 11.2 g/dl, creatinine 1.10 mg/dl, LDH 387 U/l, estimated clearance 72.5 ml/min, azotaemia 54 mg/dl, sodium 138 mEq/l, potassium 3.9 mEq/l, calcium 8.9 mg/dl. Oral corticosteroids and aspirin 100 mg were prolonged.

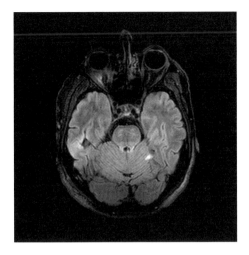

**Figure 3.4.1** FLAIR-weighted axial MR image, showing a small and hyperdense area in the left cerebellum.

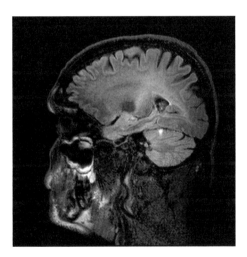

**Figure 3.4.2** FLAIR-weighted sagittal MR image, showing a small and hyperdense area in the left cerebellum.

## Clinical presentation for thrombotic thrombocytopenic purpura (TTP)

Age = 20–50 years; gender = F:M 3:1; age of onset = 20–50 years; form of the disease = acquired type (99%), congenital type (Schulman–Upshaw syndrome) (1%); Etiological forms = primary (idiopathic) (80%), secondary (drug-associated TTP, pregnant and postpartum patients, HIV and systemic autoimmune disease-associated) (20%)

Pentad of clinical features (1966): (a) microangiopathic hemolytic anemia, (b) severe thrombocytopenia, (c) neurologic symptoms, (d) fever, (e) renal involvement

Triad of clinical features: (a) microangiopathic hemolytic anemia, (b) thrombocytopenia, (c) neurologic symptoms

| System | Clinical manifestations of Moschkowitz syndrome |
| --- | --- |
| Neurologic | Headache, dizziness, altered state of consciousness, abnormal behavior, visual hallucinations, aphasia, dysarthria, cortical blindness, homonymous hemianopsia, cranial nerve palsies, gaze-evoked nystagmus, ataxia, paresis, sensory disturbances and focal and/or generalized seizures |
| Cardiac | Angina, myocardial infarctions, fatal arrhythmias and cardiac failure |
| Respiratory | Cough, pleuritic chest pain, acute respiratory distress syndrome, pulmonary embolism and pulmonary infarcts |
| Renal | Arterial hypertension, hematuria, acute and chronic renal failure |
| Gastrointestinal | Nausea and/or vomiting, abdominal pain, (bloody) diarrhoea, mesenteric ischemia, acute pancreatitis and gastrointestinal bleeding |
| Hematological | Petechiae, ecchymoses, hemorrhagic cutaneous lesions, epistaxis, gingival bleeding, and menorrhagia |
| Skeletal | Pathologic fractures |
| Other | Fever, fatigue, claudication, myalgia and arthralgia |

| General laboratory thresholds related to the classic TTP pentad | |
| --- | --- |
| Thrombocytopaenia | Mean platelet count: 10,000–30,000/µl |
| Hemolytic anemia | Microangiopathic hemolytic anemia: mean hemoglobin range 8-10g/dl; presence of schistocytes; increased levels of indirect bilirubin, lactate dehydrogenase and reticulocytes; significantly decreased levels of haptoglobin and negative direct Coombs test |
| Renal failure | Mean serum creatinine level is<2 mg/dl |
| Fever (30–72%) | Mild (37–39°C) or high fever (>39 °C) |
| Neurologic symptoms | Range of neurologic involvement 50–79% |

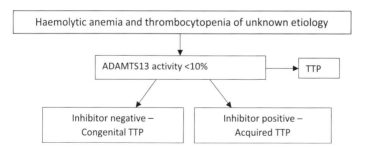

**Brain MR** is more sensitive than CT in revealing the presence of small multiple acute brain infarctions. For Moschkowitz syndrome, these lesions have been reported in the basal ganglia, thalamus, cerebellum, cortex, but more often in the subcortical white matter, with a high signal on diffusion-weighted MRI and a corresponding low signal on the apparent diffusion coefficient map, due to occlusions caused by platelet-rich thrombi of the terminal arterioles and capillaries. It not

(cont.)

unusual for cortical and small subcortical acute infarcts to coexist. Single, acute cortical infarcts are far less common, often coexisting with small pre-existing infarcts that are revealed on diffusion-weighted and T2-weighted images

In Moschkowitz syndrome multiple acute hemorrhagic infarcts, evidenced on susceptibility-weighted imaging, are a very rare. Likewise, supratentorial or brainstem hematomas, petechial hemorrhages and infratentorial microbleeds are rarely observable on brain MRI

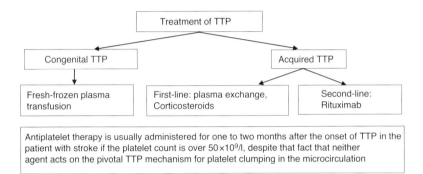

## Discussion

*Disseminated intravascular coagulation (DIC)* is an acquired syndrome characterized by intravascular activation of coagulation with loss of localization, which can arise from different causes. Likewise, DIC can originate from and cause damage to the microvasculature, and when sufficiently severe, the latter can lead to organ dysfunction[1].

Conditions associated with DIC can include sepsis and severe infection, trauma, malignancy, obstetric complications, major organ dysfunction, surgery (e.g., hip replacement), vascular disorders, toxins and/or immunologic disorders (e.g., antiphospholipid antibody syndrome).

The pathogenetic feature of DIC is its extensive and systemic generation of thrombin that can trigger microvascular thromboses. The propagation and maintenance of DIC is mediated through the inhibition of anticoagulation pathways and the dysregulation of inflammatory pathways.

The diagnosis of DIC is based on a combination of clinical features, underlying conditions and laboratory testing. The underlying cause of DIC can influence its neurologic manifestations, resulting in either cerebral thromboses or bleeding.

The neurologic manifestations in ischemic strokes can range from mild encephalopathy to coma, with or without focal neurological signs. Seizures, hemiparesis aphasia and visual field disorders are common clinical signs. The mechanism of intracranial hemorrhages resulting from DIC is thought to be due to excessive thrombin production, leading to a consumption of platelets and coagulation factors, concomitant inhibition of coagulation and accelerated fibrinolysis.

Besides low levels of fibrinogen and thrombocytopenia, patients with DIC also have both prolonged prothrombin and activated partial thromboplastin times. Furthermore, levels of D-dimer and fibrin split products are increased. The combination of prothrombin time, activated partial thromboplastin time, D-dimer, platelet count and fibrinogen levels correlates with organ dysfunction and mortality in a dose-dependent manner. However, each parameter is neither sensitive nor specific for the diagnosis of DIC.[1]

In the treatment of DIC, the first step would be to treat the underlying causes along with thrombotic or hemorrhagic complications. Replacement therapy with platelets and coagulation factors should be administered to patients with severe/active bleeding and those who are undergoing invasive procedures. Fresh frozen plasma and antifibrinolytic agents may be indicated for patients with DIC. Treatment with low-molecular-weight heparin in DIC may be preferred to unfractionated heparin with thrombotic complications. Other anticoagulants such as antithrombin and recombinant human activated protein C may be considered in the treatment of DIC, but not routinely recommended.[2]

*Thrombotic thrombocytopenic purpura (TTP)* is the most common type of thrombotic microangiopathy; the annual incidence ranges from 6 to 11 cases per million. TTP affects females more often, with a sex ratio of 3:1, although this predominance may disappear after the age of 60. The onset of TTP usually occurs between the ages of 20 and 50 years.[3] Acquired TTP (Moschkowitz syndrome) is the most common form of the disease, whereas the congenital type accounts for only 1% of all TTP cases. Primary or idiopathic TTP (without underlying disorders) affects 80% of patients with a TTP diagnosis.[4] The causes of secondary Moschkowitz syndrome can be drug-associated (either by acute immune-mediated reaction or dose-dependent toxicity), pregnant and postpartum patients, and those with HIV and/or systemic autoimmune diseases.

The pathophysiology of Moschkowitz syndrome is combined with an increase in von Willebrand factor (vWF) as a consequence of a congenital or acquired deficiency of its cleaving metalloprotease (ADAMTS13). Severe (<10%) deficiency in ADAMTS13 activity can be due to two mechanisms: (1) the acquired development of autoantibodies (neutralizing or inhibiting, and non-neutralizing) against ADAMTS13 protease, which inhibits its activity and/or accelerates its plasma clearance, (2) mutations in the gene that encodes the protease. Ultralarge vWF multimers precipitate systemic platelet aggregation and adhesion, which results in widespread thrombi in arterioles and capillaries, intravascular hemolysis from fibrin deposition and mechanical trauma.[4]

The clinical presentation of Moschkowitz syndrome is quite heterogeneous and fluctuating due to changes in microcirculation. The diagnostic pentad of clinical manifestations, proposed by Amorosi and Ultman,[5] including microangiopathic hemolytic anemia, severe thrombocytopenia, neurologic symptoms, fever and renal involvement, was subsequently replaced by a triad of clinical features consisting of microangiopathic hemolytic anemia, thrombocytopenia and neurologic symptoms.

Up to 79% of TTP patients may present with neurologic manifestations at the onset, and virtually all patients exhibit neurologic involvement during the disease. The neurologic manifestations may be transient or permanent and may precede the appearance of remarkable clinical and laboratory hematologic abnormalities by days or even years (in the literature described as atypical TTP in young and middle-aged women without cardiovascular risk factors).[6] Generalized (headache, altered state of consciousness ranging from confusion to coma, seizures) and focal stroke symptoms may be the presenting features in TTP patients.

Brain CT or MRI usually reveal small and multiple ischemic lesions, involving different arterial territories in both anterior and posterior circulations. Occasionally, large-vessel involvement is possible, resulting from branch occlusion of the middle cerebral arteries or posterior cerebral arteries or, more rarely, of the entire MCA territory.

If a patient presents with a reduced platelet count and hemolytic anemia of unknown cause, the clinician should measure ADAMTS13 activity. If the activity level is <10%, the patient is diagnosed with TTP. If the patient is positive for anti-ADAMTS13 autoantibodies, the patient is diagnosed with acquired TTP. Clinicians should be aware that patients may present with anti-ADAMTS13 autoantibodies even if they are negative for inhibitory autoantibodies.[7] The severity of thrombocytopenia is usually correlated with the level of ADAMTS-13 activity.

Plasma exchange therapy (grade of recommendation: 1A) using fresh-frozen plasma is conducted in patients with acquired TTP to supplement ADAMTS13 and remove anti-ADAMTS13 autoantibodies. To suppress autoantibody production, corticosteroid therapy (grade of recommendation: 1B) may be administered in conjunction with plasma exchange. Recent reports show that the monoclonal anti-CD-20 antibody rituximab (grade of recommendation: 1B) is effective in patients with refractory or relapsed TTP. Antiplatelet drugs (grade of recommendation: 2B) may be prescribed when the platelet count recovers to >50,000/μl. However, its impact on preventing TTP relapse has yet to be determined. Oral aspirin may be prescribed at a dose range of 81–100 mg once daily in the morning until the termination of corticosteroid use.[6]

# References

1. Scientific Subcommittee on Disseminated Intravascular Coagulation (DIC) of the International Society on Thrombosis and Haemostasis (ISTH), Taylor FB Jr, Toh CH, Hoots WK, et al. Towards definition, clinical and laboratory criteria, and a scoring system for disseminated intravascular coagulation. *ThrombHaemost*. 2001;**86**: 1327–1330.

2. Wada H, Matsumoto T, Yamashita Y. Diagnosis and treatment of disseminated intravascular coagulation (DIC) according to four DIC guidelines. *J Intensive Care*. 2014;2(1): 15.

3. Sarode R, Bandarenko N, Brecher ME, et al. Thrombotic thrombocytopenic purpura: 2012 American Society for Apheresis (ASFA) consensus conference on classification, diagnosis, management, and future research. *J Clin Apher*. 2014;**29**(3): 148–167.

4. Moncayo-Gaete J, Correa P. Thrombotic thrombocytopenic purpura. In: Caplan LR, Biller J (Eds). *Uncommon Causes of Stroke*. Cambridge: Cambridge University Press; 2018. 347–355.

5. Amorosi E, Ultmann J. Thrombotic thrombocytopenic purpura: report of 16 cases and review of the literature. *Medicine (Baltimore)*. 1966;**45**: 139–159.

6. Rojas JC, Banerjee C, Siddiqui F, Nourbakhsh B, Powell CM. Pearls and oy-sters: acute ischemic stroke caused by atypical thrombotic thrombocytopenic purpura. *Neurology*. 2013;**80**(22): e235–e238.

7. Matsumoto M, Fujimura Y, Wada H, et al. Diagnostic and treatment guidelines for thrombotic thrombocytopenic purpura (TTP) 2017 in Japan. *Int J Hematol*. 2017;**106**(1): 3–15.

# Immunoglobulin A Vasculitis (Henoch–Schönlein Purpura)

## 3.5

Sarah M. Heldner, Barbara Goeggel Simonetti,
Mirjam R. Heldner

## Case Presentation

Sokol et al. reported the case of a 15-year-old girl presenting with aphasia and right-sided weakness associated with lethargy.[1] Ten days prior to the onset of these symptoms, she had been admitted to hospital with fever, joint and abdominal pain, nausea, vomiting, and a maculopapular rash involving the lower extremities and buttocks following upper respiratory tract symptoms.

MR imaging showed a periopercular ischemic stroke with a hemorrhagic component involving the left lenticular nucleus and caudate nucleus, with a normal magnetic resonance angiogram. The cerebrospinal fluid showed $198/mm^3$ white blood cells (93% polymorphonuclear cells, 5% monocytes and 2% lymphocytes) and $12/mm^3$ red blood cells, with normal glucose and protein content, negative viral and bacterial cultures, and negative herpes polymerase chain reaction (PCR) test.

Blood analysis showed a sedimentation rate of 118 mm in the first hour, 11.8g/dl hemoglobin, $204,000/mm^3$ platelets, and $17.9/mm^3$ white blood cells (93% polymorphonuclear cells, 7% lymphocytes). Antinuclear antibodies (ANA) were less than 1:40, levels of complement factors C3 and C4 were normal, Venereal Diseases Research Laboratory (VDRL) test and rapid plasma reagent were non-reactive. Serology immunoglobulin A (IgA) and G (IgG), but not immunoglobulin M (IgM) were increased. CSF immunoglobulins were not obtained. Urinalysis showed proteinuria (> 300 mg/dl) and hematuria (large hemoglobin).

Biopsy of the skin rash revealed a leukoclastic vasculitis with the presence of IgA within the vessel walls. The finding of the leukoclastic vasculitis, abdominal pain, renal dysfunction and cerebral infarct led to the diagnosis of IgA vasculitis with neurologic involvement.

Additional serologic testing for antiphospholipid antibodies (aPL) showed 12 multiples of the mean of IgA antiphosphatidylethanolamine antibody (aPE) levels, with all other aPL isotypes negative. IgA and IgG aPE were also present in the CSF.

On corticosteroids the patient improved, developing complex partial seizures controlled with phenytoin.

On follow-up at two months, serum, and at five months, both serum and CSF, samples showed no aPL reactivity. No anticoagulant therapy was used as the aPE was transient.

# Diagnostic and Treatment Algorithm

## Clinical suspicion

Children ⋙ Adults, ♂ > ♀

Tetrad of clinical manifestations (variable in their presence and order of presentation):

- Palpable purpuric (or petechial) rash with neither thrombocytopenia nor coagulopathy
- Gastrointestinal symptoms (≤80%)
- Arthralgia and/or arthritis (≤75%)
- Renal disease (≤50%)

Rarer clinical manifestations:

- Orchitis, scrotal pain and swelling
- Pulmonal hemorrhage
- Affection of the central or peripheral nervous system

## Diagnosis

1. Typically based upon clinical manifestations.
2. In patients with an atypical presentation, in case of severe renal involvement or in adults with potentially other forms of vasculitis, by biopsy of the skin and/or kidney. Predominant IgA deposition confirmatory for diagnosis.
3. Laboratory tests: Mild elevation of inflammatory parameters, thrombocytosis and mild anemia possible. Non-diagnostic. Elevated IgA levels in >50% in serum. Normal coagulation parameters [prothrombin time (PT), partial thromboplastin time (PTT) and bleeding time] and no thrombocytopenia necessary. Other investigations for evaluation of the preceding disease or trigger, or differential diagnoses.
4. Abdominal imaging or neuroimaging according to symptoms.

## Main differential diagnoses

- Immune thrombocytopenic purpura
- Thrombotic thrombocytopenic purpura
- Hemolytic uremic syndrome
- Other small-vessel vasculitis
- Systemic lupus erythematosus
- Rheumatoid arthritis
- Juvenile idiopathic arthritis
- Toxic synovitis
- Rheumatic fever
- Sjögren syndrome
- IgA nephropathy
- Vessel malformations
- Idiopathic purpura
- Mixed connective tissue disorder
- Juvenile dermatomyositis
- Antiphospholipid antibody syndrome
- Septicemia
- Disseminated intravascular coagulation
- Papular-purpuric gloves-and-socks syndrome
- Mediterranean fever
- Leukemia
- Toxic vessel damage
- Acute abdominal emergencies (e.g., appendicitis)

## Initial and long-term management

1. Primarily supportive and symptomatic therapy involving rest, pain relief with, e.g., acetaminophen or non-steroidal anti-inflammatory drugs (NSAIDs), hydration and par-/enteral nutrition.
2. Antihypertensive therapy in some patients.
3. Hospitalization with monitoring (assessment of vital signs, urine output and hematocrit, as well as serial abdominal examinations and stool examination for blood) and supportive, symptomatic and specific treatment, in case of:

   - Severe abdominal pain
   - Gastrointestinal bleeding
   - Insufficiency of oral hydration
   - Severe arthritis/arthralgia
   - Severe renal involvement
   - Altered level of consciousness, encephalopathy, ischemic stroke and/or intracranial hemorrhage.

4. Glucocorticoids and/or additional immunosuppressive agents.
5. Special considerations in renal involvement with close fluid and electrolyte management, also potentially including dialysis and renal transplantation for end-stage kidney disease.
6. Special considerations in case of rare short- or long-term sequelae.
7. Regular clinical follow-up visits with screening for urinary abnormalities and elevated blood pressure indicating significant and potentially progressive renal disease.

# Discussion

Immunoglobulin A (IgA) vasculitis, formerly called Henoch-Schönlein purpura is a non-thrombocytopenic, immune-mediated, leukocytoclastic, small-vessel vasculitis. It is the most common form of systemic vasculitis in children. In two population-based European studies, the annual incidence was around 20 per 100,000 children.[2,3] It peaks in children at around four to six years of age. Adults are less frequently affected. Most studies show a male predominance. There is a seasonal pattern with rarest occurrence in summer, probably because of the association of IgA vasculitis with infections. Immunological, genetic and environmental factors are thought to influence occurrence of IgA vasculitis. Around one in two patients shows a preceding upper respiratory tract infection, others a history of a recent vaccination, insect bite or chemical trigger.

Pathophysiologically, immune complex IgA deposition in vessel walls leads to complement activation, which causes vessel injury.

Usually, the disease manifests over days to weeks. Typically, there is a palpable purpuric (or petechial) rash in clusters, which does not blanch under pressure, symmetrically distributed, affecting gravity/pressure-dependent areas such as the lower limbs. This classic symptom is among the presenting symptoms in around three-quarter of patients without any thrombocytopenia or coagulopathy. The rash may be itchy, but is rarely painful.

Gastrointestinal symptoms (nausea, vomiting, abdominal pain, transient paralytic ileus, but also intussusception and gastrointestinal hemorrhage/ischemia), especially mild ones, are among the most frequently reported symptoms and are described in up to four in five patients.

Arthralgia/arthritis occurs in ankle and knee joints in up to three of four patients.

With a frequency of one in two, renal disease manifests more frequently in older children and in adults. Micro- or macrohematuria is common, with mild or no proteinuria. Proliferative glomerulonephritis may cause severe arterial hypertension. Also, edema may be seen.

Rarer manifestations of IgA vasculitis are orchitis, scrotal pain and swelling, or pulmonal hemorrhage.

Neurological manifestation is more frequent in other forms of vasculitis. But, neurological manifestation of IgA vasculitis is possible, but rare. However, it potentially goes along with substantial morbidity and mortality. Involvement of the central nervous system is possible and may precede or follow the rash. Headache is frequently seen. Altered level of consciousness, encephalopathic symptoms, focal or generalized epileptic seizures, focal neurological deficits including visual abnormalities, ataxia, aphasia/dysarthria and central neuropathy have been described. Also, peripheral nervous system involvement may be seen. Neuropathies (e.g., femoral, ulnar, peroneal, tibial, facial), Guillain–Barré syndrome, brachial plexopathy and mononeuritis multiplex have been demonstrated. IgA vasculitis may cause inflammation in the walls of the vasa nervorum and induce critical ischemia to nerves. However, involvement of the peripheral nervous system may sometimes also be caused by compression due to edema or hematoma.

Serum IgA levels are elevated in more than half of all patients, especially in those with renal involvement. Other blood results are unspecific and reflect the preceding disease or trigger or support a differential diagnosis. In urinalysis, proteinuria and/or hematuria are found as time goes by and usually correlate with the degree of renal injury. Furthermore, decreased levels of complement component 3 and/or 4 (C3 and/or C4) have been described in urinalysis.

Skin and renal biopsy may be helpful to confirm the diagnosis, especially in patients where the clinical presentation is atypical, in cases of severe renal involvement or in adults in which other forms of vasculitis may be clinically alike. Biopsy shows leukocytoclastic vasculitis with predominantly IgA, but also C3 and fibrin deposition within the walls of involved vessels and within endothelial and mesangial cells of the kidney.

Imaging should be performed as deemed necessary based on clinical symptoms. Neuroimaging may reveal an ischemic stroke or a primary or secondary intracranial hemorrhage. Vessel irregularities due to vasculitis, vessel-wall proliferation or thrombosis most frequently affect several vessels. Moreover, cerebral venous thrombosis and diffuse or posterior subcortical brain edema have been described. The latter has been found not only in hypertensive, but also in normotensive or just slightly hypertensive patients. In clinical practice, MR imaging is usually the neuroimaging of choice even though digital subtraction angiography is actually the gold standard for assessment of vasculitis affecting the brain-supplying arteries.

In around every second individual, EEG abnormalities including focal or generalized slow wave activity, sharp waves, focal attenuation of the voltage activity and sometimes also paroxysmal activity can be found. Adults with no known preceding disease or trigger should also be investigated for solid-organ cancers with a low threshold.

Initial management includes primarily supportive and symptomatic therapy involving rest, pain relief with, e.g., acetaminophen or non-steroidal anti-inflammatory drugs

(NSAIDs), hydration and par-/enteral nutrition. Some patients may require antihypertensive therapy. Hospitalization is indicated in cases of severe abdominal pain, gastrointestinal bleeding, insufficiency of oral hydration, severe arthritis/arthralgia, severe renal involvement, altered level of consciousness, encephalopathy, ischemic stroke and/or intracranial hemorrhage. Monitoring helps to limit the risk of short- and long-term sequelae.[4]

The use of glucocorticoids is controversial. They may facilitate timely improvement of symptoms and may be helpful in treating the underlying disease. However, there is probably no long-term benefit and an unchanged relapse rate. Glucocorticoids show common side effects like arterial hypertension, hyperglycemia, weight gain, immunosuppression and skin changes. Furthermore, they potentially mask symptoms such as fever, pain and abdominal emergencies. In patients with severe disease and renal involvement, additional immunosuppressive agents may be considered. Moreover, management of renal involvement depending on disease phase and severity needs special consideration, with close fluid and electrolyte management, also potentially including dialysis and renal transplantation for end-stage kidney disease.

In cases of central nervous system involvement, management should include timely secondary prevention measures, control of blood pressure, perfusion and seizures. Anticoagulation is recommended in cases of secondary antiphospholipid syndrome. Glucocorticoids or additional immunosuppressive agents may be indicated in cases of relevant vessel irregularities in brain-supplying arteries or their sequelae. Involvement of the peripheral nervous system is usually self-limiting without any treatment. However, with Guillain–Barré syndrome, intravenous immune globulin or plasma exchange should be initiated.

Short-term outcomes of IgA vasculitis in children are usually favorable to excellent without specific treatment. If there is no relevant renal involvement, IgA vasculitis is mostly self-limiting within one month and non-relapsing in two-thirds of children. If a relapse occurs, it is mostly shorter and/or milder than the previous manifestation.

Long-term outcomes are largely driven by renal disease, which may be progressive and potentially lead to end-stage kidney disease. Adults are at increased risk, with reported rates of end-stage kidney disease of up to one in three at 15 years. Adults are at risk for renal disease in the long term as well as early in the disease course of IgA vasculitis. To some extent, most children develop renal disease within two months of symptom onset and almost all within a few months, despite initial complete resolution of IgA vasculitis symptoms. However, a minority of the children have persistent renal manifestation in the long term. Patients should be seen in regular clinical follow-up visits with screening for urinary abnormalities and elevated blood pressure, indicating significant and potentially progressive renal disease.

# References

1. Sokol DK, McIntre JA, Short RA, et al. Henoch-Schonlein purpura and stroke: Antiphosphatidylethanolamine antibody in CSF and serum. *Neurology*. 2000;**55**: 1379.

2. Garzoni L, Vanoni F, Rizzi M, et al. Nervous system dysfunction in Henoch-Schonlein syndrome: Systematic review of the literature. *Rheumatology*. 2009;**48**: 524–529.

3. Oni L, Sampath S. Childhood IgA vasculitis (Henoch Schonlein Purpura): Advances and knowledge gaps. *Front Pediatr*. 2019;**27** (7): 257.

4. González-Gay MA, López-Mejías R, Pina T, et al. IgA vasculitis: Genetics and clinical and therapeutic management. *Curr Rheumatol Rep*. 2018;**20**: 24.

# Stroke Associated With Cancer

## 3.6

Christine Kremer, Olof Gråhamn

## Case Presentation

A 60-year-old woman presented to the emergency room with sudden onset of left-sided hemianopia and left-sided sensory loss. She had a history of migraine with visual and sensory aura, but during the previous four months she had experienced recurring episodes of left-sided visual loss that did not conform to the normal pattern of her migraine aura, which was more typical for scintillating scotomas. In addition to the hemianopia and left-sided sensory loss she complained of dizziness and vertigo.

Electrocardiography (ECG) showed sinus tachycardia and blood pressure was 173/94 mmHg. Computed tomography (CT) of the brain showed no early signs of ischemia. On CT angiography (CTA) there was an occlusion of the right P2-PCA (posterior cerebral artery); however, more distal branches of the PCA did appear perfused. CT perfusion imaging showed significantly increased thrombotic thrombocytopenia purpura (TTP) in the territory of the PCA. However, flow along the P2-segment could be identified by transcranial duplex ultrasound.

No attempts at reperfusion therapy were made, since the symptoms and findings were thought to represent a vasoconstriction phenomenon, probably related to her migraine. The patient was discharged the next day at her own request.

The patient's vision and sensation had not fully recovered in the outpatient clinic two days later. She also complained of fatigue and difficulties concentrating. The doctor prescribed acetylsalicylic acid and a statin and ordered a brain MRI which was done about ten days later, revealing restricted diffusion within the right PCA territory, including the dorsolateral part of the thalamus. More surprisingly, there were small cortical and subcortical areas with restricted diffusion bilaterally in both the posterior and anterior circulation (Figure 3.6.1).

This most likely represented scattered emboli. MR angiography was essentially in accordance with the previous CTA. Cardiac ultrasound and ambulatory ECG-recording were both unremarkable.

Three weeks later the patient was admitted with acute onset of dysarthria and right-sided sensory loss. MRI once again showed widespread areas of small embolizations. She was now treated with dual antiplatelet therapy (DAPT) (addition of clopidogrel) and low-dose low-molecular-weight heparin (LMWH) twice daily to prevent embolization of unknown source – as well as corticosteroid pulse therapy until vasculitis could be ruled out. The transthoracic echocardiogram (TTE) was normal. Cerebrospinal fluid (CSF) studies revealed no abnormalities.

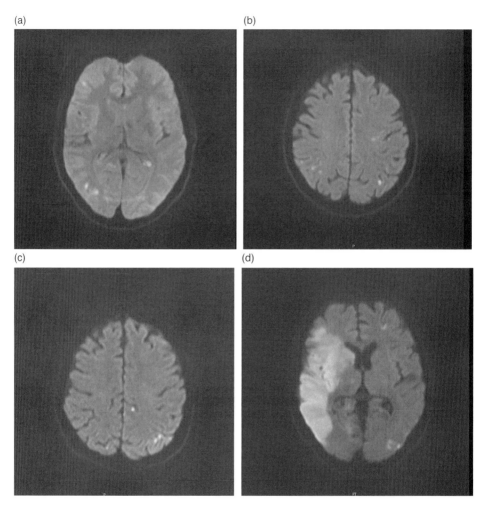

**Figure 3.6.1** MRI brain, diffusion-weighted imaging (DWI): (a) day 14, (b) day 30, (c) day 44, (d) day 64

At this time, elevation of alkaline phosphatase (ALP) was noted, causing concern for malignancy. CT of the thorax and abdomen revealed diffuse thickening along the minor curve of the gastric wall and the pyloric region and enlarged lymph nodes in the abdomen and mediastinum. Imaging with 18-F fluorodeoxyglucose (FDG)-positron emission tomography (PET) showed these regions to be very hypermetabolic, and there was also pronounced hypermetabolism in the thyroid gland. A diagnosis of gastric adenocarcinoma with spread to lymph nodes and the thyroid gland could be made by histological biopsies. Before a palliative oncologic treatment could be initiated, the patient suffered a new stroke. This time there was a large MCA infarction on the right side in addition to large numbers of scattered small emboli. The patient was transferred to a palliative care unit. She died two and a half months after initial presentation.

# Discussion

When to suspect a stroke with occult malignancy:

- Cryptogenic stroke with no evidence of cardiac or aortic source of emboli, including transthoracic echocardiogram, except patent foramen ovale (PFO)
- No other apparent plausible cause of the stroke pattern
- Imaging-based (preferably MRI) evidence of embolic-pattern of ischemic stroke:
  - o Often large number of small (< 1 cm) infarcts scattered across multiple vascular territories – and/or embolization to other organs

- Suspicion raised if recurrent embolic events or MRI evidence of emboli of varying age
- Vasculitis, connective tissue disorder, infectious disease (septic emboli) excluded

# Proposed Diagnostic Algorithm in Patient With Suspected Cancer-Associated Stroke

### Patient history

Symptoms indicative of malignancy including substantial anorexia/weight-loss, unexplained recurrent fever, excessive night sweats, dysphagia, abdominal pain, enlarged lymph nodes, persistent cough, hemoptysis, history of cancer, unexplained anemia or chronically high inflammatory markers (note: this would usually prompt evaluation for cancer regardless of stroke history)

Abdominal pain, other localized pain

Unexplained weight loss, fatigue, elevated temperature, excessive night sweats

### Clinical examination

Palpation of breast, testes, superficial lymph nodes and dermatology consultation for skin cancer

Lumbar puncture – both to make alternative diagnoses such as infectious disease and vasculitis and to find meningeal malignancy. Include cytology and flow cytometry

Organ-specific work-up according to risk-profile, findings and symptoms

### Blood tests

Complete blood count including white blood cell count differential

Prothrombin time/international normalized ratio (PT/INR), activated partial thromboplastin time (APTT), D-dimer, fibrinogen – to identify prothrombotic states, raised D-dimer in particular has been implicated as a quite specific marker for occult cancer in ischemic stroke

C reactive protein (CRP) and sedimentation rate (SR) – unspecific tests for chronic inflammation

Creatinine, urea and estimation of glomerular filtration rate (GFR) – part of routine work-up but uremia can be indicative of infrarenal obstruction in widespread malignancy

Coagulation assay (in cases of patent foramen ovale (PFO), venous coagulation disorders should be included)

Liver function tests including alkaline phosphatase (ALP) – for liver malignancies/metastasis and/or skeletal metastasis

(cont.)

## Blood tests

Lactic acid dehydrogenase (LDH) – unspecific marker of cellular demise often raised in metastatic cancer and hematologic cancer

Ionized $Ca^{2+}$ – for skeletal metastasis

Serum protein electrophoresis – for signs of chronic inflammation and hematologic malignancy

Panel for connective tissue disease including antinuclear antibodies (ANA) –systemic lupus erythematosus (SLE) especially can cause similar stroke patterns

Antibodies associated with systemic vasculitis – primarily antineutrophil cytoplasmic antibody (ANCA) when the central nervous system (CNS) is involved

Supplemental blood tests as indicated:

Anemia work-up to further differentiate

Consider serum markers of malignancy such as carcinoembryonic antigen (CEA) and cancer antigen (CA) 125 and CA19-9

## Imaging

Transesophageal echocardiography – valve vegetations or intracardiac thrombus

CT of the thorax, abdomen and pelvis (consider including neck unless previously visualized during stroke work-up) with and without intravenous contrast

Mammography

Consider 18-F FDG-PET CT to look for malignancy not apparent on standard CT

Consider MRI with vessel-wall imaging to look for signs of intracranial vasculopathy

Consider digital subtraction angiography to rule out medium and small vessel vasculopathy

## Treatment – secondary prevention

Treat underlying malignancy

Secondary stroke prevention: acetylsalicylic acid (ASA)

Consider low-molecular-weight heparin, alternatively a direct oral anticoagulant (DOAC) if a hypercoagulable state is suspected

ASA if additional atherosclerosis/vascular risk profile

Close monitoring

About one-third of the population develop malignancy within their lifetime. Stroke is the second leading cause of death globally. Of hospitalized ischemic stroke patients, 10% show an associated malignancy.[1] Since screening and treatment of cancer will improve due to extensive research and improved diagnoses in the future, the treatment of cancer-associated stroke will become more important in the long-term perspective. It can be shown that cancer increases not only the risk of venous thromboembolism but also the short-term risk of arterial thromboembolism, and therefore ischemic stroke.[2] Common cancers are gastric, pancreas, lung and breast cancers. These patients show a higher rate of cryptogenic stroke, but also higher rates of PFO due to paradox embolization and concomitant venous thromboembolization. Multifocal embolic infarcts are common, and strokes tend to be more severe. Cancer-mediated hypercoagulability has been seen as the most important mechanism. The tumors themselves can release microparticles into the bloodstream and enhance thrombosis, Pro-coagulant factors such as factor X are increased and mucins that can activate platelets and endothelial cells, are released. Cancer treatment itself can trigger vasculopathy through radiation therapy, and platinum-based chemotherapy can increase thromboembolism. Some vascular risk factors like smoking, obesity and atrial fibrillation are also more common in cancer patients. The etiology is therefore rather multifactorial. One-third of cancer patients have a recurrent thromboembolic event within three months.[3] The level of D-dimer can predict recurrence. The highest stroke risk is shortly after cancer diagnosis, with pronounced cancer activity and release of procoagulant factors, while the long-term risk can be influenced by side effects of curative or adjuvant cancer treatments. If the cancer is treated successfully, the stroke risk usually declines. The short-term clinical outcome after ischemic stroke can be favorable, with 51% good functional outcomes after three months in patients without early neurological deterioration (modified Rankin score (mRS) of 0–2).[4] Cancer patients should not be excluded per se from acute stroke treatment, such as intravenous thrombolysis and endovascular therapy, as long as their median survival time exceeds the expected stroke recovery. Intracerebral bleeding risk has not been reported to be increased. Even though no significantly increased complication rates have been reported, those treatments are still the exception and not standard. Sometimes ischemic stroke can be the initial manifestation of an occult malignancy. Given its severity and high rate of recurrence and the need for early diagnosis of an underlying cancer, a dedicated diagnostic work-up is crucial (see proposed algorithm). Additionally, secondary prevention has to be tailored, and the patient has to be closely monitored. High-grade evidence regarding secondary prevention in these patients is lacking. The choice of treatment is challenging because of the high percentage of cryptogenic strokes (>50%). Anticoagulation is recommended for cancer-associated stroke with widespread use of low-molecular-weight heparin.[5] A recently published randomized controlled trial (RCT) comparing DOACs to low-molecular-weight heparin showed that DOACs were not inferior, making them a possible alternative to subcutaneous injections.[6] The increased bleeding risk has to be taken into account, especially in patients with brain tumors/metastases and in patients with cancer in general. Injectable heparins might impose additional effort on the patients. An alternative is antiplatelet therapy with aspirin, which shows fewer side effects and usually has a higher compliance and an antineoplastic effect on cancers in the gastrointestinal tract. The disadvantage is the lack of its effect on hypercoagulability. In the absence of a large RCT, some smaller retrospective studies have shown that antiplatelet therapy was comparable to anticoagulation. More data are needed to generate evidence-based guidelines for the optimal secondary prevention of cancer-related stroke.

In conclusion, with improved survival and better quality of life for patients with cancer, cancer-related stroke is likely to increase. Stroke associated with malignancy accounts for 10% of all strokes. Given its high risk of recurrence, an improved algorithm for diagnostic work-up and better evidence regarding secondary prevention are needed.

# References

1. Sanossia N, Djabiras C, Mack WJ, Ovbiagele B. Trends in cancer diagnoses among inpatients hospitalized with stroke. *J Stroke Cerebrovasc Dis.*2013,**22**:1146–1150).

2. Navi BB, Reiner AS, Kamel H, et al. Association between incident cancer and subsequent stroke. *Ann Neurol.* 2015;**77:** 291–300.

3. Navi BB, Singer S, Merkler AE, et al. Recurrent thromboembolic events after ischemic stroke. *Neurology*. 2014;**83**: 26–33.

4. Nam KW, Kim CK, Kim TJ, et al. D-dimer as a predictor of early neurological deterioration in cryptogenic stroke with active cancer. *Eur J Neurol*. 2017;**24**: 205–211.

5. Bang OY, Seok JM, Kim SG, et al. Ischemic stroke and cancer: Stroke severely impacts cancer patients, while cancer increase the numbers of strokes. *J Clin Neurol*. 2011;**7**: 53–59.

6. Raskob GE, van Es M, Verhamme P, et al. Edoxaban for the treatment of cancer - associated venous thromboembolism. *New Engl J Med*. 2018;**378**: 615–624.

# Medication-Related Stroke

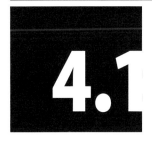

Francesca Romana Pezzella, Sabrina Anticoli,
Antonella Urso

## Case Presentation

A 53-year-old woman, with no vascular risk factors or significant previous medical history except for hysterectomy due to fibromatosis at the age of 45, was admitted to the emergency room due to sudden onset of weakness of the right limbs and speech disorder. On admission, she presented with left hemiparesis and mild aphasia accounting for an NIH stroke scale score of 5, temperature was 36.8°C, heart rate 66 beats/min, blood pressure 145/90 mm Hg and respiratory rate 22 breaths/min, with oxygen saturation of 99% on room air. Physical examination revealed no abnormalities in the head, neck, chest, abdomen or lymph nodes. On neurological exam, she demonstrated slightly decreased motor strength in her right side, predominantly upper extremity, and mild anomic aphasia with difficulties in finding words; fundoscopic examination was normal. Her medical and family history, including thromboembolism, were normal. She had no history of use of any drug apart from hormone replacement therapy (HRT) that she had started seven years before ischemic stroke onset, due to menopausal symptoms. A no-contrast-enhanced brain CT scan was performed to distinguish between hemorrhagic and ischemic stroke, and an angio CT brain and neck to identify the potential presence, location and extent of intravascular clots, stroke etiology or mechanism such as carotid atherosclerotic disease, vascular dissection or other treatable structural causes. The neuroimaging confirmed an acute ischemic stroke diagnosis; the vascular assessment did not reveal atherosclerotic disease, vascular dissection or a vascular clot treatable with endovascular therapy.

The patient was a candidate for IV tissue plasminogen activator (tPA), which was administered after verifying the absence of contraindications to IV rt-PA with a door-to-needle time of 42 minutes. During the following 24 hours of observation, the patient's clinical condition rapidly improved, no bleeding complications related to the thrombolysis were observed,\ and 24 hours after admission to the stroke unit the NIHSS was 1; sensitivity and the language had reverted to normal, right arm motor drift was present. A brain MRI was performed within 24 hours of stroke onset, showing a restriction area of diffusivity within the cortical/subcortical front left cerebral lobe, approximately 1.2 cm in maximum diameter. Regular representation of the intracranial vessels was seen (Figure 4.1.1).

During the patient's stroke unit stay, a medical history was taken, including a detailed family history with specific annotations on each family member, a thorough physical examination was done, including a careful evaluation of the patient's general appearance, which did not identify any joint laxity, or abnormalities

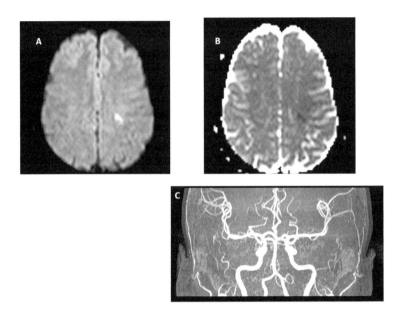

**Figure 4.1.1** (A,B). Brain MRI showed a restriction area of diffusivity within the cortical/subcortical front left cerebral lobe, approximately 1.2 cm in maximum diameter. (C) Regular representation of the intracranial vessels was seen. Neuroimages are courtesy of Professor Enrico Cotroneo, Director of the Neuroradiology Department, San Camillo Forlanini Hospital

of the skin, eyes and heart. After performing cerebral and neck vascular imaging, and considering the age, the patient underwent a full "stroke in the young" diagnostic work-up with transthoracic echocardiogram with bubble study and transesophageal echocardiogram, telemetry monitoring, 48 hours extended cardiac monitoring, basic risk factors blood work, such as lipid panel, hemoglobin A1c, thyroid functions, erythrocyte sedimentation rate, C-reactive protein, rapid plasma reagin, HIV and toxicology screen, as well as extensive coagulation testing for hypercoagulable states, including inherited thrombophilias: homocystine, factor V Leiden mutation, pro-thrombin gene mutation, protein C deficiency, protein S deficiency, and antithrombin deficiency.

All test results were normal; the patient was discharged after one week and she had a full recovery from neurologic symptoms. Therapy at discharge was aspirin 100 mg, and hormone replacement therapy was interrupted after blood hormone testing and gynecological consultation. The patient attended a neurovascular clinic, no stroke recurrences or TIAs were reported in 3.5 years of follow-up, no vascular risk factors emerged during controls; she maintained a healthy lifestyle and good adherence to antithrombic therapy. In this patient hormone replacement therapy was the only clinical key finding related to stroke that we could detect during hospital admission and follow-up; therefore, in this case we assumed the ischemic cerebrovascular event was related to it.

**Clinical suspicion of HRT-related ischemic stroke**

Healthy postmenopausal women – no history of vascular risk factors – history of hormone replacement therapy

Clinical manifestations: acute onset-focal neurological deficit

Type of ischemic stroke: PACS-LACS

**Diagnostic work-up**

Neuroimaging: Brain CT and brain and neck CTA: no atherosclerotic disease, vascular dissection or cardioembolic vascular clot

Full cardiac assessment: transthoracic echocardiogram with bubble study and transesophageal echocardiogram, telemetry monitoring, 48 hours extended cardiac monitoring – all tests should not reveal any abnormality such as PFO, cardiac arrhythmia or potential cardioembolic condition

The following laboratory studies should not demonstrate potential cause of ischemic stroke:

- o Inflammatory and coagulopathy panel: antinuclear antibody, rheumatoid factor, anti-neutrophilic cytoplasmic autoantibody, HLAB27, serum angiotensin-converting enzyme (ACE), lupus anticoagulant, antithrombin, protein S, protein C, factor VIII levels, homocysteine levels, antiphospholipid antibodies, factor V leiden mutation and activated protein C resistance
- o Lipid panel

# Discussion

Drugs commonly used in clinical practice may be associated with a slight increase in stroke risk, both ischemic and hemorrhagic. However, data on these associations are often controversial, and individualized management of patients is recommended, including the evaluation of comorbidities, and a careful risk–benefit assessment. It is also of importance that patients be provided with information to build awareness about therapy potential benefits and harms.

Hormone replacement therapy for post-menopausal syndrome is an example. There is evidence from clinical trials and observational research that indicates that standard-dose hormone therapy increases stroke risk for postmenopausal women by about one-third, and that increased risk may be limited to ischemic stroke.[1] However, for women less than 60 years of age, the absolute risk of stroke from standard-dose hormone therapy is rare, about two additional strokes per 10,000 person-years of use. Newer studies have examined the timing of HRT initiation and the dosing and routes of administration of HRT; studies support initiation of HRT earlier after menopause and using low-dose estrogen and transdermal HRTMRT at the lowest feasible dosage and shortest duration.[2] Current guidelines recommend limiting the use of HRT to short periods during the menopausal transition, primarily for menopausal symptoms. Counseling postmenopausal women on the prescription of HRT requires an assessment of their individual risk for cardiovascular disease (CVD) and discussion on their quality of life and long-term follow-up. Table 4.1.1 summarizes an approach to assessing women for HRT based on their individual CVD risks.[3]

Testosterone replacement (TRT) is used to treat men with hypogonadism but also has cardiovascular effects. There is some evidence that in men aged ≥45 years with low

**Table 4.1.1** Assessment for HRT based on CVD risks

| | |
|---|---|
| Higher risk/avoid HRT | Known atherosclerotic cardiovascular disease/coronary artery disease/peripheral artery disease |
| | Known venous thrombosis or pulmonary embolism |
| | Known stroke/TIA or myocardial infarction |
| | Known clotting disorder |
| | Known breast cancer |
| | 10 years atherosclerotic cardiovascular disease risk >7.5% |
| Definite risk for CVD/ caution with HRT | Diabetes |
| | Smoking |
| | Uncontrolled hypertension |
| | Obesity/sedentary/limited mobility |
| | Migraine with aura/systemic lupus erythematosus/rheumatoid arthritis |
| | High triglycerides or uncontrolled cholesterol levels |
| | 10 years atherosclerotic cardiovascular disease risk >5–7,4% |
| Lower risk/acceptable for HRT | Recent menopause, normal weight, normal blood pressure, active life, healthy lifestyle |
| | 10 years atherosclerotic cardiovascular disease risk >5–7,4% |

testosterone levels and no hypogonadotropic or testicular disease there is an increased risk of ischemic stroke, transient ischemic attack and myocardial infarction associated with current use of TRT, and this risk seems to be highest in the first six months to two years of TRT use.[4] Nevertheless, clinical studies have shown discrepant results for testosterone replacement in men with hypogonadism at different age classes, resulting in controversy over its clinical use, largely concerning variances in cardiovascular event rate and the ability of these studies to generate reliable data on this endpoint. Testosterone treatment is not without side effects and risks, and individualized management of patients is recommended, including the evaluation of comorbidities and CVD risk, and careful risk–benefit assessment, not the general prescription of testosterone therapy to all aging men with low testosterone.

Both antidepressants and non-steroidal anti-inflammatory drugs (NSAIDs) have been reported to affect platelet aggregation, blood pressure and heart rate. There is evidence suggesting an increased risk of ischemic stroke with the current use of rofecoxib,[5] while diclofenac[5,6] is associated with both ischemic and hemorrhagic stroke, and meloxicam[6] only with hemorrhagic stroke. Both selective serotonin reuptake inhibitors and tricyclic antidepressants are associated with an increased risk of any stroke type.[7] Recently, the effect of medications with anticholinergic (antimuscarinic) activity on stroke risk has been investigated. These medications are prescribed frequently in older adults, for example for chronic obstructive pulmonary disease. Observations highlight a possible dose-response relationship between anticholinergic medications and risk of incident stroke and stroke mortality in a large, general population[8].

Individualized therapeutic plan balancing risks and benefits, comorbidities and patients choice is recommended to reduce stroke burden, especially in patients needing polytherapy.

# References

1.  Bushnell C, McCullough LD, Awad IA, et al. Guidelines for the prevention of stroke in women: A statement for healthcare professionals from the American Heart Association/American Stroke Association. *Stroke*. 2014;**45**: 1545–1588.

2.  Renoux C, Dell'aniello S, Garbe E, Suissa S. Transdermal and oral hormone replacement therapy and the risk of stroke: A nested case-control study. *Br Med J*. 2010;**340**: c2519.

3.  Lundberg GP, Wenger NK. Menopause hormone therapy: What a cardiologist needs to know. Expert analysis. American College of Cardiology. 2019. www.Menopause Hormone Therapy: What a Cardiologist Needs to Know - American College of Cardiology (acc.org) (accessed February 2022).

4.  Loo SY, Azoulay L, Nie R, et al. Cardiovascular and cerebrovascular safety of testosterone replacement therapy among aging men with low testosterone levels: A cohort study. *Am J Med*. 2019;**132**(9): 1069–1077.e4.

5.  Varas-Lorenzo C, Riera-Guardia N, Calingaert B, et al. Stroke risk and NSAIDs: a systematic review of observational studies. *Pharmacoepidemiol Drug Saf*. 2011;**20**(12): 1225–1236.

6.  Cooper C, Chapurlat R, Al-Daghri N, et al. Safety of oral non-selective non-steroidal anti-inflammatory drugs in osteoarthritis: What does the literature say? *Drugs Aging*. 2019;**36**(Suppl 1): 15–24.

7.  Trajkova S, d'Errico A, Soffietti R, Sacerdote C, Ricceri F. Use of Antidepressants and Risk of Incident Stroke: A Systematic Review and Meta-Analysis. *Neuroepidemiology*. 2019;**53**(3–4): 142–151.

8.  Gamble DT, Clark AB, Luben RN, et al. Baseline anticholinergic burden from medications predicts incident fatal and non-fatal stroke in the EPIC-Norfolk general population. *Int J Epidemiology*. 2018;**47**(2): 625–633.

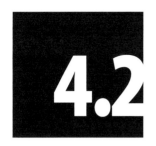

# Illicit-Drug-Related Stroke

Francesca Romana Pezzella, Marilena Mangiardi

## Case Presentation

A 42-year-old man was admitted in the emergency room because of acute onset of loss of strength in his right limbs and consciousness disorder on waking. At admission, body temperature was 36.0°C, heart rate 85 beats/min, blood pressure 140/85 mmHg and respiratory rate 22 breaths/min, with oxygen saturation of 98% on room air, NIH Stroke Scale score was 17. No family history of stroke of either vascular risk factors, or recent head and/or neck trauma.

Contrast angio-computed tomography (CT) brain scan showed no acute hypo/hyperdense lesions, and no intracranial artery stenosis, aneurysm, arteriovenous malformation or sinus thrombosis were detected . Brain magnetic resonance imaging (MRI) diffusion and T2/FLAIR-weighted images showed acute ischemic lesions in the left occipital, frontal and rolandic cortices, left post-central parietal cortex and semi-oval center (Figure 4.2.1).

Electroencephalography did not reveal epileptiform discharges.

The patient was not eligible for intravenous thrombolytic therapy due to the timing from clinical onset (wake-up stroke with positive FLAIR hyperintensity). He was admitted to the stroke unit for further clinical investigations. During his hospital, stay the acute neurological clinical picture spontaneously improved, with the NIHSS score decreasing to 7. An early rehabilitation and speech program was started and the patient benefited from it.

The patient underwent a full "stroke in the young" diagnostic work-up, which also included analysis for illicit drugs. Laboratory screening tested the urinary presence of opiates, amphetamines and cocaine. Cardiological screening (electrocardiogram and echocardiogram) highlighted negative T waves in V5-V6, D2, D3 and AVF, and the presence of irregular thrombus in the apical segment of the left ventricle with widespread ventricular walls hypokinesia (40% of left ventricular ejection fraction) (Figure 4.2.2).

The patient had been asymptomatic for chest pain and breathing discomfort before the stroke and during the hospital stay. A coronarography study did not reveal critical coronary artery stenosis and cardiac MRI confirmed the presence of a left ventricular thrombus (Figure 4.2.3).

We concluded on a diagnosis of recent myocardial infarction with intact coronary arteries and subacute ischemic stroke due to illicit drug abuse. The patient was fully informed about his diagnosis and the risks related to illicit drug use, received a full psychological counseling and was started on oral anticoagulant therapy and low-dose antiplatelets. The clinical course during hospitalization was regular, no clinical complications were observed and he was discharged to rehabilitation center.

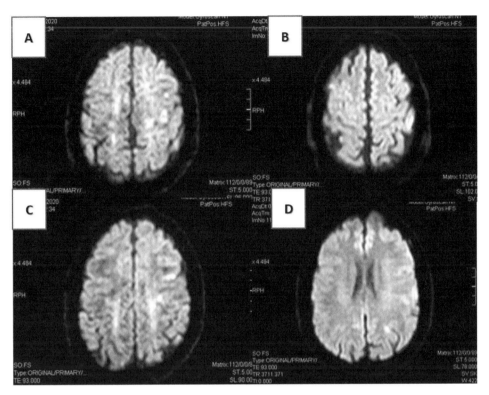

**Figure 4.2.1** Brain MRI DWI sequences. Multiple recent ischemic lesions appear in the left occipital cortex, left frontal and rolandic cortices, left parietal cortex and left semi-oval center. Neuroimages are courtesy of Professor Enrico Cotroneo, Director of the Neuroradiology Department, San Camillo Forlanini Hospital.

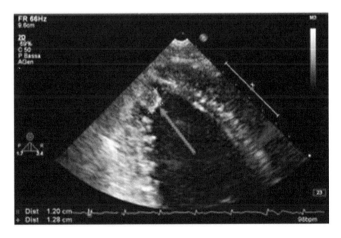

**Figure 4.2.2** Transesophageal echocardiogram showed a rounded thrombotic formation adhering to the left ventricle apical segment with irregular borders. Neuroimages are courtesy of Professor Enrico Cotroneo, Director of the Neuroradiology Department, San Camillo Forlanini Hospital.

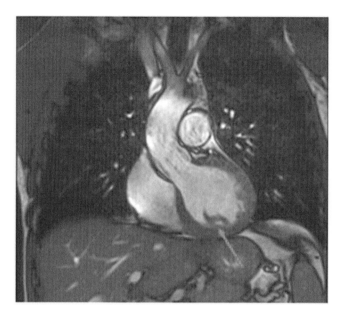

**Figure 4.2.3** Cardiac MRI showed preserved size and morphology of the left ventricle with reduced global systolic function, and previous inferior and apical ischemic necrosis, with apical thrombosis. Neuroimages are courtesy of Professor Enrico Cotroneo, Director of the Neuroradiology Department, San Camillo Forlanini Hospital.

# Clinical Suspicion of Illicit-Drug-Related Stroke

Cerebrovascular disorders contribute to the morbidity and disability associated with illicit drug use, which may be the most common predisposing condition for stroke among patients under 35 years of age. In fact, drug abusers aged 15–44 years are 6.5 times more likely to have a stroke (both ischemic and hemorrhagic) than non-drug-users.[1] The illicit drugs most commonly associated with stroke are psychomotor stimulants, in particular amphetamine and cocaine. Less commonly implicated are ecstasy, opioids and psychotomimetic drugs, including cannabis. We have added to this list anabolic androgenic steroids, which are prescribed for the treatment of several disorders, such as hypogonadism, but can also be used for ergogenic or recreational purposes (i.e., improvement of physical condition and athletic performance) and the doses are usually 5–15 times higher than those recommended for therapeutic use. At such high levels, anabolic androgenic steroids can cause a number of serious side effects, including liver dysfunction, renal disorders, cardiotoxicity and potentially stroke. In Table 4.2.1 we summarize the mechanisms of stroke related to illicit drug use for each type of stroke.[2] Even if 85–90% of strokes associated with the use of illicit drugs occur in the third or fourth decade, the age range reported in the literature is from neonatal/perinatal to old age.[1] Symptoms may occur over a background of chronic abuse, overdose, "binge" use, re-exposure after a prolonged abstinence or even first exposure to the illicit drug. Symptoms frequently occur during or within minutes to several hours/days (in case of chronic exposure) after administration of drug by any of the following routes: intravenous, intranasal, inhalational, oral, intramuscular, subcutaneous or inadvertent intra-arterial. Some individuals may take drugs by multiple routes. Presenting neurologic symptoms include focal neurologic deficits, seizures, headaches, altered mental status, depressed level of consciousness or coma. Patients might be hypertensive or normotensive or have cardiac arrhythmias when first seen. Drug use, especially cocaine use, has been commonly associated with a history of migraine headaches.[3] The relationship between stroke subtype and specific drugs depends on the substance-specific mechanisms (see Table 4.2.1). Most drugs have been

**Table 4.2.1** Stroke mechanisms by illicit drug and stroke type[1,2,4,5]

| Drug | Mechanism | Notes |
|------|-----------|-------|
| **Ischemic stroke related to illicit drug use** | | |
| Cocaine | • Enhanced platelet aggregation<br>• Vasospasm<br>• Vasculitis<br>• Accelerated atherosclerosis<br>• Cardioembolism<br>  ◦ Arrhythmias with thrombosis<br>  ◦ Cardiomyopathy<br>  ◦ Myocardial infarction (with thrombosis)<br>  ◦ Septic embolism | Intranasal administration can lead to ischemic lesions of globus pallidus |
| Opiates/heroin | • Cardioembolism<br>  ◦ Atrial ectopic, atrial fibrillation, idioventricular rhythm or malignant ventricular arrhythmias<br>  ◦ Endocarditis<br>  ◦ Foreign bodies accidentally injected<br>  ◦ Adulterants in drugs<br>• Arteritis/Vasculitis<br>• Hypotension/Hypoxemia<br>• Heroin-induced hypereosinophilia<br>• Opioid- induced increase plasma fibrinogen levels | |
| Cannabis - | • Cerebral vasoconstriction<br>• Changes in cerebral autoregulation/ impaired cerebral vasomotor function<br>• Hypotension<br>• Vasospasm<br>• Fluctuations in blood pressure | |

**Table 4.2.1** (cont.)

| Drug | Mechanism | Notes |
|------|-----------|-------|
| **Ischemic stroke related to illicit drug use** | | |
| | Hyperaggregation of platelet | |
| | • Cardioembolism | |
| | ∘ Arrhythmia | |
| | ∘ Myocardial infarction | |
| Synthetic cannabinoid | • Hyperaggregation of platelet | |
| | • Reduction of blood supply with Hypoxia | |
| | • Cardioembolism | |
| | ∘ Arrhythmias | |
| Amphetamines | • Cardioembolism | |
| | ∘ Arrhythmias with thrombosis | |
| | ∘ Cardiomyopathy | |
| | • Vasculitis | |
| | • Microinfarcts from blood vessel injury and accelerated atherosclerosis | |
| LSD- lysergic acid diethylamide | • Vasospasm | |
| | • Arterial vasoconstriction | |
| | • Vasculopathy Arteritis | |
| | • Direct vasoconstrictive effect of Serotonin | |
| Anabolic steroids | • Induce prothrombotic profile | |
| | ∘ Hyperaggregation of platelet | |
| | ∘ Increased erythropoiesis- polycythemia- elevated hematocrit- thromboembolism | |
| | ∘ Increase of plasma levels of factor VIII and IX | |

- Cardioembolism
  ∘ Arrhythmia
- Enhanced atherogenesis – decreased HDL levels, increased LDL levels, hypertension
- Hemorheologic effect – impaired endothelial function, increased viscosity

Ecstasy
- Cardioembolism
  ∘ Arrhythmias
  ∘ Cardiomyopathy
- Vasospasm → Vessel wall damage
- Direct vasoconstrictive effect of Serotonin
- Hyperthermia→Clotting cascade/DIC → microinfarcts

## Hemorrhagic stroke related to illicit drug use

Cocaine
- Hypertensive spikes
- Underlying aneurysm or arteriovenous malformation rupture
- Vasculitis
- Changes in cerebrovascular autoregulation

Cannabis
- Hypotension
- Vasospasm
- Cerebral vasoconstriction syndrome
- Vasculitis

Synthetic cannabinoid
- Transient vasospasm

Amphetamines
- High blood pressure/hypertensive surge
- Vasoconstriction

The risk of stroke is four times higher in amphetamine users than in non-users and hemorrhagic stroke may occur twice as often

**Table 4.2.1** (cont.)

## Hemorrhagic stroke related to illicit drug use

| | |
|---|---|
| Ecstasy | • Hypertensive surge<br>• Vasodilation from decreased serotonin from chronic use<br>• Consumptive coagulopathy = spontaneous bleed |
| Opiates/heroin | • Hemorrhage determined by pyogenic arteritis<br>• Rupture of a mycotic aneurysm<br>• Hemorrhagic transformation of ischemic infarction |
| Anabolic steroids | • Acute hypertension |

## Subarachnoid hemorrhage related to illicit drug use

| | |
|---|---|
| Cocaine | • Aneurysm rupture from hypertensive surges<br>• Facilitation of aneurysm formation |
| Amphetamines | • Direct toxic effect of amphetamines on cerebral vessels – necrotizing vasculitis<br>• Aneurysm formation and rupture |
| Ecstasy | • Aneurysm formation and rupture |
| Opiates/heroin | • Rupture of a mycotic aneurysm |

associated with more than one stroke subtype. Some drugs are preferentially related to certain stroke subtypes. For example, heroin is most often associated with cerebral ischemia; it has rarely been linked to subarachnoid hemorrhage or intracerebral hemorrhage, not due to infective endocarditis, renal or liver disease. Cocaine use by various routes is strongly associated with both ischemic and hemorrhagic stroke.[4]

## Neuroimaging and Diagnostic Work-Up

In a stroke patient who is less than 50 years old and without stroke risk factors, a suspicion for drug use or abuse should be considered.[1] The patient, family members and friends should be questioned for a history of drug use by all possible routes. We suggest looking for associated physical signs of drug use, such as hypertension, cardiac arrhythmias, needle marks, other cutaneous signs, other organ system signs (nephropathy), and signs of endocarditis. The patient should be evaluated by toxicologic screens. The duration of detectability is generally about four urinary half-lives, typically up to two to three days, but it may vary according to the route of drug-taking, if the drug use is chronic or acute, and any comorbidities.[3]

For ischemic stroke patients, an appropriate neuro-diagnostic evaluation, including CT scan, MRI scan, selected cardiologic investigations (cardiac enzymes, electrocardiogram, echocardiography, including contrast and transesophageal and Holter monitoring) and non-invasive vascular tests (carotid and or transcranial Doppler), should be performed to determine the stroke mechanism and choose appropriate therapy.

For patients with intracerebral hemorrhage and subarachnoid hemorrhage, an appropriate neuro-diagnostic evaluation, including CT and MRI scans, should be planned, and cerebral angiography is strongly recommended in cases of suspicion for saccular aneurysm or arteriovenous malformation, especially in cocaine users and those with sympathomimetic abuse. For intravenous drug users, human immunodeficiency virus (HIV) testing is strongly recommended.[3,5]

## Therapy

Patients with ischemic stroke may be considered for intravenous thrombolytic therapy or mechanical thrombectomy, and appropriate antithrombotic/anticoagulation therapy for secondary prevention. Patients with intracerebral hematomas and subarachnoid hemorrhage can additionally be treated with empiric or standard medical and surgical or interventional neuroradiologic techniques, or both, as appropriate. Multiprofessional care of these patients aimed at discontinuing the abuse of illicit drugs is strongly recommended as soon as its use is recognized.[1,3,5]

## References

1. Esse K, Fossati-Bellani M, Traylor A, Martin-Schild S. Epidemic of illicit drug use, mechanisms of action/addiction and stroke as a health hazard. *Brain Behav.* 2011;**1**(1): 44–54.

2. Tsatsakis A, Docea AO, Calina D, et al. A mechanistic and pathophysiological approach for stroke associated with drugs of abuse. *J Clin Med.* 2019;**8**(9): 1295.

3. Sloan MA. Illicit drug use/abuse and stroke. *Handb Clin Neurol.* 2009;**93**: 823–840.

4. Cheng YC, Ryan KA, Qadwai SA, et al. Cocaine use and risk of ischemic stroke in young adults. 2016;**47**(4): 918–922.

5. Fonseca AC, Ferro JM. Drug abuse and stroke. *Curr Neurol Neurosci Rep.* 2013;**13** (2): 325.

# Genetic Collagen Disorders
## 5.1.a Ehlers–Danlos Syndrome

Pietro Caliandro, Giuseppe Reale, Aurelia Zauli

## Case Presentation

A 32-year-old female without previous significant medical history was admitted to the emergency department with recent onset (six hours) of acute dysphagia and partial paralysis of the right lower face. In addition, she reported severe neck pain in the previous days.

On arrival she was alert and oriented, temperature was 36.6 °C, heart rate, 80 beats/min, blood pressure, 130/70 mmHg and oxygen saturation, 98% on room air. The neurological examination showed mild dysarthria and dysphonia, along with a right lower face palsy and hypoesthesia to temperature and pain of the left side of the face and the upper left arm. She also had Horner's syndrome, consisting of mild ptosis, miosis and enophthalmos of the right eye.

A brain and neck computed tomography (CT)-angiography was performed, showing an occlusive dissection of the right vertebral artery extending from its distal extracranial section to almost 5 mm from its confluence into the basilar artery (Figure 5.1.1).

In addition to that, a saccular aneurysm of the right internal carotid artery (dimensions 9 mm x 14 mm) at 4 cm from its origin (Fig. 5.1a.2) and a focal dilatation (3 mm) of the left internal carotid artery in its distal extracranial section were found.

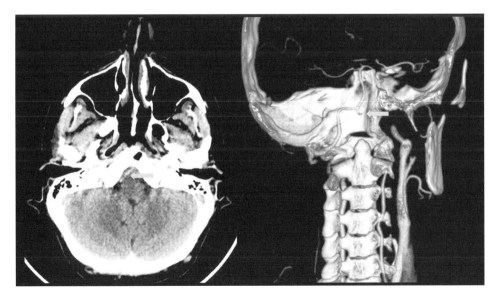

**Figure 5.1.1** On the left, basal brain CT showing hyperdensity of the intracranial tract of the right vertebral artery (arrow). On the right, brain CT-angiography 3d reconstruction documenting occlusion of the intracranial tract of the right vertebral artery.

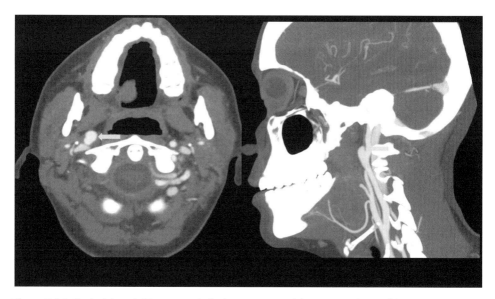

**Figure 5.1.2** On the left, neck CT-angiography finds an aneurysm of the extracranial tract of the right carotid artery (arrow). On the right, the aneurysm is showed in the sagittal plane by neck CT-angiography multiplanar reconstruction.

Brain magnetic resonance imaging (MRI) revealed a posterior right bulbar area of hyperintensity in diffusion-weighted image (DWI) sequences, which was compatible with a recent ischemic lesion in the ipsilateral vertebral artery territory (Figure 5.1.3). The patient was then started on antiplatelet medication with aspirin.

Laboratory tests, including an inflammatory and coagulopathy panel with antinuclear antibodies, extractable nuclear antigen (ENA), anti-DNA antibodies, anti-neutrophilic cytoplasmic autoantibodies, lupus anticoagulant, antithrombin, protein S, protein C, factor VIII levels, C3 and C4 levels, antiphospholipid antibodies, and activated protein C resistance, were negative. Holter electrocardiogram (ECG) and echocardiography were unremarkable.

A thorough physical examination revealed joint hyperlaxity involving particularly the knee, the elbow, the wrist and the interphalangeal joints, bilaterally. The patient also had a particular facial appearance with prominent eyes and a thin face and nose. No familiality for hyperlaxity, facial abnormalities, sudden death, abdominal hemorrhage or ischemic or hemorrhagic stroke at a young age was reported. The aforementioned physical characteristics, combined with the vertebral artery dissection and the other vascular abnormalities shown by angiography, raised suspicion of vascular Ehlers–Danlos syndrome (vEDS) or Loeys–Dietz syndrome. A blood test was carried out for DNA analysis, which resulted positive for the c.2060G>T (p.Gly687Val) mutation in one allele of the COL3A1 gene, confirming the diagnosis of vEDS. Therefore, a CT scan of the chest and the abdomen was performed to rule out any other potentially life-threatening vascular anomalies. Once the diagnosis was made, aspirin was suspended 90 days after ischemia because the risk of bleeding in vEDS patients overweighs the potential benefit of long-term antithrombotic therapy.

During the hospital stay, the patient had a moderate improvement in dysphagia with recovery of oral feeding. She was finally discharged with slight dysphagia, dysphonia, ptosis and thermo-pain hypoesthesia.

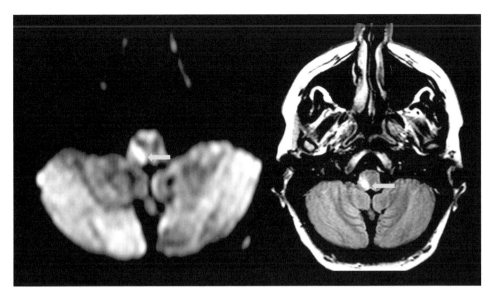

**Figure 5.1.3** Brain MRI shows the acute ischemic lesion (arrows) in the right bulb both in DWI sequences (on the left) and in FLAIR sequences (on the right).

# Discussion

Ehlers–Danlos syndrome comprises a group of inheritable connective tissue disorders. Ehlers–Danlos Syndrome Type IV, or vEDS, has an autosomal dominant pattern of inheritance. Mutations of the COL3A1 gene are responsible for vEDS and determine a defect in type III collagen synthesis, subsequently making blood vessels and organs prone to tearing and rupture. In 50% of cases, the mutation is de novo and patients do not report any familial history. The incidence of vEDS is about 1/100,000/year.[1]

Vascular complications of vEDS are typically arterial ruptures that can occur virtually in every segment of the vascular tree, but especially in the aortic, mesenteric, iliac, renal and cerebral segments. In addition, arterial dissections are also frequently reported.[2]

A high percentage of patients with vEDS will likely present with vascular and visceral complications. Spontaneous colon rupture is one of the most frequently reported event. During pregnancy, the gravid uterus might be involved too.

As with other Ehlers–Danlos syndrome types, vEDS might cause joint hypermobility, especially of distal joints. A common cutaneous finding in vEDS is translucent skin and easy bruising with subsequent atrophic scars.

Moreover, patients may have large eyes, a thin nose and face, and lobeless ears.

Diagnostic criteria have been proposed to help identify this rare disorder, as shown below (Table 5.1.1)[3]; however, the definite diagnosis still needs to be confirmed by molecular sequencing of the COL3A1 gene in search of the causative mutation of one allele.

An extensive imaging study of the vascular tree is strongly suggested at the time of diagnosis, in order to detect any asymptomatic vascular abnormality. Regular follow-ups should be programed, possibly using non-invasive measures, such as ultrasound, MRI and

**Table 5.1.1** Diagnostic criteria

| Major criteria | Minor criteria | Minimum criteria suggestive of vEDS |
|---|---|---|
| 1. Family history of vEDS with documented causative variant in COL3A1<br>2. Arterial rupture at a young age<br>3. Spontaneous sigmoid colon perforation in the absence of known diverticular disease or other bowel pathology<br>4. Uterine rupture during the third trimester in the absence of previous C-section and/or severe peripartum perineum tears<br>5. Carotid-cavernous sinus fistula (CCSF) formation in the absence of trauma | 1. Bruising unrelated to identified trauma and/or in unusual sites such as cheeks and back<br>2. Thin, translucent skin with increased venous visibility<br>3. Characteristic facial appearance<br>4. Spontaneous pneumothorax<br>5. Acrogeria<br>6. Talipes equinovarus<br>7. Congenital hip dislocation<br>8. Hypermobility of small joints<br>9. Tendon and muscle rupture<br>10. Keratoconus<br>11. Gingival recession and gingival fragility<br>12. Early-onset varicose veins (under age 30 and nulliparous if female) | A family history of the disorder, arterial rupture or dissection in individuals less than 40 years of age, unexplained sigmoid colon rupture or spontaneous pneumothorax in the presence of other features consistent with vEDS should all lead to diagnostic studies to determine if the individual has vEDS. Testing for vEDS should also be considered in the presence of a combination of the other "minor" clinical features listed above. |

CT scan. At present, there is no consensus on the timing follow-ups, so each case should be addressed according to clinical and radiological findings[4]

It is also highly recommended to maintain blood pressure within a normal or low normal range to reduce the risk of arterial dissection or rupture. This can be achieved through both lifestyle interventions and antihypertensive drugs. Furthermore, blood-thinning medications should be used carefully, thoroughly balancing the risks and benefits for every single patient.

Regarding vascular complications, arterial ruptures usually need urgent repair while many dissections do not cause severe symptoms and might not require invasive or minimally invasive treatment. However, arterial dissection might cause ischemia in the related vascular territory (stroke, gastrointestinal ischemia, limb ischemia).

Because of the frequent aforementioned complications, life expectancy is shorter than that of the general population (median age of death: 48 years). Thus, primary and secondary prevention have a key role, and it is crucial to educate the patient to pay attention to all the symptoms that may underlie a critical condition.

Differential diagnosis usually comprises the diseases reported in Table 5.1.2.

**Table 5.1.2** Differential diagnosis for vEDS

| Features | vEDS | Loeys–Dietz syndrome | Marfan syndrome | Arterial tortuosity syndrome |
|---|---|---|---|---|
| Clinical | Translucent skin, easy bruising, acrogeria, hypermobility of small joints, gingival recession, atrophic scars | Hypertelorism, bifid uvula, cleft palate, translucent skin, atrophic scars, dural ectasia | Joint hypermobility, tall stature, arachnodactyly, pectus carinatum, hindfoot valgus, ectopia lentis, dolichocephaly, scoliosis, dural ectasia | Hyperextensible skin, joint hyperlaxity, hypertelorism, long face, downslanting palpebral fissures |
| Radiological | Arterial aneurysms and dissections | Aortic and other arterial aneurysms and dissections, arterial tortuosity | Aortic root dilatation | Medium and large arterial tortuosity |
| Complications | Vascular dissection and rupture, ischemic events, organ rupture | Aortic dissection, rupture of arterial aneurysms, ischemic events | Aortic dissection, spontaneous pneumothorax | Vascular aneurysms, dissections, ischemic events |
| Genetics | COL3A1; AD | TGFBR1,TGFBR2, TGFB2; AD | FBN1; AD | SLC2A10; AR |

AD: autosomal dominant; AR: autosomal recessive

**Stroke of undetermined etiology occurring in a young patient**

**Clinical features suggestive of a collagenopathy**

- ❖ Joint hypermobility
- ❖ Arachnodactyly
- ❖ Pectus carinatum
- ❖ Dolichocephaly
- ❖ Scoliosis
- ❖ Thin, translucent skin with increased venous visibility
- ❖ Characteristic facial appearance: i.e., prominent eyes, thin nose and lips, sunken cheeks, small chin
- ❖ Acrogeria
- ❖ Easy bruising unrelated to identified trauma and/or in unusual sites
- ❖ Ectopia lentis
- ❖ Tendon and muscle rupture
- ❖ Keratoconus
- ❖ Gingival recession and gingival fragility
- ❖ Early-onset varicose veins

**Common radiological findings in collagenopathies**

- ❖ Carotid-cavernous sinus fistula (CCSF) formation in the absence of trauma
- ❖ Aortic root dilatation
- ❖ Aortic dissection
- ❖ Arterial aneurysms
- ❖ Spontaneous vascular dissections
- ❖ Arterial tortuosity

**Main genetic diagnoses**

- ❖ Marfan Syndrome: FBN1 gene (chrom. 15q21.1), encoding protein fibrillin 1
- ❖ Vascular Ehlers–Danlos syndrome: COL3A1 gene (chrom.2q31) encoding Type III procollagen
- ❖ Loeys–Dietz syndrome: TGFBR1 and TGFBR2 (chrom. 9q22 and 3p22, resp.) encoding transforming growth factor beta receptor 1 or 2

**Therapeutic approach and overall management of vEDS**

- ❖ Long-lasting antithrombotic therapy is contraindicated
- ❖ Blood pressure should be maintained in the normal range and hypertension should be treated aggressively
- ❖ Surveillance of the vascular tree via Doppler ultra-sound, CT or MRI should be performed once a year

# Conclusions

Stroke in young adults is uncommon, but its incidence is increasing.[5] Alongside modifiable risk factors, drug abuse, patent foramen ovale and arterial cervical dissection, many strokes are due to genetic causes. Although Fabry disease is the leading genetic cause among young adults with stroke, other genetic conditions must be ruled out.[6]

As this case showed, when evaluating a case of spontaneous dissection of a vessel causing stroke in a young patient with the above-described radiological and physical features, vEDS should be ruled out, even in the absence of major diagnostic criteria. This is important because vEDS diagnosis and the associated high risk of bleeding contraindicate long-term antithrombotic therapy, which is the standard secondary prevention in post-stroke patients.

In conclusion, the peculiar appearance of our patient, together with the etiology of her stroke, led us to the hypothesis of an underlying collagenopathy and made us reconsider the radiological findings in a different frame, making the final diagnosis of a rare but life-threatening condition such as vEDS.

# References

1. Pope FM, Nicholls AC, Jones PM, et al. EDS IV (acrogeria): New autosomal dominant and recessive types. *J R Soc Med*. 1980;**73**(3): 180–186.

2. Pepin M, Schwarze U, Superti-Furga A, Byers PH. Clinical and genetic features of Ehlers-Danlos syndrome type IV, the vascular type. *N Engl J Med*. 2000;**342** (10): 673.

3. Malfait F, Francomano C, Byers P, et al. The 2017 international classification of the Ehlers-Danlos syndromes. *Am J Med Genet C Semin Med Genet*. 2017;**175**(1): 8–26.

4. Byers PH, Belmont J, Black J, et al. Diagnosis, natural history, and management in vascular Ehlers-Danlos syndrome. *Am J Med Genet C Semin Med Genet*. 2017;**175** (1): 40–47.

5. Bhatt N, Malik AM, Chaturvedi S. Stroke in young adults Five new things. *Neurol Clin Pract*. 2018;**8**(6): 501–506.

6. Bersano A, Markus HS, Quaglini S, et al. Clinical pregenetic screening for stroke monogenic diseases: Results from Lombardia GENS Registry. *Stroke*. 2016;**47** (7): 1702–1709.

# 5.1.b Marfan Syndrome

Turgay Demir, Filiz Koç

## Case Presentation

A 44-year-old male, with heart valve and lens subluxation surgery, presented to the outpatient clinic with complaint of weakness on the left side. He was receiving anticoagulant treatment. His parents were second-degree relatives, and his 16-year-old son had aortic valve regurgitation and lens subluxation (Figure 5.1.4).

Physical examination: the patient was extremely tall (192 cm) and thin, with typical musculoskeletal features of Marfan syndrome. These included pectus excavatus deformity, ulnar deviation in both hands, as well as swan neck deformity, long fingers, joint hypermobility and right-sided scoliosis.

A neurological examination revealed an irregular pupil on the right, left-sided hemiparesis (modified Rankin scale (mRS) grade 2), hyper-reflexia and pyramidal signs on the left side.

Laboratory tests: hemogram, biochemical profile including fasting glucose, liver and renal functions, lipid profile, homocysteine, thyroid hormones, vitamin B12 and folic acid were normal. An electrocardiogram revealed atrial fibrillation. A transthoracic echocardiogram showed a mitral prosthetic valve, dilatation of the aortic root and left atrium, left ventricular hypertrophy, left ventricular wall motion and systolic dysfunction, mild aortic

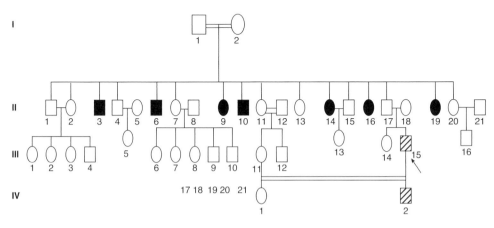

■ ● Seven relatives died in the first year of the life (etiology?)

▨ Patients

**Figure 5.1.4** Family tree of the patient showing the proband siblings and consanguinity of the parents.

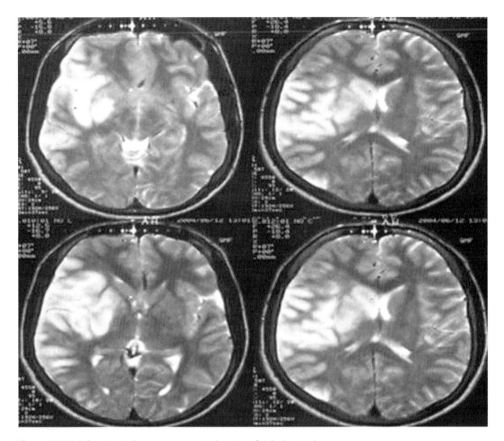

**Figure 5.1.5** Infarction in the temporo-parietal region of right hemisphere.

valve regurgitation and the ejection fraction was 42%. Brain magnetic resonance imaging showed infarction in the temporo-parietal region of the right hemisphere (Figure 5.1.5). Multiple collaterals were seen from the supraclinoid segments of the internal carotid arteries bilaterally, which give a "puff of smoke" appearance (Figure 5.1.6). Reduced calibre of the right internal carotid artery was also seen compared to the left side.

## Discussion

Marfan syndrome (MFS) is a genetically inherited systemic disease of connective tissue, usually characterized by skeletal, cardiovascular and ocular involvement. The disease was first described by Antonin Marfan, a French pediatrician, in 1896 in a 5.5-year-old girl.[1] Since the disease mainly affects connective tissues, multiple organ and system involvement is common, especially in the musculoskeletal system, respiratory system, eyes, heart and circulatory system. However, typically, patients with Marfan syndrome have long arms and legs compared to body height, muscle development is weak, and cardiac involvement is often characterized by aortic aneurysm and related complications. Autosomal dominantly inherited disease is caused by a fibrillin-1 (FBN1) gene defect localized on chromosome 15q21.1.[2] It should not be

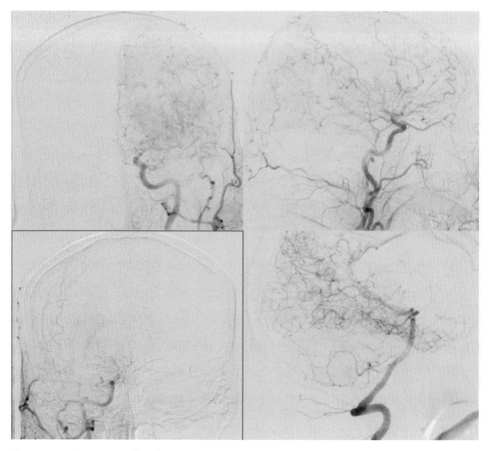

**Figure 5.1.6** Moyamoya collaterals were seen in the supraclinoid segments of the internal carotid arteries bilaterally.

forgotten that the most important supporting feature in the diagnosis is a positive family history showing the hereditary transmission.

Clinical findings in Marfan syndrome become more pronounced with age. The most common symptom in patients is myopia, and 60% of the patients have ectopia lentis. Also the patients are at risk for cataract development, retinal detachment and glaucoma.[3] The skeletal symptoms are joint laxity, dolichostenomelia, pectus excavatum or pectus carinatum, and scoliosis.[4] Tall stature, overgrowth of long bones (i.e., dolichostenomelia) and digits (i.e., arachnodactyly) compared to the trunk, reduced upper segment to lower segment ratio for age and ethnicity, chest wall deformities (pectus carinatum, pectus excavatum), joint hypermobility, joint contractures, scoliosis and thoracolumbar kyphosis, pes planus, hindfoot valgus and forefoot adductus or varus, protrusio acetabuli are skeletal anomalies that can be seen in Marfan syndrome. Aortic root dilatation and mitral valve prolapse are correlated with ocular findings in cardiovascular system involvement, which is the most life-threatening involvement. Spontaneous pneumothorax and apical blebs are seen with respiratory system involvement; inguinal hernias, incisional hernias, and striaea trophycae are found with skin and integument involvement; and attention deficit disorder, hyperactivity, dural ectasia, intracranial aneurysms are central nervous system involvement patterns. Patients with Marfan syndrome have dysmorphic facial features in the form of dolichocephaly with a long and narrow face, malar hypoplasia, micrognathism, macrognathism, enophthalmos and down-slanting palpebral fissures.[5–7]

# Epidemiology

The estimated prevalence of the disease is 1 in 10,000 to 20,000 individuals.[3] The estimated incidence ranges from 1 in 5000 to 2–3 in 10,000 indiviuals.[2] The disease does not differ in gender, ethnicity or geography.

# Pathophysiology

An FBN-1 gene mutation is thought to be the main cause of the disease, the pathophysiology of which has not been fully understood. Fibrillin protein, the product of the FBN-1 gene, plays a critical role in providing structural support in the formation of elastic fibers in the connective tissue. As a result of fibrillin protein deficiency, weakness occurs in the connective tissues of organs rich in elastic fibers, especially the aorta, lungs and eye balls.

# Differential Diagnosis

Non-specific connective tissue disorder, potential Marfan syndrome, MASS syndrome (mitral valve prolapse, myopia, borderline and non-progressive aortic enlargement, and non-specific skin and skeletal findings), mitral valve prolapse, familial ectopia lentis syndrome, velo-cardio-facial syndrome (Shprintzen–Goldberg syndrome), Loeys–Dietz syndrome, arterial tortuosity syndrome, congenital contractural arachnodactyly (Beals syndrome), familial thoracic aortic aneurysm and dissection syndrome, homocystinuria, hereditary progressive arthro-ophthalmopathy (Stickler syndrome), Ehlers–Danlos syndrome, fragile-X syndrome.[8–10]

# Diagnosis

For the diagnosis of Marfan syndrome, findings in the ocular, skeletal, sibling and genetic systems defined in the Ghent criteria are taken as the basis (Table 5.1.3).[5] Major criteria in at least two different organ systems and the involvement of a third system are required for the diagnosis.[4,10,11]

**Table 5.1.3** Scoring of systemic findings[5]

| | |
|---|---|
| Wrist and thumb sign | +3 |
| Pectus carinatum deformity | +2 |
| Pectus excavatum or chest asymmetry | +1 |
| Hindfoot deformity | +2 |
| Plain pes planus | +1 |
| Pneumothorax | +2 |
| Dural ectasia | +2 |

**Table 5.1.3** (cont.)

| | |
|---|---|
| Protrusio acetabuli | +2 |
| Reduced upper segment/lower segment ratio and increased arm/height ratio and severe scoliosis | +1 |
| Scoliosis (>20°) or thoracolumbar kyphosis | +1 |
| Reduced elbow extension | +1 |
| Skin striae | +1 |
| Mitral valve prolapse (all types) | +1 |
| Myopia> 3 diopters | +1 |
| Facial features (3/5)<br>dolichocephaly<br>enophthalmos<br>down-slanting palpebral fissures<br>malar hypoplasia<br>retrognathia | +1 |
| Score of ≥7 points indicates systemic involvement | Total: 20 points |

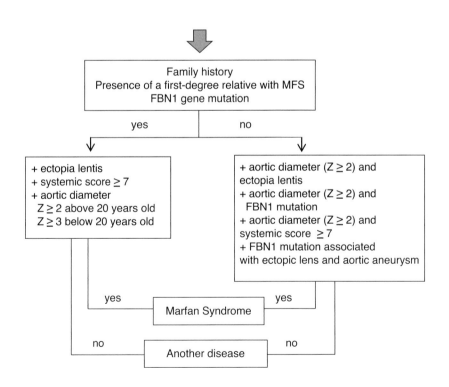

## Treatment and Prognosis

Treatment is mostly supportive and multidisciplinary, and includes managing clinical findings and preventing complications. Management of cardiovascular manifestations includes both medical and surgical therapy. Beta-blockers are standard care for MFS. Angiotensin II receptor blockers type 1 (losartan) and angiotensin-converting enzyme (ACE) inhibitors are alternatives. Prophylactic surgery should be done for dilated aortic segments to prevent aortic dissection. Lifestyle changes are necessary to avoid activities that worsen the risk of aortic dissection. Psychological and social support is important for anxiety and depression accompanying MFS. Physical therapy and, if necessary, orthopedic surgery should be considered for musculoskeletal abnormalities.[8–10,12]

Today, patients with Marfan syndrome who are diagnosed early and are given the proper medical treatment in time, have a lifespan that is almost the same as the general population.

## References

1. Meester JAN, Verstraeten A, Schepers D, et al. Differences in manifestations of Marfan syndrome, Ehlers-Danlos syndrome, and Loeys-Dietz syndrome. *Ann Cardiothorac Surg.* 2017;**6**(6): 582–594.

2. Sakai LY, Keene DR, Renard M, De Backer J. FBN1: The disease-causing gene for Marfan syndrome and other genetic disorders. *Gene.* 2016;**591**(1): 279–291.

3. Yuan S-M, Jing H. Marfan's syndrome: an overview. *Sao PaoloMed J.* 2010;**128**(6): 360–366.

4. Pepe G, Giusti B, Sticchi E, et al. Marfan syndrome: current perspectives. *Appl Clin Genet.* 2016;**9**: 55–65.

5. Loeys BL, Dietz CH, Braverman AC, et al. The revised Ghent nosology for the Marfan syndrome. *J Med Genet.* 2010;**47**(7): 476–485.

6. Kumar A, Agarwal S. Marfan syndrome: an eyesight of syndrome. *Meta Gene.* 2014;**2**: 96–105.

7. vonKodolitsch Y, De Backer J, Schüler H, et al. Perspectives on the revised Ghent criteria for the diagnosis of Marfan syndrome. *Appl Clin Genet.* 2015;**8**:137–55.

8. Tinkle BT, Saal HM, and Committee on Genetics. Health supervision for children with Marfan syndrome. *Pediatrics.* 2013;**132**(4):e1059–72.

9. Ozyurt A, Baykan A, Argun M, et al. Early onset Marfan syndrome: Atypical clinical presentation of two cases. *Balkan J Med Genet.* 2015;**18**(1): 71–76.

10. CSANZ Cardiovascular Genetics Working Group, Ades L. Guidelines for the diagnosis and management of Marfan syndrome. *Heart Lung Circ.* 2007;**16**(1): 28–30.

11. Pyeritz R. Evaluation of the adolescent or adult with some features of Marfan syndrome. *Genet Med.* 2012;**14**(1): 171–177.

12. Ha HI, Seo JB, Lee SH, et al. Imaging of Marfan syndrome: Multisystemic manifestations. *Radiographics.* 2007;**27**(4): 989–1004.

# 5.1.c Fibromuscular Dysplasia

Otgonbayar Luvsannorov, Baigali Gongor

## Case Presentation

A 52-year-old male was admitted to the stroke unit with a severe headache, nausea, vomiting and imbalance, which had been bothering him for the previous three days. The headache was located in the occipital region radiating to the neck. On admission, he was conscious with a normal mental state. His temperature was 36.5°C, heart rate, 65 beats/min, blood pressure, 140/100 mmHg and respiratory rate, 22 breaths/min, with oxygen saturation of 96% on room air. No abnormalities in the head, neck, chest, abdomen or lymph nodes were revealed by physical examination. On neurological examination, slight neck stiffness and end-position nystagmus with normal motor strength in his extremities were demonstrated.

The patient had suffered from periodic severe headaches since the age of 32. Over the past two years he had been complaining of dizziness, which was getting worse. His blood pressure had increased up to 180/100 mmHg over the past five years and was poorly controlled.

Family history: he was the youngest in his family, 10 out of 13 siblings in the family died in childhood. The causes of mortality were not known as the family lived in a rural region with poor medical services. Both parents suffered from high blood pressure; his father and his older brother had suffered strokes. He had been a heavy smoker over the last 30 years (one box of cigarettes a day). He took antihypertensive medications, but not regularly.

Considering the patient's age, clinical features and family history, a brain CT was performed and revealed a subarachnoid hemorrhage (SAH) (Figure 5.1.7)

Carotid duplex sonography and magnetic resonance imaging/angiography (MRI-MRA) were performed to rule out vascular abnormalities such as aneurysm or dissection of cranial arteries. Carotid duplex sonography revealed thickening of the wall of both the common carotid, internal carotid arteries and carotid bifurcation, and marked stenosis of the left vertebral artery (VA) (Figure 5.1.8).

Subacute SAH, predominantly in the posterior circulation, and a "pseudoaneurysm" in the left vertebral artery were observed on brain MRI-MRA (Figure 5.1.9).

Laboratory studies, including total peripheral blood count, biochemical screen, HbA1c, erythrocyte sedimentation rate, C-reactive protein, renal and hepatic functions, were normal.

The results of the investigations were suggestive of fibromuscular dysplasia (FMD) affecting the vertebral and internal carotid arteries; therefore, catheter-based angiography was carried out to support the diagnosis. Contrast-enhanced catheter-based

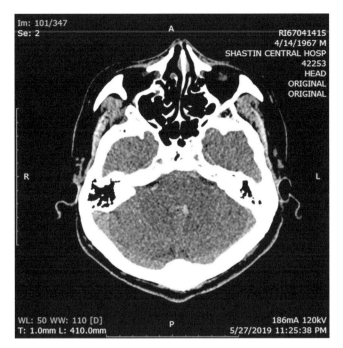

**Figure 5.1.7** Brain CT showing subarachnoid hemorrhage.

angiography revealed a "string of beads" pattern in the long cervical segments of the left VA, which was consistent with FMD (Figure 5.1.10).

In order to identify other areas of FMD, as well as to screen for occult aneurysms and dissections, contrast-enhanced computed tomography angiography (CTA) of all the vessels in the body was performed and revealed ostioproximal short-segment stenosis in the left subclavian artery (SA) and diffuse long-segment moderate stenosis in the left radial artery (RA).

On the basis of all the above-described angiographic investigations, the patient was diagnosed with multifocal FMD. The SAH most likely developed due to the rupture of a small-sized aneurysm (pseudoaneurysm), and the patient was successfully treated medically and discharged from the hospital with antiplatelet therapy and a recommendation of follow-up.

(a)

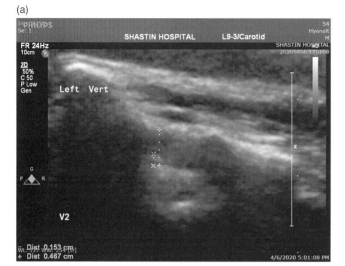

(b)

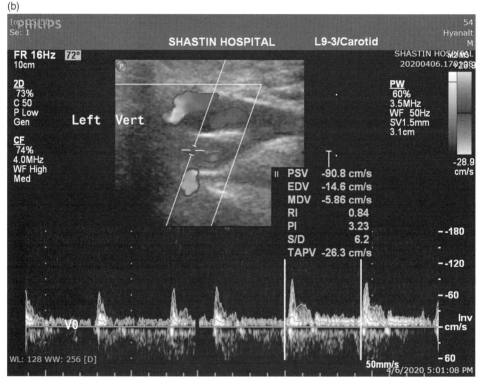

**Figure 5.1.8** (a,b) Carotid duplex sonography revealed thickening of the wall of both the common carotid, internal carotid arteries and carotid bifurcation, and marked stenosis of the left vertebral artery (VA).

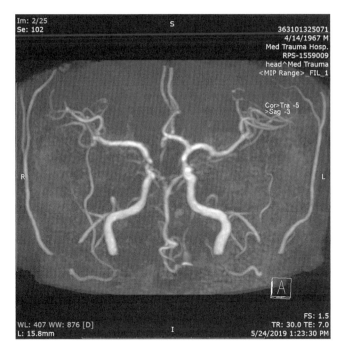

**Figure 5.1.9** Subacute SAH predominantly in the posterior circulation and "pseudoaneurysm" in the left vertebral artery was observed on brain MRI-MRA

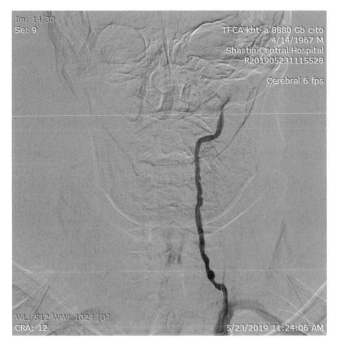

**Figure 5.1.10** Contrast-enhanced catheter-based angiography revealed a "string of beads" pattern in the long cervical segments of the left VA, which was consistent with FMD.

Clinical manifestation of FMD

Age = ± 53 ; Gender = F>M (80–90% women) Cardinal symptoms of cerebrovascular FMD : (a) chronic, mostly migraine-type headache (60%), (b) pulsatile tinnitus (32%), (c) neck pain, non-pulsatile tinnitus and dizziness (20%–26%), (d) cervical bruit on exam (22.2%) , (e) unilateral head/neck pain or focal neurologic findings (e.g., partial Horner's syndrome with ipsilateral ptosis and miosis) (f) as a consequence of FMD: TIA (13.4%), stroke (9.8%), subarachnoid hemorrhage (aneurism) ( 3% and 49%), amaurosis fugax (5.2%), cervical artery dissection (12.1%)

Non-specific neurological manifestaions

5.6% of patients with no symptoms may identify FMD incidentally on imaging

Diagnostic approach to cerebrovascular FMD

**Duplex ultrasound** = An increase in velocity (peak systolic velocity 250 cm/s, EDV 100 cm/s), turbulence and tortuosity in the mid to distal internal carotid artery and the vertebral arteries with associated turbulence of color flow or spectral Doppler signal

**Catheter-based angiography** = Alternating dilatation and constriction (string of beads), focal concentric or tubular stenosis of the middle and distal segments of the internal carotid and vertebral arteries; aneurysm, dissection and vessel tortuosity of medium-sized arteries

**CTAngiography or MR Angiography** = Dissections, non-ruptured cerebral aneurysms of the extracranial and intracranial cerebral vessels

Confirmed FMD–etiological investigations

**Genetics**
FMD appears to be both sporadic and familial in a subset of patients, with autosomal dominant inheritance suggested in some families (1.9–7.3%)
There are currently no genetic tests that are specific to FMD

**Environmental factors**
Female hormones (contraceptive use, hormone therapy)
Lifetime mechanical stress
Tobacco use (37.2%)

Differential diagnosis of FMD

| Systemic arterial mediolysis | Arterial spasm | Atherosclerosis | Large-vessel vasculitis (e.g., Takayasu, giant-cell arteritis) | William's syndrome | Neurofibromatosis type 1 |
|---|---|---|---|---|---|
| Non-inflammatory, non-atherosclerotic disease. Manifests as spontaneous arterial dissection, rupture, occlusion or aneurysm, most often in the abdominal visceral arteries. May be indistinct from multifocal FMD on angiographic imaging. Definitive diagnosis requires histopathological examination demonstrating vacuolar degeneration of the artery media | Benign radiologic findings due to medication induced or catheter-related vasospasm. Transient flow-related physiologic changes in the artery resulting in regular oscillations distinct from multifocal FMD (beading of varying size) | Cardiovascular risk factors: older age, hypertension, hyperlipidemia, tobacco use, obesity, diabetes, etc. Predominantly affects the origin and proximal artery branching points; can affect any arterial bed. Plaques with or without calcification may be visualized on CTA, MRA, or duplex ultrasound | Clinical: fevers, weight loss, pain over the affected arteries; elevated inflammatory markers, anemia, thrombocytopenia. Imaging: focal or tubular stenosis and/or aneurysm of the aorta and branch vessels at the origin or proximal arterial segment. | Clinical: "Elfin fac" (broad forehead, upturned nose, pointed chin); developmental delay; hypercalcemia; garrulous personality; congenital heart defects. Imaging: supravalvular aortic stenosis, mid-aortic syndrome, renal artery or pulmonary artery stenosis, coronary artery dilation Associated gene: ELN | Clinical: freckling, cafe' au lait spots, peripheral neurofibromas, optic gliomas, central nervous system neoplasms, soft tissue sarcomas, skeletal abnormalities, learning disabilities, renovascular hypertension. Imaging: renal artery stenosis, intracranial stenosis, including moyanoya (rare). Associated gene: NF1 |

| Treatment of FMD | | | | | |
|---|---|---|---|---|---|
| **Medical therapy** | | | | **Interventional therapy** | |
| **Antihypertensive** All antihypertensive medication can be prescribed, angiotensin-converting enzyme inhibitors or AT1 blockers (ARB) recommended. Beta-blockers may have a protective effect for migraine headache | **Antiplatelet** Aspirin 75–100 mg daily is reasonable for patients with FMD to prevent thrombotic and thromboembolic complications | **Management of headache and pulsatile tinnitus** Particular caution is advised in prescribing tryptans, ergots and other vasoconstrictive agents for treating headache, especially for patients with a prior history of CeAD or SCAD, in whom these agents may be contraindicated. Some antihypertensive medications (i.e. betablockers, calcium channel blockers, ARBs) may also be effective for prevention of migraine. Consultation with audiology and otolaryngology for patients with tinnitus, reassurance and education, sound or cognitive behavioral therapy | | **Endovascular therapy** For arterial stenosis angioplasty with or without stenting, for dissection stents, for aneurysms (coiling with or without additional devices) | **Surgery** Surgical clipping of aneurism |

**Additional considerations**

Smoking cessation

Physical limitations (chiropractic neck manipulation, rollercoaster rides, etc.)

Patients with unruptured intracranial aneurysm are often advised to undergo follow-up imaging to monitor for aneurysm growth

# Discussion

Fibromuscular dysplasia (FMD) is an uncommon, idiopathic, segmental, non-atherosclerotic and non-inflammatory disease of the musculature of arterial walls, leading to stenosis of small and medium-sized arteries.[1] The cause of FMD and its prevalence in the general population are not known. Arterial lesions in FMD should be classified according to the angiographic appearance as focal FMD or multifocal FMD. The disease primarily affects women and involves intermediate-sized arteries in many areas of the body, including cervical and intracranial arteries. Although often asymptomatic, FMD can also be associated with spontaneous dissection, severe stenosis that compromises the distal circulation or intracranial aneurysm, and is therefore responsible for cerebral ischemia or SAH. FMD has been reported in virtually every arterial bed but most commonly affects the renal and carotid or vertebral arteries (in ≈65% of cases).

The clinical signs of cerebrovascular FMD are non-specific. There is an average delay from the time of the first symptom or sign to diagnosis of FMD of four to nine years. The most common symptom of cerebrovascular FMD is headache, which is often of the migraine type (60%). Pulsatile tinnitus (27.5%) is a very common symptom and described by patients as a "swishing" or "whooshing" sound in the ears. The most serious sequelae of cerebrovascular FMD include TIA, stroke, SAH and cervical artery dissection. Focal neuro-logical events may be related to the following mechanisms: severe stenosis producing cerebral hypoperfusion, embolization, thrombosis, dissection and aneurysm rupture.[2]

The diagnosis of FMD is typically based on angiographic appearance, mostly CTA or contrast-enhanced MRA as the initial imaging modality. CTA and MRA allow a detailed evaluation of the extracranial and intracranial ostio to identify FMD, dissections and cerebral aneurysms. CTA is a reasonable screening tool for non-ruptured aneurysms because endovascular or surgical treatment is not generally performed unless the aneurysm is >5 mm. Advantages of MR-based technology are the lack of radiation and the lack of iodinated contrast agents, which may make it a reasonable screening tool in younger patients. For the evaluation of carotid FMD, it is reasonable to start with a carotid duplex exam, although this modality is inadequate to assess the vertebral and intracranial arteries for FMD. Duplex ultrasound findings consistent with carotid FMD include the identifica-tion of velocity shifts, turbulence and tortuosity in the mid to distal internal carotid artery and the vertebral arteries.[3]

Catheter-based angiography remains the gold standard for the diagnosis of FMD, but it is generally reserved for symptomatic patients in whom intervention is contemplated or for cases in which there is uncertainty about the patient's diagnosis or severity of disease. Angiography may also be required for the accurate determination of intracranial aneu-rysms, which cannot be evaluated by non-invasive imaging. Angiographic patterns consist-ent with FMD are a string-of-beads pattern, smooth tubular or focal lesions consistent with focal FMD and smooth lesions with associated outpouching (aneurysm).

Advances in imaging, medical and endovascular therapies have made the treatment of patients with FMD less invasive, safer and more effective. Treatment may include medical therapy and surveillance, endovascular therapy for stenosis (angioplasty with or without stenting), dissection (stents) or aneurysms (coils, stents), or surgery. Therapeutic decisions depend on the nature and location of vascular lesions (stenosis vs dissection vs aneurysm), the presence and severity of symptoms, prior vascular events related to FMD, the presence and size of aneurysms, and comorbid conditions.[4]

There are no trials assessing the utility of medical therapy in FMD or prospectively comparing medical therapy to intervention in this population. As patients with FMD may present with thrombotic and thromboembolic events, even in the absence of dissection or aneurysm, antiplatelet agents (i.e., aspirin 75–100 mg daily), are reasonable for both symptomatic and asymptomatic FMD. Older age, concomitant coronary artery disease, prior vascular intervention and isolated cerebrovascular FMD were factors associated with higher rates of antiplatelet use. Medical therapy for the care of a patient with FMD should also address hypertension and common symptoms of headache and pulsatile tinnitus that may have an impact on quality of life. Treatment may include lifestyle modification to avoid triggering factors, preventive therapies and medications to abort migraines. Particular caution is advised in prescribing triptans, ergots and other vasoconstrictive agents for patients with a prior history of cervical artery dissection (CeAD) or spontaneous coronary artery dissection (SCAD).[5]

Patients with FMD should be seen at follow-up at least annually. Follow-up includes clinical assessment and imaging. The timing of follow-up imaging should be customized to each patient's pattern and severity of disease, including the need for monitoring of aneurysms or dissections, or following revascularization, as well as local imaging resources and experience.

# References

1. Olin JW, Gornik HL, Bacharach JM, et al. Fibromuscular dysplasia: State of the science and critical unanswered questions. A scientific statement from the American Heart Association. *Circulation*. 2014;**129**: 1048–1078.

2. Gornik HL, Persu A, Adlam D, et al. First international consensus on the diagnosis and management of fibromuscular dysplasia. *Vasc Med*. 2019;**24**(2): 164–189.

3. Touze E, Oppenheim C, Trystram D, et al. Fibromuscular dysplasia of cervical and intracranial arteries. *Int J Stroke*. 2010;**5**: 296–305.

4. Harriott AM, Zimmerman E, Singhal AB, et al. Cerebrovascular fibromuscular dysplasia. *Neurol Clin Pract*. 2017;**7**: 225–236.

5. Varennes L, Tahon F, Kastler A, et al. Fibromuscular dysplasia: What the radiologist should know. A pictorial review. *Insights Imaging*. 2015;**6**: 295–307.

# 5.1.d  Neurofibromatosis Type 1

Zuhal Yapici, Çağla Turan, Oğuzhan Obuz

## Case Presentation

During the newborn period, our patient had café-au-lait spots diagnosed as neurofibromatosis type 1 (NF1) at six months. She also had bone deformities in the lower extremities, which were followed by the orthopedics department. At age 2, it was noticed that she had started to use her right hand less often than the left, so the child neurology department was consulted.

The case was the first child of the mother and delivery was vaginal, at term and spontaneous. Birth weight was 2750 g. No pre-, peri- or postnatal problems were encountered. Motor and mental developmental steps were completely normal. There were no complaints or symptoms related to the neurological systems. The mother and her father had widespread café-au-lait spots along with neurofibromas and were being followed for NF.

Examined at age 2, the patient was found to have more than six café-au-lait spots (one of which was larger than 15 mm), a congenital compound nevus and a number of solitary neurofibromas, as well as one plexiform neurofibroma. Lisch nodules or axillary/inguinal freckles were not detected. Compared to that of the right, the distance between the knee and ankle of the left lower extremity was 3 cm longer (Figure 5.1.11).

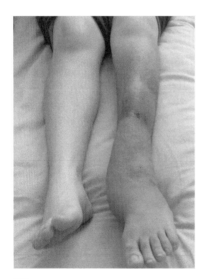

**Figure 5.1.11** Hyperplastic left lower limb.

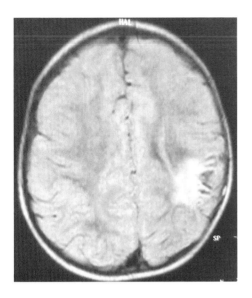

**Figure 5.1.12** Axial FLAIR image shows left parietal chronic infarction. Cortical cerebral parenchymal loss, sulcal widening and peripheral gliosis can be seen.

In addition to mild thoracic scoliosis, there was also bone deformity in the right anterior hemithorax. Neurological examination revealed that cranial nerves were normal, muscle strength was 4/5 in the right upper extremity and normal in the right lower, deep tendon reflexes were hyperactive in the right upper extremity and plantar reflex was flexor, bilaterally. Other neurological systems were within normal limits.

Cranial magnetic resonance imaging (MRI) performed at age 2 revealed a cortico-subcortical encephalomalacic area (chronic-stage infarct) in the left temporo-parietal region, at the level of the pre- and postcentral gyri (Figure 5.1.12).

Examination of this region made it possible to determine an increase in the depth of the sulcus, loss of volume and signal differences, suggesting a surrounding gliotic lesion. Other findings were mildly dilated occipital horn of the left lateral ventricle and increased signals in the periventricular deep white matter in T2-weighted (T2 W) and fluid-attenuated inversion recovery (FLAIR) images, which was suggestive of gliosis. In addition, marked hyperintense heterogeneous areas in both the dentate nuclei were detected in T2 W and FLAIR images (Figure 5.1.13).

This was probably indicative of a hamartoma. Magnetic resonance angiography (MRA) showed thin calibre and an irregular contour in the left middle cerebral artery and subdivision branches emerging from it (Figure 5.1.14).

Results obtained from the orbital MRIs performed for optic glioma were within normal limits.

Lower extremity direct radiographs showed that the left tibia was 3 cm longer than the right, and there was bowing and cortical thinning. MRI of the cruris made it clearly visible that there was a subcutaneous soft tissue mass penetrating between the muscles in the left cruris. The mass was hyperintense in T2 W and showed a pattern of diffuse contrast in the postcontrast T1 W series. Compared to the right, the left tibia and fibula were longer. There was widening and cortical thickening in the medullary canal of the distal metadiaphysis. These were considered to support plexiform neurofibroma and fibrodysplasia. Excisional

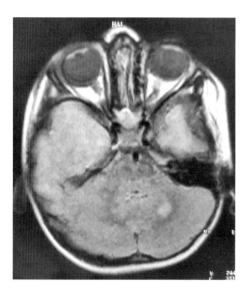

**Figure 5.1.13** T2 W axial image shows cerebellar dentate nucleus hamartomas, which are more prominent on the left.

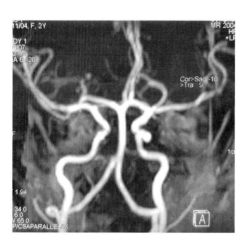

**Figure 5.1.14** MRA image: there are contour irregularities and thinning on the left MCA and its subdivision branches. Other cerebral vessels are normal.

biopsy performed on the lesion was suggestive of a congenital compound nevus. Repeated abdominal ultrasound examination and chest X-rays did not disclose the existence of any lesions. Brainstem evoked-response audiometry test gave normal results. No Lisch nodules were detected during ophthalmological examinations.

Clinico-radiological follow-up of the case has been continued for 13 years. During this time, the patient has had no neurological complaints, and neuroimaging tests have not revealed any new lesions. MRI performed at the age of 13 showed that the lesion had become more chronic, and the infarct area appeared to be completely cystic encephalomalacia (Figure 5.1.15).

During the physical examination carried out at that time, it was noticed that the number of café-au-lait spots increased from 6 at age 2 to 21 at age 12, and their diameters were enlarged (two had a diameter larger than 15 mm). Lisch nodules were not detected, but axillary or inguinal freckles were (Figure 5.1.16). Orbital MRI was not indicative of optic glioma.

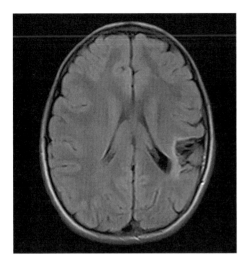

**Figure 5.1.15** Axial FLAIR image: widening can be seen on the left side of a temporoparietal late-phase cortico-subcortical infarction and in the ventricle occipital horn. Slight periventricular gliosis has occurred.

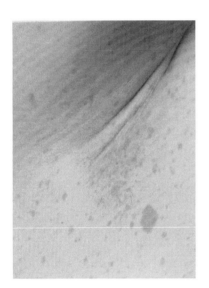

**Figure 5.1.16** Axillary freckles on the patient.

# Clinical Features

NF1 is the most common of the neurocutaneous syndromes, transmitted by autosomal dominant trait.[1] The clinical manifestations are highly variable, and it can involve not only the nervous systems and the skin but also some bones, as well as the ophthalmological, gastrointestinal, endocrine and vascular systems. The syndrome occurs in approximately 1 in 3,000 individuals.

# Diagnostic Algorithm

> The most common symptoms are milky brown spots on the skin. When observed, these spots call for the examination of the patient to see if he or she meets the diagnostic criteria in the framework below

> 1. Six or more café-au-lait macules more than 5 mm in greatest diameter in prepubertal children, and more than 15 mm in greatest diameter in postpubertal children
> 2. Two or more neurofibromas of any type or one plexiform neuroma
> 3. Freckling in the axillary or inguinal regions
> 4. Optic pathway glioma
> 5. Two or more Lisch nodules (iris hamartomas)
> 6. A distinctive osseous lesion, such as sphenoid dysplasia or thinning of long bone cortex, with or without pseudarthrosis
> 7. Diagnosis of NF1 in a first-degree relative (parent, sibling or offspring) according to the foregoing criteria
>
> According to the decision taken in the Consensus Meeting held in 1997, the existence of at least 2 out of 7 criteria listed above are necessary so that the clinical diagnosis of NF1 can be made.

Only about half of children with NF1 with no known family history of NF1 meet the above criteria for diagnosis by age 1, but almost all do by age 8.[1] Café-au-lait macules are the most frequently seen skin lesions, and skin-fold freckling is usually the second sign to appear, which begins in the inguinal region in children at 3 to 4 years of age and eventually appears in the axillae. In mild cases, café-au-lait spots and subcutaneous neurofibromas are the only features. Plexiform neurofibromas often represent tumors that contain a longitudinal section of the nerve. There are developmental and neoplastic disorders of the nervous system in severely affected individuals. In 8–13% of cases of NF1, there is a malignant peripheral nerve-sheath tumor,[3] which usually presents with pain or sudden growth. Various other neoplastic disorders, such as leukemia and pheochromocytoma, occur more frequently in patients with NF1 than in the general population. NF1 causes distinctive anomalies in the whole skeletal system. Scoliosis and deformities on the thorax wall have been reported to occur in 10–40% of patients.[3] Bowing of the tibia, fibula and other long bones can be present in early life, paving the way for spontaneous future fractures at the junction of the middle and distal thirds of the bone shaft.

*Ophthalmologic features* of NF1 include Lisch nodules, glaucoma and optic glioma.[1,3] Iris Lisch nodules are melanocytic hamartomas and are highly specific to NF1. Optic pathway gliomas are found in approximately 15% of patients. Though most are asymptomatic, these tumors can manifest with decreased visual acuity, visual field defects or precocious puberty. Visual symptoms do not necessarily correlate with the size or growth of the tumor detected radiographically. Glioma can involve the optic nerves, chiasm, optic radiations and hypothalamus. Optic gliomas are pilocytic astrocytomas, but are usually slow-growing.

In general, primary CNS abnormalities in NF1 include *hamartomas*, vascular abnormalities, intraspinal neurofibroma and dural ectasias.[1,3] Astrocytomas of the cerebrum, brainstem and cerebellum are the most common intracranial tumors encountered in NF1.[3] The symptoms of intracranial tumors depend on the region where they appear; however, they can often be detected by MRI during the asymptomatic phase. NF1 exhibits the characteristics of overgrowth syndromes, such as macrocephaly, various tumors and even asymmetric hyperplasia of the extremities and/or fingers. Both megalocephalia, in which the volume of white matter increases, and macrocephaly without hydrocephalus are seen in NF1.[3] The incidence of macrocephaly can be as high as 50%.

*Vascular abnormalities* in NF1 can occur in peripheral or cerebral vessels, and pathologically include regions of intimal proliferation and fibromuscular changes in small arteries.[3] According to the location of vascular involvement in the nervous system, variable neurological symptoms can be seen. Stenosis of the internal carotid artery can lead to moyamoya disease and stroke, although lesions are often asymptomatic. Strokes may be caused by either aneurysms or vessels affected by stenosis, or hypertension complications.[3] Renal artery stenosis can lead to hypertension in both children and adults, and involvement of other vessels can cause vascular insufficiency or hemorrhage as a result of arterial wall dissection. Another significant aspect of NF1 is that it increases the risk of early-onset cerebrovascular diseases. However, the pathogenesis of how NF1 leads to these diseases has not yet been clarified.[4] Health-care professionals treating NF1 patients must be aware of the high risk of stroke in this population.

Moyamoya syndrome (MMS) is the most common cerebral vasculopathy among children with NF1.[3,5] It has been demonstrated that the features of MMS were similar in patients with NF1 and those without.[5] Additionally, the phenotype-genotype features of NF1 were similar between children with MMS and those without. Diagnosis of MMS may assist in properly addressing that of NF1 in very young children who do not fulfill the diagnostic criteria.[5] No associations were found between vasculopathy and common clinical features of NF1, including optic pathway glioma, plexiform neurofibroma, skeletal abnormalities, attention-deficit hyperactivity disorder (ADHD) or suspected learning disability.[6]

*Epileptic seizures* and headaches are the most commonly seen neurological symptoms of NF1.[3] Seizures occur in approximately 6–10% of patients, are often focal and may be associated with structural changes in the brain. Children with NF1 manifest an increased frequency of migraine, which may be accompanied by abdominal pain, nausea and vomiting. The most common neuropsychiatric involvement is a learning disability, which has been reported in up to 70% of individuals.[1,3] The profile may include impulsiveness, easy distractibility and visual-motor incoordination. Other consequences of the disease include both verbal and non-verbal disabilities and attention-deficit disorder, as well as expression and language problems.[3] Those with attention-deficit disorder do tend to respond to stimulant medication. Problems with motor coordination and balance are also seen, and correlate with the presence of other neurocognitive dysfunctions. There is also an increased frequency of symptoms consistent with autism spectrum disorders.

# Genetics

Inherited as an autosomal-dominant trait, NF1 has an estimated prevalence of 1 in 3,000 in all populations, and about half of the cases are new mutations.[1,3] The NF1 gene is located at 17q11.2, and the abnormal protein product is neurofibromin, which functions as a tumor suppressor. NF1 exhibits a wide range of variability of expression and complete penetrance.

Because of the high penetrance of the disorder, unaffected parents of a sporadically affected child have a low risk of recurrence in a subsequent child.[3] Genetic testing for diagnosis of NF1 is available on a clinical basis. Cases with a mutation in the SPRED1 gene may have multiple café-au-lait macules, freckles and macrocephaly. However, they do not develop neurofibromas or other tumors related to NF1. This condition is called Legius syndrome. A child with multiple café-au-lait spots is often first screened for a mutation in the NF1 gene and second for a mutation in the SPRED1 gene.

## Imaging

MRI helps reveal areas of increased T2 and FLAIR signal intensities in the basal ganglia, cerebellum, brainstem and subcortical white matter, which are usually indicative of hamartomas.[1] Positron emission tomography (PET) scanning may be helpful in distinguishing a malignant peripheral nerve-sheath tumor from plexiform neurofibroma.[3] MR-angiography and digital angiography may be recommended according to the stroke symptomatology.

## Management

Management is primarily supportive:

1. Anticonvulsant drugs for seizures, surgery for accessible tumors and orthopedic procedures for bony deformities.[1]
2. Affected persons should be followed on a regular basis by a physician who is familiar enough with the disorder to recognize treatable complications early and to provide anticipatory guidance and counseling. The value of the "baseline" examination is questionable because most of the lesions in NF1 are slow-growing and can be followed both clinically and by imaging once they come to attention.[3] Yearly examinations, on the other hand, provide guidance for strategically locating some hamartomas. Regular ophthalmological examinations are needed due to the risk of optic pathway gliomas, seen in approximately 15% of patients with NF1.
3. Surgical procedures are recommended when gliomas or fibromas are symptomatic, causing mass effects, medically intractable pain or cosmetic problems. Neurofibromas of the peripheral nerves need not be removed unless they are subject to repeated trauma or develop signs of malignant change.[3]
4. Neuropathic pain associated with spinal neurofibromas may be treated with gabapentin 20–60 mg/kg/day, or pregabalin 2–8 mg/kg/day. Amitriptyline and duloxetine can be helpful as adjunctive therapies for pain management.
5. Malignant peripheral nerve-sheath tumors tend to be highly malignant, so early diagnosis is essential. Patients with unexplained pain or growth of a neurofibroma should be evaluated, with consideration of biopsy. Malignant tumors are managed with appropriate surgical measures and often with radiation therapy and chemotherapy.
6. Surgical revascularization has been shown to be effective in preventing ischemic episodes in instances of internal carotid stenosis.[3] It has been shown that despite radiographic evidence of progressive stenosis in 48% of patients, nearly all demonstrated stable or improved neurological status after surgical revascularization.[3,7] Surgical revascularization in children appears safe and is protective against further ischemic and neurological damage.[7]

# Acknowledgement

We would like to thank Mr. Cüneyt Bademcioğlu for his contribution in the preparation of the chapter.

# References

1. Pina-Garza JE, James KC. Psychomotor Retardation and Regression (Chapter 5). In: Pina-Garza JE, James KC. (Eds). *Fenichel's Clinical Pediatric Neurology, 8th Edn.* Philedelphia: Elsevier; 2019. 134–137.

2. Gutmann DH, Aylsworth A, Carey JC, et al. The diagnostic evaluation and multidisciplinary management of neurofibromatosis 1 and neurofibromatosis 2. *J Am Med Assoc.* 1997;**278**: 51–57.

3. Thiele EA, Korf BR. Phakomatoses and allied conditions (Chapter 45). In: Swaiman KF, Aschwal S, Ferriero DM, et al. (Eds). *Swaiman's Pediatric Neurology.* China: Elsevier; 2017. 362–372.

4. Rukavina K, Töpper R, Kunze A, et al. Early-onset stroke in two siblings with neurofibromatosis type 1. *Eur J Med Genet.* 2019;**62**: 103710.

5. Santoro C, Giugliano T, Kraemer M, et al. Whole exome sequencing identifies MRVI1 as a susceptibility gene for moyamoya syndrome in neurofibromatosis type 1. *Am J Med Genet A.* 2017;**17**: 1521–1530.

6. Kaas B, Huisman TAGM, Tekes A, et al. Spectrum and prevalence of vasculopathy in pediatric neurofibromatosis type 1. *J Child Neurol.* 2013;**28**: 561–569.

7. Koss MK, Scott RM, Irons MB, Smith ER, Ullrich NJ. Moyamoya syndrome associated with neurofibromatosis type 1: Perioperative and long-term outcome after surgical revascularization. *J Neurosurg Pediatr.* 2013;**11**: 417–425.

# 5.1.e Hereditary Hemorrhagic Telangiectasia

Paola Santalucia, Mariangela Piano

## Case Presentation

In 2011, a 10-year-old boy came to the ER for recurrent epistaxis. His medical history showed frequent episodes of headache and epistaxis; otherwise, he had a regular life, good school profile and practiced regular physical activity. His father, affected by cerebral arteriovenous malformation (AVM), has been diagnosed with hereditary hemorrhagic telangiectasia (HHT – also called Osler–Weber–Rendu syndrome). On admission, he was asymptomatic and his blood work was within normal limits. He underwent a diagnostic work-up including brain computed tomography (CT) and CTA (CT angiography), which showed multiple bilateral ischemic lesions and the presence of two AVMs, one right frontal-mesial with pseudoaneurismal-adjacent venous dilation and the other left frontal opercular. He also underwent a lung radiography and CT that showed multiple arteriovenous fistulae (AVF) in the right lung, apex and base (Figure 5.1.17).

The cerebral angiography showed multiple cerebral AVMs, besides the right frontal-mesial and the left frontal-opercular, localized at the left cerebellar hemisphere, right anterior frontal lobe and left rolandic area (Figure 5.1.18).

A genetic test confirmed the diagnosis of HHT. Between 2012 and 2020, the patient underwent surgical treatment of one pulmonary AVM (PAVM) along with endovascular

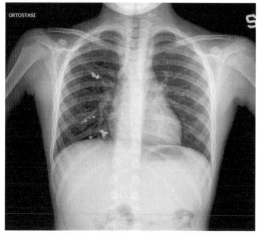

**Figure 5.1.17** Chest X-ray showing pulmonary AVF occlusions.

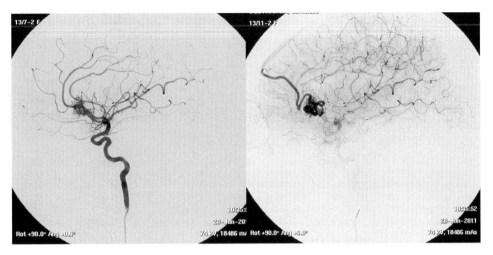

**Figure 5.1.18** Left internal carotid artery(ICA) digital subtraction angiography(DSA) lateral view of frontal opercular AVM.

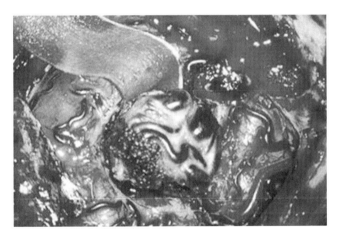

**Figure 5.1.19** Intraoperative picture of right frontal AVM resection.

embolization of four other PAVMs, followed by surgical clipping and radiosurgery with a gamma knife of the cerebral AVMs (Figure 5.1.19).

Regular MRI and cerebral angiographic follow-up showed resolution of the treated lesions (Figure 5.1.20).

He was treated for symptomatic epileptic episodes right after the cerebral AVM treatment and for a long period presented certain sleep disturbances requiring medical attention.

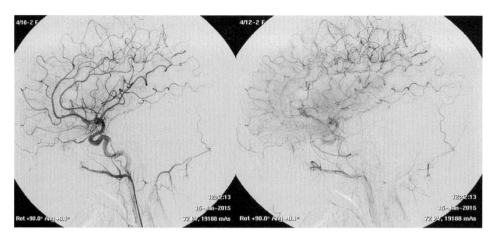

**Figure 5.1.20** Left ICA DSA lateral view of the frontal operculum at four-year follow-up post gamma-knife treatment.

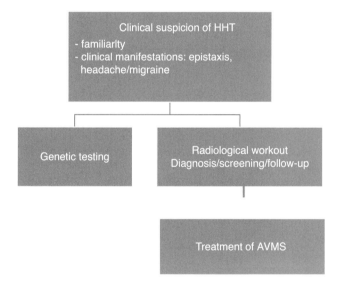

# Clinical Suspicion of HHT

- Familiality
- Clinical manifestations: epistaxis (the most common clinical manifestation due to telangiectasia of the nasal mucosa)
- Headache/migraine

# Genetic Testing

## Diagnostic Screening and Follow-Up for Asymptomatic AVMs

- Cranial CT that shows multiple ischemic lesions
- Neuroimaging based on brain MRI and MRA for diagnosis before and follow-up after procedures for cerebral AVMs
- Cerebral angiography

## Therapeutic Approach to AVMs

- Surgical treatment of PAVMs
- Surgical treatment of cerebral AVMs
- Radiosurgery with gamma knife for cerebral AVMs

## Disease Description

Hereditary hemorrhagic telangiectasia (HHT), also known as Osler–Weber–Rendu syndrome, is a vascular disorder inherited as an autosomal dominant trait with varying penetrance and expression. Three major disease-associated genes have been identified:

- ENG-HHT1 caused by pathogenic variants in ENG (protein product, endoglin, OMIM#187300)
- ACVRL1-HHT2 caused by pathogenic sequence variants in ACVRL1 (protein product: activin receptor-like kinase 1, ALK1, OMIN #600376)
- SMAD4-JPHT is a juvenile polyposis-HHT overlap syndrome that accounts for approximately 1% of HHT cases and is due to pathogenic sequence variants in SMAD4, OMIN #175050).

In addition, more than 600 different pathogenic variants in HHT genes have been described.

The HHT genes all encode proteins involved in the transforming growth factor beta (TGF-β) signaling pathway necessary for the development and maintenance of blood-vessel wall integrity.

As a result of this encoding dysfunction, patients can present with a variety of lesions in different vascular districts, including AVMs, AVFs and telangiectasias.

Epidemiologic studies suggest prevalence rates between 1:5000 and 1:8000 cases with approximately 85,000 individuals affected in Europe;[1] however, HHT is likely underreported worldwide, with geographic variability.

HHT as medical entity can be recognized by the presence of a combination of epistaxis, gastrointestinal bleeding and iron deficiency anemia associated with telangiectasia on the lips, oral mucosa and fingertips.[2]

The majority of patients experience only epistaxis and present mucocutaneous telangiectasia; sometimes they develop iron deficiency anemia secondary to blood loss.

At least half of HHT patients have PAVMs, placing them at risk of early onset and preventable strokes. About 10% have cerebral involvement with varying vascular abnormalities.

The majority of children in HHT families have recurrent epistaxis and sometimes become symptomatic from AVMs. In a series of 44 children screened in a multidisciplinary HHT center, 52% had hepatic AVMs, 45% PAVMs and 16% cerebral AVMs.[3]

*Epistaxis* is usually the earliest sign of disease, pulmonary AVMs generally become apparent after puberty although they may be present during childhood and cerebral AVMs develop during childhood.

Recurrent *gastrointestinal bleeding*, due to telangiectasias localized in the GI tract, more commonly stomach and duodenum than colon, occurs in up to one-third of patients, most commonly over 40 years of age.

*PAVMs* are often asymptomatic for respiratory symptoms; however, they are at risk for complications, mostly stroke due to paradoxical embolism. PAVM bleeding is a rare event that can present with hemoptysis or hemothorax due to vessel rupture into the bronchus or the pleural cavity.

An increased prevalence of migraine has been described in association with PAVMs in the presence of right-to-left shunting due to patent foramen ovale (PFO).

*Cerebral vascular abnormalities* range from benign developmental venous abnormalities and cavernous malformations at low hemorrhagic risk to AVMs and high-flow cerebral AVFs, affecting about 10% of HHT patients. The clinical presentation and prognosis of cerebral vascular malformations depend on the type and location (VASCERN: European Reference Network on Rare Multisystemic Vascular Diseases).

*Hepatic AVMs* may occur in up to two-thirds of patients, potentially symptomatic for left-to-right shunting with increased cardiac output, portal hypertension and hepatic encephalopathy.

HHT patients are also at risk for *venous thromboembolism* and *arterial thrombosis*.

Laboratory findings are usually within normal range, except in cases of sideropenicanemia due to chronic or severe bleeding from AVMs, and are not specific.

Life expectancy is generally good, although there are circumstances, such as pregnancy, in which HHT lesions could result in increased morbidity and mortality due to bleeding of PAVMs, cerebral hemorrhage and thrombotic complications in women previously considered healthy.

# Diagnosis

The presence of HHT may be suspected in patients with the above clinical manifestations, particularly if there is a first-degree relative with HHT.

The Second International Guidelines on HHT[2] recommends the use of the international consensus diagnostic criteria based on the following four findings:

– Spontaneous and recurrent epistaxis
– Multiple mucocutaneous telangiectasias at characteristic sites
– Visceral involvement (pulmonary and/or cerebral and/or hepatic AVMs)
– A first-degree relative with HHT.

These criteria define:

– definite HHT (three or more criteria)
– suspected HHT (two criteria)
– unlikely (one criterion).

The diagnosis may be confirmed by genetic testing, the second International Guidelines on HHT recommend genetic testing for all individuals with HHT, as it may facilitate further investigations and screening for vascular malformations.

## Therapy

Medical therapy is according to the possible clinical complications (e.g., anemia, stroke, venous thromboembolism).

Vascular malformations are treated according to their specific location and risk of complications.

## References

1. Shovlin CL, Buscarini E, Kjeldsen AD, et al. European Reference Network for Rare Vascular Diseases (VASCERN) outcome measures for hereditary haemorrhagic telangiectasias (HHT). *Orphanet J Rare Dis.* 2018;**13**: 136.

2. Faughnan ME, Mager JJ, Hetts SW, et al. Second international guidelines for the diagnosis and management of hereditary hemorrhagic telangiectasia. *Ann Intern Med.* 2020;**173**(12): 989–1001.

3. Giordano P, Lenato GM, Suppressa P, et al. Hereditary hemorrhagic telangiectasia: Arteriovenous malformation in children. *J Pediatr.* 2013;**163**: 179.

# Genetic Small-Vessel Diseases

## 5.2.a Cerebral Autosomal Dominant (Recessive) Arteriopathy with Subcortical Infarcts and Leukoencephalopathy: CADASIL and CARASIL

Yasemin Akinci, Adnan I. Qureshi

## Case Presentation

A 65-year-old woman was admitted to our clinic for evaluation of a new ischemic stroke presenting with right hemiparesis three months ago. She was struggling with left hemiparesis, dysphagia, memory difficulties and gait impairment, which were residual effects from previous strokes. She needed assistance with some daily activities, such as dressing and toilet activities, and was able to ambulate with the help of a walker. The patient had developed migraine with aura at the age of 10 years that resolved at the age of 50 years. She had her first minor ischemic stroke at the age of 56, followed by two additional ischemic strokes at age 58 and 60 years. She later developed absence and complex focal seizures at the age of 62 years. Unfortunately, she suffered another ischemic stroke at the age of 64, followed by the current episode. In the family history, her father died of a stroke at the age of 75 and one of her sons had a history of migraine headaches.

On admission, the neurological examination was notable for mild dysarthric speech, left hemiparesis and evidence of cognitive impairment with a score of 21 out of 30 on the Montreal cognitive test. Systemic examination revealed skin macular erythematous lesions more extensive at elbow joints (see Figure 5.2.1).

Magnetic resonance imaging (MRI) demonstrated chronic encephalomalacia from multifocal chronic ischemic infarctions in the left posterior parietal, parieto-occipital regions and the pons (see Figure 5.2.2).

Magnetic resonance angiography (MRA) revealed attenuation of both vertebral arteries with irregular signal and a tortuous basilar artery. The posterior cerebral arteries were not adequately visualized. A cerebral angiogram that was performed for further examination demonstrated hypoplastic intracranial vertebral and basilar arteries with minimal filling of the right posterior cerebral artery from the basilar artery (see Figure 5.2.3).

Based on the history of migraine and recurrent strokes, examination and imaging findings, a diagnosis of cerebral autosomal dominant arteriopathy with subcortical infarcts and leukoencephalopathy (CADASIL) was suspected. The patient underwent NOTCH3 testing. An analysis of the protein sequence of the NOTCH3 gene did not demonstrate any alterations characteristic of CADASIL disease. However, instead of characteristic alterations, a deoxyribonucleic acid variant with transversion of alanine with tyrosine and

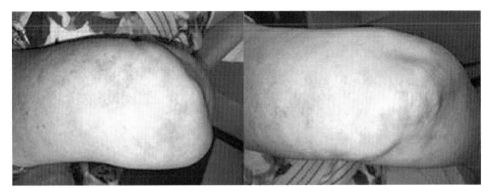

**Figure 5.2.1** Macular erythematous skin lesions on the extensor surface of elbows.

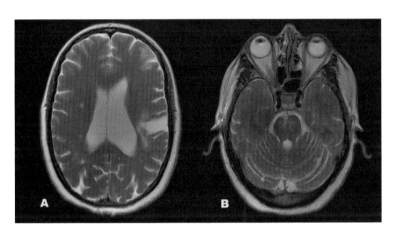

**Figure 5.2.2** T2-weighted axial MR images showing right chronic lacunar infarcts within the subcortical white matter and left parietal encephalomalacia (A), and chronic infarcts in the pontine region (B)

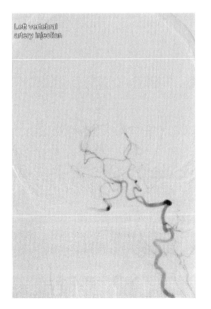

**Figure 5.2.3** Cerebral angiogram shows hypoplastic intracranial vertebral and basilar arteries with minimal filling of the right posterior cerebral artery from the basilar artery.

change of histidine to leucine at nucleotide position 3782 and codon position 1215 was detected. A skin biopsy also did not show any characteristic granular deposits in the basal lamina of small blood vessels on electron microscopy. Ultimately, the patient was diagnosed with a new sporadic variant of CADASIL-like disease.

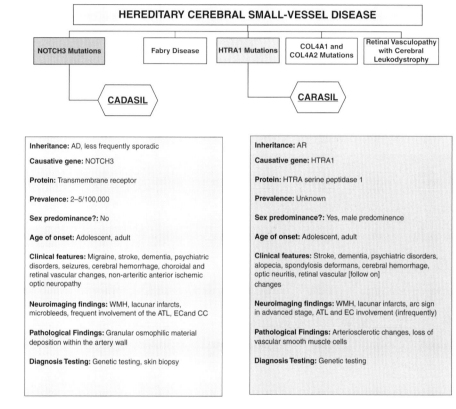

## Discussion

Brain infarction due to cerebral small-vessel disease (SVD) accounts for up to 25% of all ischemic strokes.[1] Approximately 5% of cerebral SVD is considered hereditary.[2] CADASIL and a phenotypically similar condition, cerebral autosomal recessive arteriopathy with subcortical infarcts and leukoencephalopathy (CARASIL), are among the monogenic hereditary cerebral SVDs. Herein, we report a case of sporadic CADASIL-like disease and provided information about CADASIL and CARASIL, two of the most common of inherited SVDs that are usually overlooked.

# CADASIL

CADASIL, the cause of about 2% of lacunar infarcts and leukoaraiosis seen under the age of 65 years, is the most common hereditary cerebral SVD.[3,4] It is autosomally dominantly inherited; however, de novo mutations are possible. Mutations in the NOTCH3 gene located on chromosome 19p13.1 result in accumulation of the Notch3 extracellular domain in arterial walls followed by vascular smooth muscle cell degeneration and subsequent fibrosis and stenosis of arterioles. The majority of the more than 230 different mutations reported are missense mutations, which cause either substitution of a wild-type cysteine with another amino acid or vice versa. However, patients that presented a CADASIL-like phenotype with a non-cysteine mutation in NOTCH3 have also been reported, as seen in our patient.[5–7]

Cardinal manifestations of the disease are migraine with and without aura, transient ischemic attacks and stroke (usually lacunar syndromes, rarely large-vessel stroke), cognitive decline and subcortical vascular-type dementia, and psychiatric disorders (most commonly apathy and major depression). Epileptic seizures usually due to strokes, spontaneous and anticoagulant-related subcortical hemorrhage, acute reversible and self-limiting encephalopathy, choroidal and retinal vascular involvement and non-arteritic anterior ischemic optic neuropathy are other reported clinical manifestations. The mean age of onset of clinical manifestations is 41 years (±9.2 years), but the age of onset of different manifestations varies. For instance, the average age of onset for migraine, the earliest feature of the disease, was reported to be about 30 years, while for stroke it was 40–50 years. Patients usually become bedridden at an average age of 62.1 and 66.5 years in men and women, respectively.[2,4,7–9]

Cerebral MRI shows lacunar infarcts, extensive white-matter hyperintensities (WMH), with frequent involvement of the anterior temporal pole, external capsule (EC) and corpus callosum. Dilated perivascular spaces, brain atrophy and cerebral microbleeds are other findings. Among these anterior temporal lobe (ATL) involvement is a sensitive and relatively specific marker for CADASIL. MRI findings are detectable from the age of 20 and are present in all patients by the age of 35.[2]

MRA can show both congenital and acquired abnormalities (fenestrations, vertebral artery hypoplasia and agenesis, common trunk and fetus posterior cerebral artery, stenosis, prolongation or tortuosity). Cerebral angiography shouldn't be performed as it does not contribute to the diagnosis, and complications are common (in ~ 69% of patients undergoing cerebral angiography), or patients should be closely monitored if it needs to be done.[10]

Mutation testing is the gold standard for the diagnosis. If the diagnosis is strongly suspected and the mutation testing is negative, skin biopsy, which detects granular osmophilic material deposition within the artery wall, can be used.[4]

Currently, there is no effective and specific treatment for CADASIL. Treatment options include genetic counseling, supportive care, symptomatic treatments for migraine and psychiatric disorders, and secondary prevention of stroke. The effectiveness of antiplatelets used by most neurologists after an ischemic attack has not been proven. Anticoagulants should be avoided due to reported rare cases of subcortical hemorrhage associated with anticoagulants; if this is not possible, patients should be carefully monitored.

# CARASIL

This is the second most common hereditary cerebral SVD following CADASIL. The prevalence of this extremely rare disease is currently unknown. The disease is mostly reported in Japan and China; however, cases from Europe, Turkey, India, America and Africa have also been described.[11,12] CARASIL is linked to single gene mutation in the high-temperature requirement A serine peptidase 1 (HTRA1) gene on the long arm of chromosome 10. Due to the mutation, increased expression of the TGF-β family within the tunica intima and media of cerebral small vessels causes arteriolosclerosis-like changes to occur. Patients homozygous for mutations in HTRA1 manifest symptoms consistent with classic CARASIL, while patients heterozygous for mutations in HTRA1 manifest mild signs and symptoms of CARASIL.[13]

Cardinal clinical features of CARASIL are adult early-onset subcortical infarcts, stepwise deterioration of brain functions, early-onset progressive dementia, progressive gait disturbance, behavioral and mood changes, and extraneurologic symptoms, including lumbago associated with spondylosis and disk degeneration, and diffuse alopecia. Seizures, cerebral hemorrhage, optic neuritis and retinal vascular changes are other reported clinical manifestations. CARASIL patients have a more rapid progression of symptoms compared to CADASIL patients, becoming bedridden around the age of 40 years.[7,12-14]

Cerebral MRI shows confluent WMH, lacunar infarctions and atrophy. ATL and EC involvement, that are characteristic early signs in CADASIL, may be seen in some patients. The "arc sign," an arc-shaped hyperintense lesion from the pons to the middle cerebellar peduncle is characteristic of advanced-stage CARASIL. Spondylosis and disk degeneration become observable on cervical and lumbar MRI around the age of 30 years.[2,15]

Histopathological findings include intense arteriosclerosis, mainly in the small penetrating arteries, and loss of vascular smooth muscle cells.[7] The diagnosis is made by the presence of an HTRA1 gene mutation. Skin biopsy is not useful for diagnosis, unlike CADASIL.

Like CADASIL, there is currently no effective specific treatment for patients with CARASIL. Treatment options include genetic counseling, secondary prevention of stroke, supportive care, medications for dementia and psychiatric disorders, medications (tizanidine or baclofen) for spasticity, standard treatment for spinal spondylosis, and a wig or hairpiece for alopecia. The roles of antithrombotic and anticoagulant drugs are still uncertain.

# References

1. Petty GW, Brown RD Jr, Whisnant JP, et al. Ischemic stroke subtypes: a population-based study of incidence and risk factors. *Stroke*. 1999;**30**(12): 2513–2516.

2. Søndergaard CB, Nielsen JE, Hansen CK, Christensen H. Hereditary cerebral small vessel disease and stroke. *Clin Neurol Neurosurg*. 2017;**155**: 45–57.

3. Dong Y, Hassan A, Zhang Z, et al. Yield of screening for CADASIL mutations in lacunar stroke and leukoaraiosis. *Stroke*. 2003;**34**(1): 203–205.

4. Di Donato I, Bianchi S, De Stefano N, et al. Cerebral Autosomal Dominant Arteriopathy with Subcortical Infarcts and Leukoencephalopathy (CADASIL) as a model of small vessel disease: Update on

clinical, diagnostic, and management aspects. *BMC Med.* 2017;**15**(1): 41.

5. Dichgans M, Ludwig H, Müller-Höcker J, et al. Small in-frame deletions and missense mutations in CADASIL: 3D models predict misfolding of Notch3 EGF-like repeat domains. *Eur J Hum Genet.* 2000;**8**(4): 280–285.

6. Joutel A, Monet M, Domenga V, Riant F, et al. Pathogenic mutations associated with cerebral autosomal dominant arteriopathy with subcortical infarcts and leukoencephalopathy differently affect Jagged1 binding and Notch3 activity via the RBP/JK signaling Pathway. *Am J Hum Genet.* 2004;**74**(2): 338–347.

7. Tikka S, Baumann M, Siitonen M, et al. CADASIL and CARASIL. *Brain Pathol.* 2014;**24**(5): 525–544.

8. Opherk C, Peters N, Herzog J, et al. Long-term prognosis and causes of death in CADASIL: a retrospective study in 411 patients. *Brain.* 2004;**127**(Pt 11): 2533–2539.

9. Rufa A, De Stefano N, Dotti MT, et al. Acute unilateral visual loss as the first symptom of cerebral autosomal dominant arteriopathy with subcortical infarcts and leukoencephalopathy. *Arch Neurol.* 2004;**61**(4): 577–580.

10. Dichgans M, Petersen D. Angiographic complications in CADASIL. *Lancet.* 1997;**349**(9054): 776–777.

11. Oluwole OJ, Ibrahim H, Garozzo D, et al. Cerebral small vessel disease due to a unique heterozygous *HTRA1* mutation in an African man. *Neurol Genet.* 2019;**6**(1): e382.

12. Yu Z, Cao S, Wu A, et al. Genetically confirmed CARASIL: Case report with novel HTRA1 mutation and literature review. *World Neurosurg.* 2020;**143**: 121–128.

13. Nozaki H, Nishizawa M, Onodera O. Features of cerebral autosomal recessive arteriopathy with subcortical infarcts and leukoencephalopathy. *Stroke.* 2014;**45**(11): 3447–3453.

14. Fukutake T. Cerebral autosomal recessive arteriopathy with subcortical infarcts and leukoencephalopathy (CARASIL): From discovery to gene identification. *J Stroke Cerebrovasc Dis.* 2011;**20**(2): 85–93.

15. Nozaki H, Sekine Y, Fukutake T, et al. Characteristic features and progression of abnormalities on MRI for CARASIL. *Neurology.* 2015;**85**(5): 459–463.

# 5.2.b Retinal Vasculopathy with Cerebral Leukoencephalopathy and Systemic Manifestations (RVCL-S)

Janika Kõrv

## Case Presentation

A 46-year-old male was admitted to the emergency department with a generalized tonic-clonic seizure. After the seizure, neurological examination revealed left-sided hemiparesis and facial weakness. Brain computed tomography (CT) showed a diffuse low-density area in the right frontal white matter and non-specific calcifications. Mild anemia and mildly impaired renal and liver function were found on routine laboratory tests.

On the next day, magnetic resonance imaging (MRI) showed a rim-enhancing lesion with mass effect and surrounding edema in the right frontal white matter. Mild cognitive decline was diagnosed in addition to left-side hemiparesis. His family reported that the left-side weakness had progressed slowly over the last year; anxiety and signs of cognitive decline were also noted. At the age of 35 he had complained of blind spots in his visual field and poor visual acuity. Retinal vasculopathy was diagnosed and the patient underwent pan-retinal photocoagulation for retinal bleeding. Raynaud's phenomenon was diagnosed in his twenties.

A brain tumor was suspected, and he underwent a biopsy of the right hemispheric lesion. The biopsy showed necrotic tissue without a definite diagnosis. High-dose IV methylprednisolone was initiated, and his hemiparesis somewhat improved.

The patient's father had complained of headaches and decreased visual acuity at the age of 38. He was diagnosed with a brain tumor 20 years later, but the biopsy showed only reactive gliosis, focal necrosis and calcifications, and perivascular lymphocytosis. Corticosteroids provided some clinical improvement, but the patient subsequently developed progression of limb paresis, apraxia and dementia. He died at the age of 64 because of sepsis.

The patient's younger sister was diagnosed with Raynaud's syndrome and retinal vasculopathy in her twenties. Pan-retinal laser photocoagulation was applied, but vitreous hemorrhage occurred, and she became blind in her right eye. Chronic kidney disease was diagnosed in her thirties. From the age of 41, she suffered from frequent attacks of migraine with aura.

Based on clinical findings and family history, there was suspicion for retinal vasculopathy with cerebral leukoencephalopathy and systemic manifestations (RVCL-S). Genetic testing demonstrated a TREX1 gene mutation in the patient and his younger sister. Three months after the initial diagnosis and corticosteroid treatment, the right frontal lesion on MRI had diminished in size, and enhancement was only minimal. However, the edema and gliosis remained as a large zone of confluent T2 hyperintensities with small nodular foci, with and without enhancement. The patient deteriorated over five years with severe cognitive decline, right-side weakness and aphasia. MRI was not repeated. He died at the age of 52 after being bedridden and incontinent.

**Clinical suspicion of RVCL-S**

Age of symptom onset: middle age (35–50 years)

**Major features:**
(a) Retinal vasculopathy (typically decreased visual acuity and/or visual field defects until blindness). Signs: telangiectasias, microaneurysms, and cotton wool spots (early stages), and perifoveal capillary obliterations and neovascularizations (later stages); complications of vascular retinopathy: macular edema and neovascular glaucoma.
(b) Focal brain dysfunction (neurologic features: hemiparesis, facial weakness, aphasia, etc.) and/or global brain dysfunction (progressive cognitive impairment), and brain MRI abnormalities in white matter: (i) focal, non-enhancing T2-hyperintense lesions scattered throughout the periventricular and deep white matter (at an age when nonspecific age-related white matter hyperintensities are infrequent); (ii) punctate T2-hyperintense white matter lesions with nodular enhancement; (iii) hyperintense mass lesions on T2 and hypointense lesions on T1-weighted images, enhanced with gadolinium contrast, and often surrounded by extensive edema. Occasionally, restricted diffusion (most often centrally) referred to as a "pseudotumor." Lesions mostly reported in later stages, frequently localized in the frontoparietal lobe, occasionally in other regions; often lead to displacement of adjacent structures and sulci effacement; can increase in size, remain stable or diminish;
(c) positive family history: autosomal dominant inheritance pattern (absence of a known family history does not preclude the diagnosis)

**Evaluations following initial diagnosis (follow general standards)**

Ophthalmologic: signs of retinopathy, macular edema, glaucoma
Cardiovascular: blood pressure
Renal function: Serum creatinine, BUN and urinalysis (including creatinine and protein content)
Liverfunction: Liver enzymes (AST, ALT, ALP, GGT), serum albumin consideration of serum LDH levels, coagulation studies, bilirubin concentration
Neurologic: cognitive function, migraine, EEG if seizures, focal neurologic symptoms and signs
Endocrinologic: thyroid function (TSH and free T4)
Hematologic: complete blood count (for anemia)
Rheumatologic: Raynaud phenomenon
Psychiatric: depression, [follow on] psychosis, anxiety or other psychiatric diagnoses
Biopsies: not required

**Supportive features:** (a) calcifications on brain CT; (b) non-specific MRI white matter lesions (more frequently than expected given the age of the individual); (c) microvascular liver disease (modest elevations of ALP and GGT; (d) Microvascular kidney disease (typically mild-to-moderate increase in serum creatinine/proteinuria until severe/fatal); (e) psychiatric symptoms (depression, psychosis, anxiety and others)

**Likely associated features:** (a) anemia (typically normocytic and normochromic); (b) microscopic gastrointestinal bleeding; (c) hypertension; (d) migraine with or without aura; (e) Raynaud phenomenon (typically mild); (f) subclinical hypothyroidism; (g) avascular necrosis of the femoral head; (h) macular skin rash and punctate skin lesions

**Confirmed RVCL-S**

Molecular genetic testing (heterozygous C-terminal frameshift mutations in TREX1 gene): (a) single-gene testing (sequence analysis of TREX1); (b) multigene panel (includes TREX1 and other genes of interest for differential diagnosis)

**Management of RVCL-S**

No established treatment, no evidence of efficacy of immunosuppressive therapy and antiplatelet therapy; avoid IV tPA for acute ischemic stroke; standard treatment for most systemic manifestations; [follow on] genetic counselling

# Discussion

RVCL-S is a very rare genetic multiorgan small-vessel disease affecting the retina and brain, but also other highly vascularized organs, mostly the kidneys and liver. Before the identification of the gene responsible, the disease was known as cerebroretinal vasculopathy (CRV), hereditary vascular retinopathy (HVR), hereditary endotheliopathy, retinopathy, nephropathy and stroke (HERNS) and hereditary systemic angiopathy (HSA).[1]

RVCL-S is inherited in an autosomal dominant manner and is caused by heterozygous C-terminal frameshift variants in the TREX1 (Three Prime Repair Exonuclease 1) gene.[2] De novo mutations may be possible, although none have been reported to date. Penetrance seems high.[3] The exact molecular mechanism whereby RVCL-S variants cause the disease is unknown.[4] The onset and severity can vary within the same family.

Clinically, RVCL-S has remained under-recognized and its prevalence is unknown. The clinical phenotype is largely based on details from a study of 78 members of 11 unrelated families.[3]

The mean age of diagnosis is usually between 35 and 50 years.[3] Clinical manifestations vary, but are predominantly in the retina and brain.[3–5] The features of RVCL-S are progressive blindness due to vascular retinopathy, followed by neurological manifestations of focal and diffuse brain dysfunction, and white matter hyperintensities and intracerebral mass lesions on neuroimaging.[3,5]

Most mutation carriers (90%) have clinical manifestations of brain disease, including focal neurological deficits (68%), migraine (59%), cognitive impairment (56%), psychiatric disturbances (depression, anxiety and others) (42%) and seizures (17%).[3] Additional systemic features include liver disease (78%), anemia (74%), nephropathy (61%), hypertension (60%), mild Raynaud's phenomenon (40%), and gastrointestinal bleeding (27%). Bone disease and subclinical hypothyroidism have also been described.[4]

Vascular retinopathy and Raynaud's phenomenon present from the age of 20 onwards.[1,3] Kidney disease manifests from around age 35 and liver disease, anemia, migraine and subclinical hypothyroidism, from age 40. Cerebral and cognitive deficits usually start mildly around age 50, associated with white matter and intracerebral mass lesions, and become severe around age 60–65, leading to death. The causes of death are pneumonia or sepsis.

Punctate, hyperintense, white-matter lesions, with or without nodular enhancement, have been detected on MRI in 97%, rim-enhancing mass lesions in 84% and calcifications in the white matter on CT in 52% of mutation carriers.[3] Although a non-specific finding, punctate hyperintense non-enhancing white-matter lesions should raise suspicion of RVCL-S, if combined with retinopathy or a positive family history.[3] A clinical manifestation can also be a large enhancing lesion mimicking a tumor with pronounced mass effect or tumefactive inflammation[4] (Figure 5.2.4). Focal deficits can be associated with the development of contrast-enhancing lesions on MRI, which can become large and confluent, sometimes with perilesional edema. Lacunar strokes are not common.[4]

The differential diagnosis based on MRI findings showing rim-enhancing mass lesions include tumefactive multiple sclerosis, central nervous system tumors and metastases.[3] Early white matter lesions can be confused with multiple sclerosis, multi-infarct dementia, vasculitis and other hereditary small-vessel diseases with prominent white matter lesions, such as CADASIL (cerebral autosomal dominant arteriopathy with subcortical infarcts and leukoencephalopathy).[3,5] Diffusion restriction observed in the center of some mass lesions

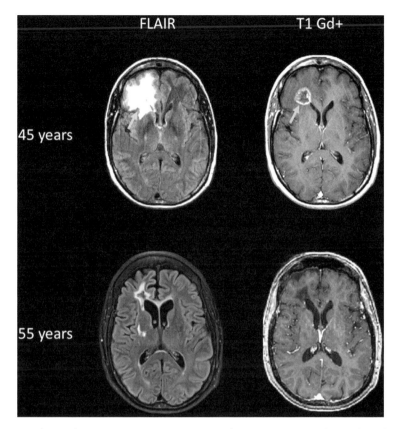

**Figure 5.2.4** Evolution of magnetic resonance imaging (MRI) changes in a patient with retinal vasculopathy with cerebral leukoencephalopathy and systemic manifestations. Pseudotumor adjacent to the right frontal horn (arrows on top images) with surrounding vasogenic edema. The lesion demonstrates ring enhancement following gadolinium contrast. An MRI scan a decade later demonstrates that the previous pseudotumor is inactive, without contrast enhancement or significant vasogenic edema. Additional white-matter hyperintensities have developed, without contrast enhancement (arrows on lower images). (With thanks to the team of Associate Professor Andria Ford and Professor John Atkinson, Washington University School of Medicine.) FLAIR, Fluid Attenuated Inversion Recovery. Reprinted with permission from reference[4].

as marker of cytotoxic edema on MRI has led to the diagnosis of ischemic stroke in patients with acute focal neurological deficits.[3]

Diagnostic criteria have been proposed by Stam, et al.[3] and an update suggested by Pelzer et al.[1]

## Major Diagnostic Criteria

- Vascular retinopathy (which in the early phases is associated with retinal hemorrhages, intraretinal microvascular abnormalities and/or cotton wool spots)
- Features of focal and/or global brain dysfunction associated on MRI with: (i) punctate T2 hyperintense white-matter lesions with nodular enhancement and/or (ii) larger T2 hyperintense white-matter mass lesions with rim-enhancement, mass effect and surrounding edema

- Family history of autosomal dominant inheritance with middle-age onset of disease manifestations. (De novo mutations may be possible although none have been reported to date)
- Demonstration of a C-terminal frameshift mutation in TREX1 to genetically confirm the diagnosis.

## Supportive Features

- On CT, focal white-matter calcifications and/or on MRI non-enhancing punctate T2 hyperintense white-matter lesions at an age that non-specific age-related white-matter hyperintensities are infrequent
- Microvascular liver disease (nodular regenerative hyperplasia)
- Microvascular kidney disease (arterio- or arteriolonephrosclerosis, glomerulosclerosis)
- Anemia consistent with blood loss and/or chronic disease
- Microscopic gastrointestinal bleeding
- Subclinical hypothyroidism.

## Possibly Associated Features

- Raynaud's phenomenon (typically mild)
- Migraine with or without aura (typically relatively late onset)
- Hypertension.

The clinical and histopathologic findings are consistent with the hypothesis that RVCL-S is a systemic small-vessel vasculopathy caused by an endotheliopathy that disrupts the vascular basal membrane and leads to progressive loss of microvascular blood flow.[3] The pathology is non-specific, except the basement membrane changes, and should point to RVCL-S when present in combination with characteristic clinical and neuroimaging features of RVCL-S.[3]

The diagnosis of RVCL-S is established by molecular genetic testing showing C-terminal frameshift mutations in TREX1.[2] How TREX1 mutations lead to RVCL-S is unknown. The TREX1 mutations that cause RVCL-S preserve the enzymatic function of the TREX1 protein, but alter its intracellular localization because the C-terminus that anchors the protein to the endoplasmic reticulum is absent.[2] RVCL-S displays no features of vasculitis and does not seem to be primarily an autoimmune disorder.[3]

There is no established treatment for RVCL-S.[4] There is no evidence of efficacy of immunosuppressive therapy and antiplatelet therapy in RVCL-S. A phase I trial with aclarubicin is ongoing.

Some authors would advise against intravenous (IV) tissue-type plasminogen activators for acute ischemic stroke, because of the risk of secondary hemorrhage.[5]

The treatment of manifestations is not specific for RVCL-S.[5] For visual impairment, retinal laser therapy can prevent and slow down the progression of retinal involvement. Bevacizumab has been proposed by some authors for macular edema.[5] Renal replacement therapy (including transplantation) may be considered in severe cases. In patients with liver function abnormalities, monitoring to prevent complications associated with liver fibrosis and to exclude other causes has been suggested. Corticosteroids can temporarily reduce cerebral vasogenic edema but have no effect on the underlying lesions (IV methylprednisolone followed by an oral corticosteroid treatment).[3,5]

There are currently no consensus guidelines for monitoring individuals with RVCL-S; however, close monitoring is recommended.[5] The frequency depends on the manifestations and rate of disease progression.

It is appropriate to offer genetic counseling (including discussion of potential risks to offspring and reproductive options) to young adults who are affected or at risk.[5]

# References

1. Pelzer N, Hoogeveen ES, Haan J, et al. Systemic features of retinal vasculopathy with cerebral leukoencephalopathy and systemic manifestations: a monogenic small vessel disease. *J Intern Med.* 2019;**285**: 317–332.

2. Richards A, Van Den Maagdenberg AMJM, Jen JC, et al. C-terminal truncations in human 3'-5' DNA exonuclease TREX1 cause autosomal dominant retinal vasculopathy with cerebral leukodystrophy. *Nat Genet.* 2007;**39**: 1068–1070.

3. Stam AH, Kothari PH, Shaikh A, et al. Retinal vasculopathy with cerebral leukoencephalopathy and systemic manifestations. *Brain.* 2016;**139**: 2909–2922.

4. Mancuso M, Arnold M, Bersano A, et al. Monogenic cerebral small-vessel diseases: Diagnosis and therapy. Consensus recommendations of the European Academy of Neurology. *Eur J Neurol.* 2020;**27**: 909–927.

5. de Boer I, Pelzer N, Terwindt G. Retinal vasculopathy with cerebral leukoencephalopathy and systemic manifestations. Sep 19 2019: In *GeneReviews®* *[Internet]* (Adam MP, Ardinger HH, Pagon RA, et al., Eds): Seattle (WA): University of Washington, Seattle, 1993–2020.

# Genetic Metabolic Diseases

## 5.3.a  Fabry Disease

Natan M. Bornstein, Yasemin Akıncı, Derya Uludüz

## Case Presentation

In August 2018, a 21-year-old male presented with sudden-onset left-sided weakness lasting about 12 hours. His medical history revealed that one year ago he had a first attack of left-sided weakness and numbness and was admitted to another hospital. During that time his magnetic resonance imaging (MRI) showed ischemic infarction involving the right posterior limb of the internal capsule (Figure 5.3.1).

Detailed etiological investigations were performed, including cerebrospinal fluid which had a positive oligoclonal band of systemic IgG synthesis (pattern 4). Antiplatelet treatment was started, his symptoms and signs resolved within 15 days and the discharge report revealed that the diagnosis was young ischemic stroke with cryptogenic etiology; however, demyelinating disease could not be excluded.

The patient was admitted to our clinic for his current complaints. He denied alcohol, drug or tobacco use. He was the first child of healthy parents (second-degree relatives). On admission his temperature was 36.5 °C, heart rate 65 beats/min, blood pressure 120/70 mmHg and respiratory rate 20 breaths/min with oxygen saturation of 99% on room air. His physical examination was normal and neurological examination revealed left-sided mild hemiparesis. A brain MRI demonstrated a new stroke in the right pons with chronic multiple asymptomatic ischemic lesions (Figures 5.3.2 and 5.3.3).

There were no vascular abnormalities on magnetic resonance angiography (MRA) images. Laboratory studies, including total peripheral blood count, blood glucose, liver and kidney functions, Fe, ferritin, glycated hemoglobin, vitamin B12, folic acid, erythrocyte sedimentation

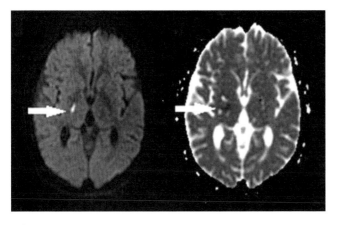

**Figure 5.3.1** Diffusion-weighted axial MR images showing acute ischemic infarction involving the right posterior limb of the internal capsule.

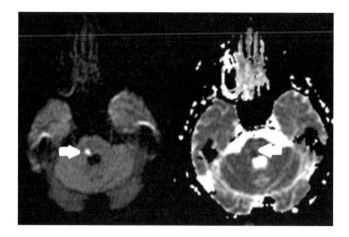

**Figure 5.3.2** Diffusion-weighted axial MR images showing acute right pontine infarction (August 2018).

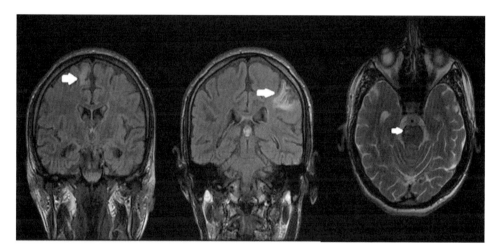

**Figure 5.3.3** T2-weighted coronal and axial MR images showing old right frontal lobe (asymptomatic), left parietal lobe (asymptomatic) and right pontine infarctions (August 2018).

rate, C-reactive protein, thyroid function tests and urine analysis, were normal. Serological screening tests for HIV, hepatitis B, hepatitis C and syphilis were negative. Autoimmune profiles (including serum angiotensin-converting enzyme, antinuclear antibody, rheumatoid factor, antineutrophil cytoplasmic autoantibodies, antiphospholipid antibodies) were negative. Electrocardiography showed sinus rhythm, 24-hour Holter electrocardiogram and transesophageal echocardiography were normal, with an ejection fraction of 82%. Additional investigations were performed for a young stroke etiology. Plasma levels of factor VIII, protein C, protein S and antithrombin III were normal. Prothrombin gene and factor V Leiden gene mutations were negative; however, he was a homozygous carrier for the C677T methylenetetrahydrofolate reductase (MTHFR) mutation.

A more detailed history revealed that the patient had been experiencing mild neuropathic pain in distal extremities and intolerance to heat that was suggestive of Fabry disease

(FD). On further examination, dermoscopy revealed a small area of red lakes (angiokeratomas) on the abdomen. His α-Gal A activities were low (0.1 nmol/h/ml; nv >1.2), and α-galactosidase A *gene* (GLA) study revealed a (c.[680G >A] (p.[R227Q])) mutation, therefore a diagnosis of FD was established. Urine analysis showed evidence of microalbuminuria, however his electromyography (EMG) findings and eye examinations were normal. Enzyme replacement therapy (ERT) with agalsidase beta was started. He was the index case of the family. Later, the patient's mother and uncle (44 and 39 years old, respectively) who were also diagnosed with FD were admitted with ischemic stroke during continued ERT.

**EVALUATION of FABRY DISEASE in YOUNG STROKE PATIENTS (< 55 years)**

**History**
**Physical Examination**

- **Personal History:** Neuropathic pain that begins in childhood, abdominal cramps, chronic diarrhea, hypohidrosis, fatigue, heat or cold intolerance, deafness, depression
- **Family History:** Young stroke, renal failure, cardiomyopathy, sudden death, no male-to-male transmission
- **Examination:** Angiokeratoma, cornea verticillata, hearing loss

**Standard Evaluation**

- Brain MRI/CT, MRA/CTA of the head and neck
- TTE, 12-lead ECG, cardiac telecardiography, 24-h Holter monitoring
- Complete blood count, peripheral blood count, PT(INR), aPTT, glucose, urea, creatinine, electrolits, liver enzymes, CRP, ESR, pregnancy test (for females), lipid panel, TSH, HbA1c, HIV and syphilis serology, urinalysis

- Proteinuria, abnormal kidney function tests
- Brain white matter hyperintensities, dilative arteriopathy of vertebro-basilar system, serebral micro-bleeding, pulvinar sign, posterior circulation stroke
- Left ventricular hypertrophy
- Shortened PR interval, AV block, high voltage of R wave, abnormal Q waves, ST-T changes[22]

**Advanced Evaluation**

- Cerebral angiography
- TEE, embolic shower test, prolonged holter monitor
- Hypercoagulability work-up (protein C-S, AT III and factor VIII activity, beta2-glycoprotein Ig G-M, anticardiolipin Ig G-M, LA, homocysteine, D-dimer, lipoprotein a, prothrombin gene mutation, MTHFR, activated protein C resistance)

- Stroke considered to be cryptogenic

**Even the patient has another etiology that can cause stroke, he/she may also have FD**

**Consider Fabry Disease**
**Male patients:** alpha-galactosidase A activity testing
**Female patients:** moleculer analysis of the GLAgene

| Secondary prevention in ischemic stroke / TIA patients with confirmed Fabry disease | | | |
|---|---|---|---|
| **ERT** | **Antithrombotics** | **Anticoagulants if indicated (e.g. cardioembolic stroke)** | **Control cardiovascular risk factors** |
| ➢ Agalsidase alpha 0.2 mg/kg IV once a week<br>**or**<br>➢ Agalsidase beta 1.0 mg/kg IV every 2 weeks | ➢ Aspirin<br>**or**<br>➢ Clopidogrel | ➢ Warfarin or NOACs<br>➢ Assess bleeding risk before treatment (careful examination for angiokeratomas, endoscopy for GI angiokeratomas) | (HT, hyperlipidemia, diabetes overweight/obesity, hyperhomocysteinemia, etc.) |
| **Follow-up care under the supervision of a multidisciplinary team** | | | |

# Discussion

Fabry disease is a rare multisystemic X-linked lysosomal storage disease characterized by lysosomal α-galactosidase A (α-Gal A) enzyme deficiency that results in globotriaosylcer-amide (Gb-3) accumulation inside the body.[1] The incidence of the disease has been estimated to be approximately 1 in 40,000 to 1 in 117,000 in the general population.[2] Accumulation of Gb-3 within many cell types damages renal and respiratory epithelium, myocardial cells, dorsal root ganglia, neurons, vascular endothelium and smooth muscle cells.[3] Clinical presentations are varied. Early changes predominantly involve the micro-vasculature, as the age increases, medium-to-large caliber involvement occurs. Male patients and symptomatic heterozygous females have symptoms including skin lesions (angiokeratomas, caused by damage to the vascular endothelial cells in the dermis), acro-paresthesia, corneal and lenticular changes, abdominal pain, chronic diarrhea, proteinuria and hypohidrosis. Later, progressive vascular involvement leads to renal insufficiency, cardiovascular dysfunction and stroke.[1,5] Because of the high penetrance of the gene, in male individuals the classic phenotype of the disease occurs and diagnosis is made by measuring α-Gal A activity. Due to random inactivation of one of the X chromosomes, variable expression appears in female individuals, in whom a diagnosis is made on the basis of molecular analysis of the GLA gene, because enzyme dosage can be normal.[5]

Stroke is a common clinical manifestation and usually occurs before diagnosis.[6] Although it is considered to occur in the end-stage of the disease, it can be seen as early as childhood.[3] In the Fabry Registry cohort, results showed that the vast majority of patients experienced their first stroke between the age of 20 and 50 years. Female patients were shown to be older at their first stroke and more likely to experience stroke.[7] Ischemic strokes and transient ischemic attacks (TIA) are most common cerebrovascular events in FD; however, intracerebral hemorrhage, subarachnoid hemorrhage, cerebral venous thrombosis and cervical carotid dissection can occur. The risk for ischemic stroke and TIA is 20 times higher in Fabry patients, compared to the general population. The stroke risk is higher in male patients.[4,8] Accumulation of Gb-3 within the endothelium of brain blood vessels, hypertension due to renal involvement, presence of a prothrombic state, cerebral blood flow abnormalities, autonomic dysfunction, increased reactive oxygen species, cardiac emboli due to cardiomyopathy, valvular disorders and arrhythmias are thought to be responsible for stroke and TIA.[3,4]

Large-vessel or small-vessel disease such as symptomatic or asymptomatic subcortical stroke and asymptomatic cerebral white-matter hyperintensity (CWMH) can be seen.[4] Stroke affects anterior and posterior circulatory systems with a predilection for the posterior circulation. Cortical and subcortical areas may be affected. Infarctions in the vertebrobasilar area are correlated with vertebrobasilar changes like dolichoectatic pathology, which can be used as an early marker of neurovascular involvement, as it was found to be present in 56% of male and 35% of female FD patients.[4,9]

Standard CNS imaging modalities (CT, MRI) can be used for detecting cerebrovascular lesions in FD patients. The MRI protocol should include T1-weighted (sensitive to the pulvinar sign; bilateral hyperintensity of the thalamic posterior area which is characteristic of FD, especially in male patients), fluid attenuated inversion recovery/T2-weighted (sensitive for CWMH, lacunar and territorial stroke), T2*/susceptibility (sensitive for hemorrhage) and diffusion-weighted imaging sequences. Time-of-flight (TOF) MRA can be useful instead of CT and MR angiography to avoid the side effects of contrast media, especially patients with serious renal involvement.[4] Three-dimensional volumetric isotropic turbo spin echo acquisition (3D-VISTA) sequences can be used to show the arterial wall thickening of the cerebral arteries, which occurs in FD patients because of smooth muscle cell proliferation and endothelial Gb-3 storage.[4,10,11] Every FD patient should have a brain MRI every three years and when clinically needed for monitoring. TOF MRI should be done at the first assessment in males aged over 21 and females over 30 and then when clinically needed.[12]

α-Gal A activity, which can be measured in plasma, leukoytes or dried blood spots, is diagnostic for males; however, for females evidence for the mutation in the GLA gene is required for the diagnosis since the plasma enzyme activity can be found to be within the normal range. Additional GLA variants or variants of unknown significance can be present in the genetic test. In such situations, clinical, biochemical, or histopathological evidence of FD is required to make the diagnosis.[12]

Treatment should include ERT and adjunctive therapies under the supervision of a multidisciplinary clinical team. ERT is available in the forms of agalsidase alpha and agalsidase beta. Agalsidase alfa is given at 0.2 mg/kg body weight by intravenous (IV) infusion every other week, agalsidase beta is administered at 1.0 mg/kg body weight by IV infusion every 2 weeks.[12] ERT has been found to improve the overall prognosis and has a beneficial effect on stroke prevention.[13] Using IV thrombolysis for acute ischemic stroke in FD patients, even in the presence of cerebral microbleeds seems safe and should be used in appropriate patients.[14,15] Antithrombotic agents (aspirin or clopidogrel) are indicated as secondary ischemic stroke prevention, however there is no available data for primary prevention.[12] Prior stroke/TIA, angiokeratoma, end-diastolic left ventricular posterior wall thickness (LVPWd) >14 mm, creatinine ≥1.0 mg/dl and global systolic strain <13.5% have been found to be independent risk factors for first or recurrent stroke/TIA in FD patients without atrial fibrillation. Although it hasn't been tested and validated with large studies, based on this data, a scoring tool called the 'Fabry-specific score' has been created. According to the tool, prior stroke/TIA is 2 points, presence of the angiokeratomas is 1 point, creatinine ≥1.0 is 1 point, LVPWd>14 mm is 1 point, GLS < 13.5% is 1 point). A total score of ≥ 2 is associated with higher risk of new-onset or recurrent stroke/TIA. It can be helpful to use this scoring tool and add therapies such as antithrombotic agents in high-risk patients to reduce future cerebrovascular events.[16] Secondary stroke prevention with anti-coagulants (warfarin or new anticoagulant drugs in absence of kidney failure), should be used if the patient has an indication, such as cardioembolic stroke.[12] However, life-threatening bleeding following anticoagulation may occur due to widespread gastrointestinal angiokeratomas. Especially patients with extensive dermal angiokeratomas should be observed carefully before and during anticoagulation. Apixaban may be preferred due to the lower risk of bleeding and because of low renal clearance in FD patients, and antiplatelet agents should be considered as an alternative.[17] The percentages for cardiovascular risk factors such as hypertension, hyperlipidemia, overweight/obesity and hyperhomocysteinemia are high in FD patients.[8] Attention should also be paid to controlling these factors for primary and secondary stroke prevention.

Due to rarity and multiple organ system involvement with non-specific symptoms, long delays between symptom onset and diagnosis are common. The average time between symptom onset and definite diagnosis was found to be 13.7 years in men, 16.3 years in women.[10] The American National Society of Genetic Counselors (NSGC) suggests considering FD in any patients with a family history of FD or corneal vercillata (whorl-like, linear opacities in the inferior part of the cornea) on a slit lamp exam. In the absence of these, NSGC advises clinicians to evaluate decreased sweating, angiokeratomas, personal and/or family history of kidney failure, personal and/or family history of acroparesthesia, personal and/or family history of exercise, heat or cold intolerance and cardiac hypertrophy. In the presence of two of these, the NSGC recommends testing the patient for FD.[18] However, there is still no definitive recommendation for stroke patients. A screening study of 721 young patients (age 18 to 55 years) with cryptogenic stroke, showed that 4.9% of males and 2.4% females had FD.[9] These findings suggest that clinicians should consider a diagnosis of FD in patients with cryptogenic stroke. A complete physical examination, detailed personal and family history, the presence of typical findings for the disease such as proteinuria, cardiomyopathy, neuropathy and vertebrobasilar dolichoectasia can be useful for suspecting the diagnosis.[19] Even if a young patient has known risk factors that can be the etiology of a stroke, FD should be considered if suspicious is high, as in our patient. Considering all the above and the fact that the disease is potentially treatable, it could be rational to screen for FD in all young stroke patients, even in the absence of family/personal history, physical examination findings, etc. This may allow earlier diagnosis and hence earlier access to effective enzyme replacement therapy before severe stroke develops.

# References

1. Desnick RJ, et al. α-Galactosidase A deficiency: Fabry disease. In: Scriver CR, Beaudet AL, Sly WS, Valle D. (Eds). *The Metabolic and Molecular Basis of Inherited Disease, 8th Edn.* New York: McGraw-Hill; 2001. 3733–3774.

2. Zarate YA, Hopkin RJ. Fabry's disease. *Lancet.* 2008;**372**: 127–135.

3. Vincent T. Fabry disease: Why stroke neurologists should care. *Eur Neurol Rev.* 2006;**2**: 94–96.

4. Kolodny E, Fellgiebel A, Hilz MJ, et al. Cerebrovascular involvement in Fabry disease. *Stroke.* 2015;**46**: 302–313.

5. Resende de Jesus PM, Martins AM, Chiacchio ND, Aranda CS. Genital angiokeratoma in a woman with Fabry disease: the dermatologist's role. *An Bras Dermatol.* 2018;**93**(3): 426–428.

6. Gündoğdu AA, Kotan D, Alemdar M, Ayas ZÖ. Fabry disease diagnosis in a young stroke patient: A case report. *Noro Psikiyatr Ars.* 2018;**55**(3): 291–292.

7. Sims K, Politei J, Banikazemi M, Lee P. Stroke in Fabry disease frequently occurs before diagnosis and in the absence of other clinical events: natural history data from the Fabry Registry. *Stroke.* 2009;**40**: 788–794.

8. Fancellu L, Borsini W, Romani I. Exploratory screening for Fabry's disease in young adults with cerebrovascular disorders in northern Sardinia. *BMC Neurol.* 2015;**15**: 256.

9. Rolfs A, Böttcher T, Zschiesche M, et al. Prevalence of Fabry disease in patients with cryptogenic stroke: A prospective study. *Lancet.* 2005;**366**(9499): 1794–1796.

10. Zhang Y-N, Guo ZN, Zhou HW, et al. Fabry disease with acute cerebral infarction onset in a young patient. *Chin Med J.* 2019;**132**(4): 477–479.

11. Qiao Y, Steinman DA, Qin Q, et al. Intracranial arterial wall imaging using three-dimensional high isotropic resolution black blood MRI at 3.0 Tesla. *J Magn Reson Imaging.* 2011;**34**(1):22–30.

12. Ortiz A, Germain DP, Desnick RJ, et al. Fabry disease revisited: Management and treatment recommendations for adult patients. *Mol Genet Metab.* 2018;**123**(4): 416–427.

13. Sheng S, Wu L, Nalleballe K, et al. Fabry's disease and stroke: Effectiveness of enzyme replacement therapy (ERT) in stroke

prevention, a review with meta-analysis. *J Clin Neurosci.* 2019;**65**: 83–86.

14. Kargiotis O, Psychogios K, Safouris A, et al. Intravenous thrombolysis for acute ischemic stroke in Fabry disease. *Neurologist.* 2019;**24**(5): 146–149.

15. Saarinen JT, Sillanpää N, Kantola I, et al. A male Fabry disease patient treated with intravenous thrombolysis for acute ischemic stroke. *J Clin Neurosci.* 2015;**22** (2): 423–425.

16. Liu D, Hu K, Schmidt M, et al. Value of the $CHA_2DS_2$-VASc score and Fabry-specific score for predicting new-onset or recurrent stroke/TIA in Fabry disease patients without atrial fibrillation. *Clin Res Cardiol.* 2018;**107**(12): 1111–1121.

17. Kang E, Kim Y-M, Kim D-H, et al. Life-threatening bleeding from gastric mucosal angiokeratomas during anticoagulation: A case report of Fabry disease. *Medicine (Baltimore).* 2017;**96**(6): e6063.

18. Laney DA, Bennett RL, Clarke V, et al. Fabry disease practice guidelines: Recommendations of the National Society of Genetic Counselors. *J Genet Couns.* 2013;**22**(5): 555–564.

19. Wu L-C, Chiang C-T, Lee K-F, et al. A case of Fabry disease presenting with young stroke and fever. *Acta Neurol Taiwan.* 2019;**28**: 52–56.

# 5.3.b Mitochondrial Diseases

Füsun Ferda Erdoğan, Duygu Kurt Gök, Halil Dönmez, İzzet Ökçesiz

## Case Presentation

We present a 12-year-old male with a drug-resistant epilepsy. The patient, whose parents are relatives was born weighing 3500 g, with normal vaginal delivery. Up to the age of six he was healthy. At the age of six, he started to have three generalized tonic-clonic seizures a day. Diagnosed with epilepsy, he was given carbamazepine. Despite an effective dose of carbamazepine, seizures were not controlled. Approximately four or five seizures a month were recorded. During the course of the disease, cognitive impairment was noticed. One year later, myoclonic seizures started, especially in the right arm and body. Levetiracetam was added, but without any change. With the above-mentioned clinical features, mental retardation and cognitive impairment got worse. Seizures became more frequent when he was eight years old, followed by a sudden onset of left hemiparesis, which led to his hospitalization. On his cranial MRI imaging, there were T2 hyperintense lesions in the right temporoparietal region. He was investigated regarding thromboembolic stroke and neurometabolic disorders, but no definitive diagnosis was reached. Clobazam was added to the existing treatment, and then, within a year, all seizures ceased. But, due to lack of medical control and poor adherence to antiepileptic therapy, his seizures started again. They were focal or generalized tonic-clonic seizures. In the next two to four weeks, in addition to seizures, other symptoms appeared, such as headache, speech and walking disturbances, due to ataxia and left hemiparesis. After each episode with speech and walking impairment and seizure accumulation, there was no return to baseline and his neurologic condition gradually worsened.

His family history revealed that his parents were in a consanguine marriage, his mother's cousin had mental retardation, drug-resistant epilepsy, and impairment of hearing and sight. The neurologic examination showed severe mental retardation, microcephaly, dysarthria, ataxic gait and pyramidal signs on both sides. In the clinical evaluation, with the presence of left hemiparesis onset with seizure accumulation, stroke-like episodes characterized by speech and walking disorders, drug-resistant epileptic seizures, severe mental retardation and progressive neurologic impairment, mitochondrial and neurometabolic diseases were investigated. Hyperintense signal changes, including cortical and subcortical areas, were observed on the brain magnetic resonance (MR) fluid-attenuated inversion recovery (FLAIR) sequences in the right frontal and parieto-occipital areas. Also, diffusion-weighted images showed restriction of diffusion in the right cerebellar hemisphere and cerebellar vermis. The axial apparent diffusion coefficient (DAC) map confirmed vasogenic edema in the right cerebellar hemisphere (Figure 5.3.4).

MR angiography was normal (Figure 5.3.5).

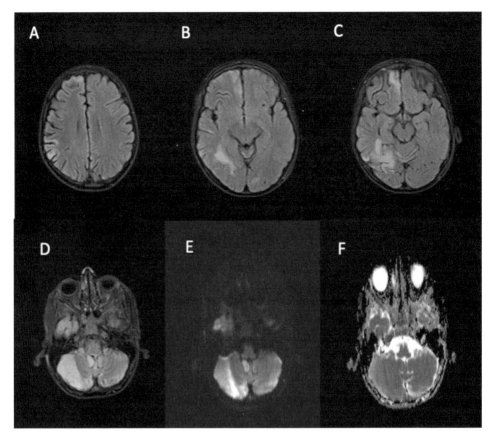

**Figure 5.3.4** Neuroimaging of the patient at the first stroke-like episode. (A–D)FLAIR images illustrating abnormal signals in the cortex and subcortical white matter of the right temporo-occipital lobe, right cerebellar hemisphere and vermis, as well as a smaller increased signal at the right frontal and parietal areas. (E) Axial diffusion-weighted images demonstrating increased diffusion in the right cerebellar hemisphere and cerebellar vermis. (F) Axial apparent diffusion coefficient (ADC) map confirming vasogenic edema in the right cerebellar hemisphere.

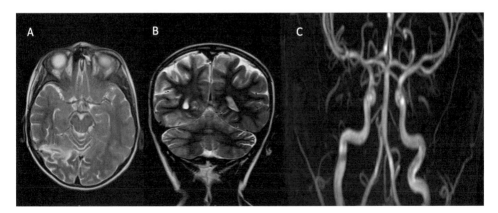

**Figure 5.3.5** Neuroimaging of the patient at the first-year follow-up after the first stroke-like episode. (A, B) Axial and coronal T2-weighted (T2 W) images show atrophic changes in the affected areas. (C) MR angiography shows no pathological findings.

Control investigations on the second year showed mild global atrophy of the supratentorial areas (Figure 5.3.6).

An increase in lactate peak was detected on MR spectroscopy (Figure 5.3.7).

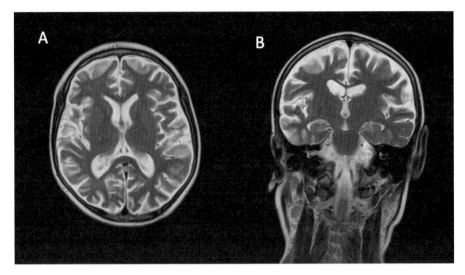

**Fig 5.3.6** Second-year follow-up (A) Axial T2 W image and (B) coronal T2 W image shows mild global atrophy of the supratentorial areas.

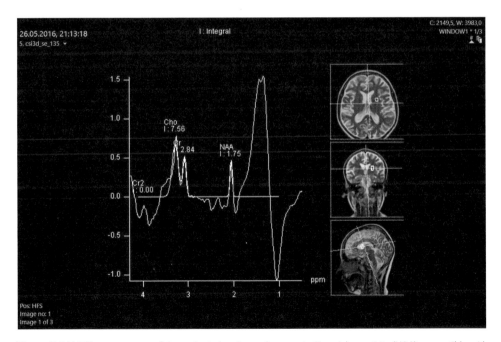

**Figure 5.3.7** MR spectroscopy of the patient showing a decrease in *N*-acetyl aspartate (NAA) compatible with neuronal destruction and an increase in lipid-lactate metabolites, which is a sign of ischemic necrosis.

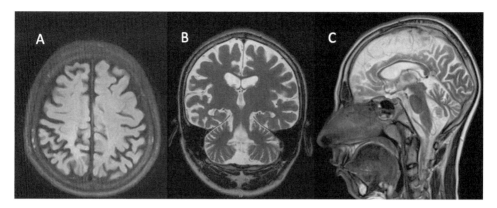

**Figure 5.3.8** Neuroimaging findings at fifth-year follow-up. (A) Axial T2 FLAIR showing diffuse cerebral cortical atrophy. (B) Coronal T2 W image showing diffuse cerebral and cerebellar atrophy. (C) Sagittal T2 showing diffuse cerebro-cerebellar atrophy with marked thinning of the corpus callosum.

Control neuroimaging findings of the patient at the fifth-year follow-up showed diffuse cerebral cortical atrophy, and cerebellar and brainstem atrophy (Figure 5.3.8).

Video-electroencephalography (EEG) monitoring revealed very frequent spike-and-wave and polyspike discharges on the left frontotemporal region and atonic generalized seizures. In non-rapid eye movement (NREM) stage 2 sleep, there were generalized epileptiform discharges, background rhythm abnormalities and left focal slowing in the frontotemporal region (Figure 5.3.9).

Routine blood and urine tests were normal. Serum urine amino acid and organic acid screening tests were normal. Lumbar puncture was performed and lactate and pyruvate levels were high in the brain cerebrospinal fluid (CSF). Hypertrophic cardiomyopathic changes were observed on echocardiography. There was no sensorineural hearing loss. On fundoscopic examination, there was retinopathy with excessive vascular structures in the retina.

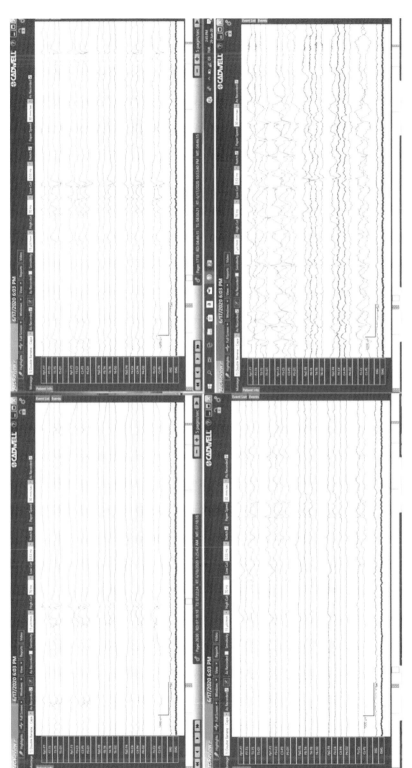

**Figure 5.3.9** Video EEG showing very frequent spike-and-wave and polyspike discharges in the left frontotemporal region.

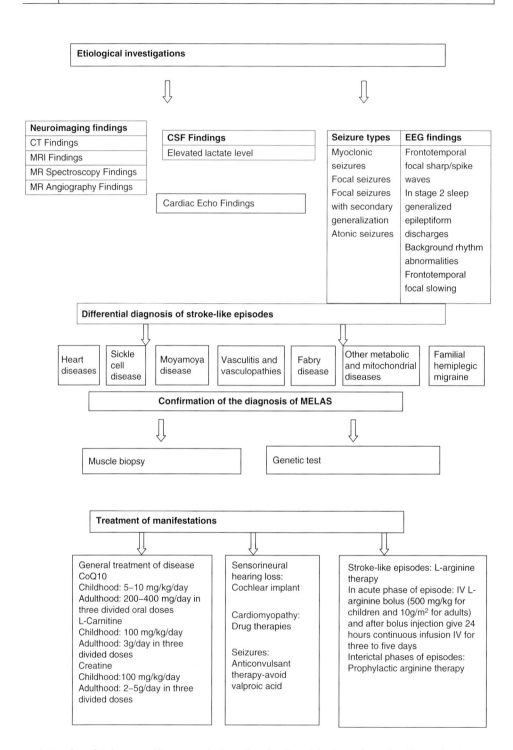

Mitochondrial myopathy, encephalopathy, lactic acidosis and stroke-like episodes are very specific clinical findings for MELAS, which is a very rare neurodegenerative disease.

This disease is maternally inherited.[1] It is bound to a defect of adenosine triphosphate (ATP) energy-production and was identified for the first time in 1984.

The molecular basis of MELAS was discovered in 1990 when adenine to guanine transition at position 3243 of mtDNA (m.3243ANG) in the MT-TL1 gene encoding tRNA Leu(UUR) was found to be related to this syndrome.[2]

In 1992, diagnostic criteria for MELAS syndrome were issued. The clinical diagnosis of this syndrome is based on the following unchanging criteria:[3]

1. stroke-like episodes before the age of 40,
2. encephalopathy characterized by seizures and/or dementia, and
3. mitochondrial myopathy evident by lactic acidosis and/or ragged-red fibers (RRF).

The diagnosis is regarded as verified if there are also at least two of the following criteria:

1. normal early psychomotor development,
2. recurrent headaches, and
3. recurrent vomiting episodes.

Criteria were published in 2012 by Yatsuga et al., by which the diagnosis is considered definitive with at least two items from category A (headache with vomiting, seizure, hemiplegia, cortical blindness or hemianopsia, acute focal lesion identified via brain imaging) and two items from category B (high lactate levels in plasma and/or cerebral spinal fluid or deficiency of mitochondrial-related enzyme activities, mitochondrial abnormalities in muscle biopsy, definitive gene mutation related to MELAS). ([4])

The prevalence of the illness is recorded as 0.2/100,000 in Japan.

MELAS has multi-organ involvement. Stroke-like episodes, dementia, epilepsy, lactic acidosis, myopathy, cardiomyopathy, recurrent headaches, hearing impairment, diabetes and short stature can all be seen in this syndrome. The symptoms and signs of MELAS in 65–70% of cases begin before the age of 40.[5]

Stroke-like episodes are the fundamental findings seen in 84–99% of cases. These attacks are seen as recurrent aphasia, hemiparesis, cortical blindness, headaches, changes in mental status and seizures. The affected areas in neuroimaging may not correlate with classical vascular boundaries. The lesions are mostly asymmetric, and the posterior brain regions tend to be more affected than anterior. As lesions are restricted to the cortical regions, they can be seen in the subcortical regions and thalamus. Very rarely, cerebellar involvement has been reported in MELAS. Cranial MRI angiography findings are usually normal. Low levels of NAA (indicating neuronal loss) and high levels of lactate picks (indicate anaerobic metabolism) are determined in MR spectroscopic (MRS) examinations. MRS can be used to follow up on prognosis and response to the treatment. An increase in the lactate peak indicates a worse prognosis.[6]

Cognitive impairments are seen in 40–90% of cases, which may be due to cortical damage. The executive cognitive dysfunctions in MELAS patients are not only due to regional involvement of the frontal cortex, but diffuse neurodegenerative impairment of the brain also implies cognitive dysfunction.

Epilepsy is one of the most frequently seen neurological findings in MELAS patients. Focal and generalized seizures can be seen. Seizures can occur alone or with stroke-like episodes. Controllable seizures in the early course of the disease become drug-resistant during the progress of the disease.[7]

Migrainous headaches are seen rather frequently in MELAS patients and can even be initial symptoms. Headaches may be accompanied by stroke-like episodes and can be more severe.

Peripheral neuropathy, sensorineural hearing loss, ataxia, myoclonus, ophthalmoplegia, pigmentary retinopathy and calcification of basal ganglia can be accompanied by other more frequent findings.[8]

Myopathy characterized by proximal muscle involvement is seen in 87–90% of MELAS cases. Exercise intolerance and easy fatiguability are very common. Lactic acid levels in the serum increase with exercise and stress. Histologic examination of muscle tissue from a patient with MELAS syndrome shows scattered vacuolated muscle fibers with an obvious surrounding rim using hematoxylin and eosin (H&E) staining. Using the Gomori trichrome stain, RRFs can indicate mitochondrial proliferation below the plasma membrane of the muscle fibers, causing the outline to become uneven. These proliferated mitochondria in RRFs also strongly stain with succinate dehydrogenase (SDH) stain giving the appearance of ragged blue fibers.[9]

Lactic acidemia is another major finding and is seen in 94% of affected cases, but is not specific for MELAS. The level of CSF lactate is also high.

Cardiomyopathy is an important finding in 18–30% of the cases. Both hypertrophic and dilated cardiomyopathies can be seen; most common is non-obstructive concentric hypertrophy. Cardiac conduction abnormalities are seen, especially Wolf–Parkinson–White syndrome.

Endocrine disorders are also seen in MELAS cases, usually diabetes mellitus or growth hormone deficiency. Growth hormone deficiency can be responsible for short stature.

Gastrointestinal complications such as recurrent vomiting and diarrhea, constipation, gastric dysmotility, pancreatitis and pseudo-obstruction are seen in MELAS patients.

Renal tubulopathies, focal segmental glomerulosclerosis, vitiligo and reticular pigmentation are rarely seen.

The pathogenesis of this disease has not been determined but many hypotheses have been put forward, including microvascular angiopathies, disrupted mitochondrial energy production and nitric oxide deficiency. The mutations found in MELAS affect complexes 1, 2 and 3 and the production of energy is disrupted. Dysfunction of ATP production leads to multiorgan failure. The reduced energy production negatively affects arginine and citrulline production from nitric oxide (NO), causing endothelial dysfunction, which is one of the major causes of vasculopathy. Finally, ischemic damage occurs causing stroke-like episodes.[10]

There is currently no disease-specific treatment for MELAS. With a multidisciplinary approach, intermittent, frequent follow-up and symptomatic treatment must be applied.

L-arginine is effective in the protective and preventive treatment of stroke-like episodes. L-arginine is a semi-essential amino acid and a precursor of NO. In the acute period, arginine has the effect of fast correction of neurological findings and in the interictal period, it lessens the severity and frequency of the attacks. As with arginine, citrulline is also effective in boosting the production of NO.[11]

Coenzyme Q10 treatment is effective for eye and cardiac involvement in MELAS cases. Idebenone is an analog of coenzyme Q10, and is more effective as it easily passes through the blood–brain barrier.[12]

L-carnitine is involved in transportation of fatty acids into the mitochondrial matrix, hence its use in the treatment of MELAS. Additionally, creatine, cytochrome C, menadione (vitamin K3), antioxidants and vitamins C, B1, B2 and B3 can be effective.[13]

Avoiding certain drugs that can cause mitochondrial dysfunction is an important part of the management of MELAS patients, valproic acid being one of the most important, but zonisamide, topiramate, ethosuximide, oxcarbazepine, carbamazepine, gabapentin, vigabatrin, phenobarbital should also be used very carefully. Nowadays, lacosamide is a recommended treatment for refractory epileptic seizures and perampanel for status epilepticus.[14]

# References

1. El-Hattab AW, Adesina AM, Jones J, Scaglia F. MELAS syndrome: Clinical manifestations, pathogenesis, and treatment options. *Mol Genet Metab.* 2015;**116**: 4–12.

2. Finsterer J, Wakil SM. Stroke-like episodes, peri-episodic seizures, and MELAS mutations. *Eur J Paediatr Neurol.* 2016;**30**: 1–6.

3. Hirano M, Ricci E, Koenigsberger MR, et al. MELAS: An original case and clinical criteria for diagnosis. *Neuromuscul Dis.* 1992;**2**(2): 125–135.

4. Hsu YHR, Yogasundara H, Parajuli N, et al. MELAS Syndrome and cardiomyopathy: Linking mitochondrial function to heart failure pathogenesis. *Heart Fail Rev.* 2016;**21**(1): 103–116.

5. Ito H, Mori K, Kagami S. Neuroimaging of stroke-like episodes in MELAS. *Brain Dev.* 2011;**33**: 283–288.

6. Koening MK, Emrick L, Karaa A, et al. Recommendations for the management of strokelike episodes in patients with mitochondrial encephalomyopathy, lactic acidosis, and strokelike episodes. *JAMA Neurol.* 2016;**73**(5): 591–594.

7. Lee S, Oh DA, Bae EK. Fixation-off sensitivity in mitochondrial encephalomyopathy, lactic acidosis, and stroke-like episodes (MELAS) syndrome. *Seizure.* 2019;**64**: 6–7.

8. Rimiano G, Vollono C, Dono F, Servidei S. Drug-resistant epilepsy in MELAS: Safety and potential efficacy of lacosamide. *Epilepsy Res.* 2018;**139**: 135–136.

9. Santa KM. Treatment options for mitochondrial myopathy, encephalopathy, lactic acidosis, and stroke-like episodes (MELAS) syndrome. *Pharmacotherapy.* 2010;**30**(11): 1179–1196.

10. Yatsuga S, Povalko N, Nishioka J, et al. MELAS: A nationwide prospective cohort study of 96 patients in Japan. *Biochim Biophys Acta.* 2012;**1820**(5): 619–624.

11. Hovsepain DA, Galat A, Chong RA, et al. MELAS: Monitoring treatment with magnetic resonance spectroscopy. *Acta Neurol Scand.* 2019;**139**(1): 82–85.

12. Malhotra K, Liebeskind DS. Imaging of MELAS. *Curr Pain Headache Rep.* 2016;**20**: 54.

13. Muramatsu D, Yamaguchi H, Iwasa K, Yamada M. Cerebellar hyperintensity lesions on diffusion-weighted MRI in MELAS. *Intern Med.* 2019;**58**(12): 1797–1798.

14. Santamarina E, Alpuente A, Maisterra O, et al. Perampanel: A therapeutic alternative in refractory status epilepticus associated with MELAS syndrome. *Epilepsy Behav Case Rep.* 2019;**11**: 92–95.

# 5.3.c Menkes Disease

Linda Azevedo Kauppila, Mariana Fonseca,
Ana Catarina Fonseca

## Case Presentation

A 4-month-old, male infant was admitted due to right focal motor seizures with secondary generalization. He was the first-born of a 32-year-old primigravida mother of Australian origin. He had been born at term. Pregnancy, labor and delivery were unremarkable. His focal motor seizures had started during the morning. He had had four episodes, over two hours prior to admission. Phenobarbital and valproic acid were given to control the seizures, with effect. On examination, he was responsive to stimulation but irritable. He had pale skin, a depressed nasal bridge and micrognathia. Also of note, he had very sparse hair, which was lightly pigmented and curly. He had spontaneous eye opening, blinked to bright light, but did not fix or follow. He occasionally reacted to noise and a poor suck reflex was noted. He had a spastic tonus in all extremities and bilateral hyper-reflexes with clonus at the ankles. He also had bilateral extensor Babinski responses. Brain magnetic resonance imaging (MRI) showed increased signal in the head of the left caudate on a diffusion-weighted sequence (DWI) suggesting infarction. The T2-weighted images showed white matter changes suggestive of mildly delayed myelination. A brain MRI angiogram revealed tortuous and irregular intracranial vessels. The serum copper level was 8 mg/dl (normal 85–150), and ceruloplasmin was 5 mg/dl (normal 25–63). The diagnosis of Menkes disease (MD) was confirmed by an elevated ratio of dihydroxyphenylalanine to dihydroxyphenylglycol. Electron microscopy of the hair showed typical changes of pili torti. Intramuscular copper-histidine therapy was initiated. The brain MRI was repeated three months later and presented new DWI signal abnormalities in the right striatum.

## Diagnostic Algorithm

### Clinically suspicious of Menkes disease

Age: infant; Gender: X-linked recessive trait, mainly males

Clinical manifestations: classical MD is the most severe form

Classic MD – Diagnosis usually three to six months of age, mostly due to "kinky hair." May also have depressed nasal bridge, pale skin, frontal or occipital bossing, micrognathia, chubby or sagging cheeks, expressionless appearance

Seizures may be the presenting symptom for stroke

Seizures are, frequently, a clinical manifestation of stroke

**Brain MRI –** Both hemorrhagic and ischemic stroke have been reported. Bilateral ischemic lesions in deep grey matter, or in the cortical areas.

Other possible findings: subdural hematomas and hygromas, cerebral white matter changes, diffuse symmetrical cerebral and cerebellar atrophy, defective myelination and ventriculomegaly

**AngioMRI –** Marked intracranial vessels irregularity and tortuosity

### Confirm diagnosis

Reduced serum copper and ceruloplasmin levels

In the neonatal period, plasma catecholamine analysis (ratio of dihydroxyphenylalanine (DOPA) to dihydroxyphenylglycol) indicative of dopamine β-hydroxylase deficiency

Final diagnostic test for MD is the establishment of a molecular defect in *ATP7A*

### Treatment

There is no cure available, but early copper-histidine treatment may help some of the neurological symptoms

Antithrombotic therapy may be considered, but it is unclear if it slows down neurologic worsening

# Discussion

Menkes disease (MD) is a rare and lethal infantile neurodegenerative multisystemic disorder of copper metabolism, inherited as an X-linked recessive trait.[1] In classic MD, patients have a serious clinical progression, with death in early childhood.[1] There are, however, less severe forms of MD: mild MD and occipital horn syndrome (OHS).[1,5] The incidence of MD is estimated to be 1 in 300,000 to 360,000,[1,4] with higher incidences reported in Australia.[1] Most patients are male. The females who have been described mostly have an X:autosome translocation, where the normal X-chromosome is preferentially inactivated.[1] MD occurs due to mutations in the *ATP7A* gene.[3] Most of these are intragenic mutations (missense, nonsense and splice-site mutations) or partial gene deletions; insertions and duplications have also been described.[1] About half of the point mutations are truncating mutations, which typically result in a non-functional truncated protein.[1] This gene encodes an energy-dependent transmembrane protein, involved in delivering copper to secreted copper enzymes and in the export of surplus copper from cells.[4] Copper is necessary for normal function of several copper enzymes that participate in important metabolic processes, such as cellular respiration, neurotransmitter biosynthesis, maturation of hormones, free-radical scavenging, cross-linking of elastin, collagen and keratin, melanin production and iron homeostasis.[1] Copper is also involved in myelination, regulation of the circadian rhythm and is required for coagulation and angiogenesis.[1] *ATP7A* is expressed in almost every organ except the liver, where *ATP7B* is predominantly expressed.[1] MD is therefore a systemic disorder.[1] Copper-dependent enzyme dysfunction causes the phenotypic findings in MD.[2] Almost all tissues will present abnormal copper levels, including low levels of cooper in the brain and liver.[1,5] In MD, copper is likely to be detained at the blood–brain barrier and the blood–cerebrospinal fluid barrier, while neurons and glial cells are copper deprived.[2]

Classical MD patients usually die before the age of three.[1] Diagnosis usually occurs at three to six months of age, mostly due to the presence of "kinky hair."[1] Clinical abnormalities may be absent or less obvious in neonates,[3,5] which makes diagnosis more difficult before two months of age, when copper deficiency becomes advanced.[3] There are usually no complications during pregnancy.[1] Premature labor and delivery may occur, but most males are born at term with suitable birth measurements.[1] Cephalohematomas and spontaneous fractures have been observed on neonates.[1,3,5] In the early neonatal period, prolonged jaundice, hypothermia, hypoglycemia and feeding difficulties may occur.[1,5] Pectus excavatum, skin laxity, and umbilical and inguinal hernias have also been described.[1,5] The first sign of MD may be the so-called "kinky hair,"[1,2] singular, sparse and matted scalp hair which resembles wool, becoming knotted on the top of the head, usually by two months of age.[1] There may also be a depressed nasal bridge,[5] pale skin, frontal or occipital bossing, micrognatia,[1] chubby or sagging cheeks, and an expressionless appearance.[1,5]

Hyperextensive joints, skin laxity and xerosis may be noticed very early on.[1,3] Seborrheic dermatitis is also a common characteristic. There is developmental regression,[1–5] which becomes more noticeable around five to six months of age.[1] Patients may develop seizures,[3] including refractory epilepsy, most commonly after three months of age.[1] Initial hypotonia is replaced by spasticity, and infants become much more limited in their motor abilities.[1] Routine ophthalmoscopy is typically normal,[1] but optic discs may be pale[5]; later on, patients often fail to follow visual stimulus, and blindness may occur.[1] The progression is typically relentless, but the speed of neurologic deterioration differs.[5] There are recurrent infections of the respiratory and urinary tracts.[5] Sepsis and meningitis are common, as well as subdural hematomas and stroke.[5] Classic MD progresses to severe neurodegeneration and death between seven months and three and a half years.[5] Mild MD patients have better psycho-motor development with autonomous walking and maintained language skills.[5] They may have muscular weakness, tremor, ataxia and head titubation, with mild intellectual disability.[5] Connective tissue symptoms may be more prominent than in classic MD, and include tortuous blood vessels and pili torti (twisted hair).[5] Life expectancy is higher than in classic MD.[5] OHS is the mildest form of MD, and its main clinical aspects concern connective tissue, including lax skin and joints.[1,5] The main characteristic is occipital horns on brain imaging.[1] These are symmetric exostoses, wedge-shaped calcifications, protruding from the occipital bone.[1,5] OHS usually presents in the school-aged child,[5] and diagnosis is normally made only around five to ten years of age.[1] Vascular anomalies, such as varicose veins, are common and arterial aneurysms have also been described.[1] No apparent correlation between genotype and MD phenotype has been definitively established.[1] This is emphasized by inter- and intrafamilial phenotypic variability in MD/OHS patients with the same *ATP7A* mutation.[1] Normally, patients with a milder phenotype (such as OHS) have a higher proportion of mutations, leading to a moderately functional protein or reduced amounts of normal protein.[1] Initial MD diagnosis is indicated by clinical features, namely, the distinctive hair, and supported by reduced serum copper and cerulo-plasmin levels.[1,2,4] Interpretation of these laboratory changes is more difficult in the neonatal period, since they may exist in healthy individuals.[1] In this period, plasma catecholamine analysis (ratio of DOPA to dihydroxyphenylglycol) indicative of dopamine β-hydroxylase deficiency might be preferred as a rapid diagnostic test.[1,5]

A definitive biochemical test for MD exists and is based on intracellular copper accumulation due to impaired efflux.[1] Accumulation is evaluated in cultured cells, mostly fibroblasts, by measuring radioactive copper retention.[1] The final diagnostic test of MD is the establishment of a molecular defect in *ATP7A*.[1] Diagnosis is most often determined in a proband by detection of a hemizygous *ATP7A* pathogenic variant in a male or a heterozygous *ATP7A* pathogenic variant in a female, with over 282 known mutations.[5] Other laboratory investigations such as arteriography, computed tomography and magnetic resonance imaging are useful in detecting different clinical features of MD. MRI is the brain imaging modality of choice.[4] Neuroimaging reports have shown several abnormalities. Both hemorrhagic and ischemic stroke have been reported. Other findings include hygromas, cerebral white matter changes,[2] diffuse symmetrical cerebral and cerebellar atrophy,[4] ventriculomegaly[5] and marked intracranial vessel tortuosity. Bilateral ischemic lesions in deep gray matter, or in the cortical areas, as a consequence of brain infarcts have been documented.[2] These patients have vasculopathy, with tortuous morphology of cerebral arteries,[2] reflecting connective tissue changes,[3] which may predispose to intracranial hemorrhage.[2] Sudden and massive cerebral hemorrhages due to vascular rupture have been described.[1,5] Subdural hematomas may also occur. Tortuous extracranial vessels have been reported.[4,5] Comparable changes are observed in the systemic vasculature,[5] and aneurysms are not uncommon.[5] They can involve the internal jugular vein, and the brachial, lumbar and iliac arteries.[5] Lysyl oxidase is a copper-dependent enzyme implicated in collagen and elastin cross-linking and vascular architecture formation. Dysfunction of this protein in MD leads to anomalous vessel structure and tortuosity.[2] Pathologic examination in MD shows fragmentation of the internal elastic lamina of the arteries, irregular vessel-wall thickness, and variation in the lumen of the arteries, resulting in erratic and turbulent blood flow, predisposing vessels to thrombotic occlusion and artery-to-artery embolism with ensuing cerebral infarction.[2,5] Increased tortuosity of the main cerebral arteries can result in distortion and occlusion of small perforating arteries, even in the absence of overt arterial stenosis.[7] A convergence of many detrimental mechanisms may contribute to infarctions of deep gray matter, including dysfunctional copper-zinc superoxide dismutase that leads to cytotoxic effects and neuronal damage, susceptibility to free-radical attack and inadequate energy supply from oxidative phosphorylation.[2] The pathophysiologic mechanism responsible for neurodegeneration is unknown, but is probably related to the impairment of copper-dependent enzymes and their role in neuronal function and vascular architecture.[2] Presently, no treatment successfully delays the neurodegeneration of MD,[2] but early diagnosis and timely start of treatment is essential.[3] MD treatment is mostly symptomatic. The goal is to offer surplus copper to tissues and copper-dependent enzymes.[1] Trials of copper and copper compounds have had inconsistent success, most likely because the defect in intracellular copper transport cannot be overcome by copper replacement therapy alone.[2] Because copper is not absorbed intestinally, it is mandatory to give it parenterally or subcutaneously.[1,5] Copper-histidine has proven to be most effective, but its positive outcome depends on timely initiation and the existence of at least partially functional *ATP7A*.[1] Well-timed parenteral copper-histidine supplementation may alter disease progression considerably.[1] Infants who started subcutaneous injections of copper-histidine as newborns had better neurologic outcome and some had normal development.[6] Infarction due to cerebral vasculopathy can be important in this matter. Antithrombotic therapy may be considered,[2] but it is unclear whether this therapy may help slow down neurologic worsening.[2] Anticoagulation may further increase the risk of intracerebral hemorrhage in these patients.[2] Concerning vessel tortuosity and irregularities, which are attributed to the decreased activity of lysyl oxidase, subcutaneous copper-histidine therapy will not ameliorate its activity because administered copper is not transported to the Golgi apparatus, where the enzyme combines with copper in order to function.[3]

# References

1. Tümer Z, Moller LB. Menkes disease. *Eur J Human Genetics* 2010;**18**: 511–518.

2. Hsich GE, Robertson RL, Irons M, Soul JS, du Plessis AJ. Cerebral infarction in Menkes' disease. *Pediatr Neurol.* 2000;**23**: 425–428.

3. Kobayashi S, Yokoi K, Kamioka N, et al. A severe case of Menkes disease with repeated bone fracture during the neonatal period, followed by multiple arterial occlusion. *Brain Dev.* 2019;**41**: 878–882.

4. Rangarh P, Kohli N. Neuroimaging findings in Menkes disease: A rare neurodegenerative disorder. *BMJ Case Rep.* 2018;**2018**: bcr2017223858.

5. Lehwald LM, Menkes JH. Menkes disease. In: Caplan L, Biller J. (Eds). *Uncommon Causes of Stroke.* Cambridge: Cambridge University Press; 2018. 250–254.

6. Kaler SG, Holmes CS, Goldstein DS, et al. Neonatal diagnosis and treatment of Menkes disease. *N Engl J Med.* 2008;**358**: 605–614.

7. Manara R, Rocco MC, D'agata L, et al. Neuroimaging changes in Menkes disease, part 2. *Am J Neuroradiol.* 2017;**38**: 1858–1865.

# 5.3.d Tangier Disease

Fatih Süheyl Ezgü

## Case Presentation

A 17-year-old female patient presented to the emergency room with sudden onset left-sided significant weakness accompanied by a severe headache. The medical history was unremarkable except for having frequent upper respiratory tract infections in the past. The family history was significant for several family members having early-onset ischemic heart disease. The parents were first cousins.

The neurological examination revealed mildly impaired consciousness. The nasolabial sulcus on the left side was shallow and there was significant weakness of the left upper and lower limbs. The deep tendon reflexes were normal and there was no pathological reflex.

Also during the physical examination the patient was noted to have yellow-orange colored tonsils, mild hepatomegaly in addition to splenomegaly, and axillar and inguinal bilateral enlarged lymph nodes.

Laboratory examinations revealed alanine aminotransferase 52 IU/l (normal 0–35), aspartate aminotransferase 48 IU/l (normal 0–35), low-density lipoprotein cholesterol (LDL-C) 128 mg/dl (normal <130), high-density lipoprotein cholesterol (HDL-C) 8mg/dl (normal > 40), total cholesterol (TC) 148 (normal <200) and platelets 142,000/mm$^3$ (normal 166,000–308,000). The C-reactive protein, erythrocyte sedimentation rate, uric acid, creatine kinase, lactate dehydrogenase, blood urea nitrogen and creatinine, hemoglobin, white blood cells, coagulation tests, urinalysis, humoral immune series, antineutrophil cytoplasmic antibody and anticardiolipin antibodies were all in the normal range.

Brain magnetic resonance imaging (MRI) was consistent with ischemic stroke in addition to minimal intraparenchymal bleeding. Digital subtraction cerebral angiography showed stenosis of the right internal carotid artery.

The patient was hospitalized and started on intensive treatment for stroke. With the clinical signs and symptoms, Tangier disease was suspected and DNA sequence analysis for the *ABCA1* gene coding for adenosine triphosphate (ATP) binding cassette transporter A1 (ABCA1) was requested, which revealed a homozygous previously defined mutation confirming the disorder.

### Clinical suspicion of Tangier disease

(a) Enlarged tonsils that are yellow and/or orange in children and young adults

(b) Peripheral neuropathy

(c) Hepatomegaly and/or splenomegaly

(cont.)

### Clinical suspicion of Tangier disease

(d) Hypersplenism (Thrombocytopenia)

(e) Corneal opacities

(f) Premature atherosclerosis (coronary artery disease, stroke)

(g) Lymphadenopathy

### Laboratory investigations

(a) Very low plasma HDL-C, typically <5 mg/dl (0.125 mmol/L), rarely 5–10 mg/dl

(b) Very low or absent apolipoprotein A-I concentration, usually <30 mg/dl (typically <5 mg/dl)

(c) Small or absent alpha band on lipoprotein electrophoresis

(d) Low plasma total cholesterol concentration, typically <150 mg/dl (4 mmol/l)

(e) Mild-to-moderate hypertriglyceridemia, up to 400 mg/dl (4.5 mmol/l)

(f) Decreased LDL-C concentration

### Confirmatory tests

DNA sequencing (90%) or deletion and duplication analysis (10%) of *ABCA1* gene

### Differential diagnosis of stroke or stroke-like episodes in inborn errors of metabolism

| | | |
|---|---|---|
| Urea cycle defects | Organic acidurias | Mitochondrial disorders (MELAS) |
| Homocystinurias | Fabry disease | Congenital defects of glycosylation (CDG) |

### Laboratory approach to differential diagnosis

Plasma and urine amino acids, acylcarnitines, urinary organic acids, blood lactic acid, pyruvic acid, ammonia, isoelectric transfocusing, enzyme assay, molecular genetic testing

### Treatment

Specific effective therapies are lacking

Atherosclerosis and cerebral infarction

- anti-platelet aggregation and statins
- improvement in the lifestyle (including weight loss, low-fat diet, increased physical activities, and smoking cessation)

Most recent medications used in few cases

- Cholesterol ester transfer protein (CETP) inhibitors
- Miglustat

# Discussion

HDL-C is synthesized in the liver and small intestine and is mainly formed by apolipoprotein A-I (ApoA-I) and apolipoprotein A-II (ApoA-II). The newly secreted ApoA-I must acquire cholesterol or phospholipids in order to form pre-βHDL. This step is mediated by ATP binding cassette transporter A1 (ABCA1).

Tangier disease is caused by mutations in the *ABCA1* gene that codes for ABCA1 transporter and is characterized by severe deficiency or absence of HDL-C in the circulation, which results in accumulation of cholesteryl esters throughout the body, particularly in the reticuloendothelial system.

The clinical signs and symptoms include hyperplastic yellow-orange tonsils, hepatomegaly and splenomegaly and peripheral neuropathy, as well as more rare complications such as corneal opacities and premature atherosclerotic coronary artery disease (ASCVD) and hematologic manifestations, such as thrombocytopenia, reticulocytosis, stomatocytosis or hemolytic anemia.[1]

It has previously been shown that monogenic diseases resulting in deficiency in HDL cause ASCVD. Tangier homozygous patients are said to have four- to sixfold increased risk for ASVD compared to age-matched controls. In heterozygotes the prevalence of cardiovascular disease is 60% higher than unaffected relatives. Tangier disease has also been shown to cause central nervous system (CNS) ischemia, stroke and sometimes bleeding. Even heterozygotes for *ABCA1* mutations were shown to have increased carotid intima-media thickness. In addition, platelet abnormalities, including thrombocytopenia, a mild bleeding tendency, altered platelet morphology and impaired platelet function, which have been reported in Tangier disease, might contribute to bleeding in the CNS.[2]

Serfaty-Lacrosniere et al. reviewed published clinical information on 51 cases of homozygous Tangier disease, reported three new cases and provided autopsy information on three cases and controls for atherosclerotic involvement. CVD was observed in 20% of Tangier patients vs 5% of controls (p< 0.05), and in those that were between 35 and 65 years of age, 44% (11 of 25) had evidence of CVD (either angina, myocardial infarction or stroke) vs 6.5% in 1533 male controls and 3.2% in 1597 female controls in this age group (p< 0.01). Of the nine patients who died, two died because of stroke at ages 56 and 69.[3]

Currently, specific effective therapies are lacking for Tangier disease. Patients with atherosclerosis and cerebral infarction can be treated with antiplatelet aggregation and statins, lipid-lowering stable plaques and other comprehensive treatments, while improving lifestyle (including weight loss, low-fat diet, increased physical activity and smoking cessation) to improve the prognosis. CETP inhibitors that increase HDL levels have been used for confirmed patients, but long-term data showing their effect on prognosis is lacking.[2]

Miglustat (Zavesca) is a small-molecule inhibitor of glycosphingolipid biosynthesis used to treat the progressive neurological symptoms of the lysosomal disease Niemann-Pick disease type C (NPC). A patient with Tangier disease was misdiagnosed with NPC, treated with miglustat and her neurological symptoms and skin lesions improved. Low HDL-C concentrations and reduced ABCA1 protein expression are seen in NPC, postulated to be due to accumulation of glycosphingolipids. Miglustat treatment of fibroblasts in Tangier patients resulted in reduced relative lysosomal volume and normalization of glycosphingolipid levels.[4]

Tangier disease should always be considered in the differential for patients with chronic inflammatory demyelinating polyneuropathy, premature myocardial infarction or stroke, especially in the presence of hepatosplenomegaly, thrombocytopenia, anemia, gastrointestinal problems and corneal opacities.

## References

1. Burnett JR, Hooper AJ, McCormick SPA, et al. Tangier disease. 2019 Nov 21. In: *GeneReviews®[Internet]*. (Adam MP, Ardinger HH, Pagon RA, et al., Eds): Seattle (WA): University of Washington, Seattle, 1993–2020.

2. Hooper AJ, Hegele RA, Burnett JR. Tangier disease: Update for 2020. *Curr Opin Lipidol.* 2020;**31**: 80–84.

3. Serfaty-Lacrosniere C, Civeira F, Lanzberg A, et al. Homozygous Tangier disease and cardiovascular disease. *Atherosclerosis.* 1994;**107**: 85–98.

4. Sechi A, Dardis A, Zampieri S, et al. Effects of miglustat treatment in a patient affected by an atypical form of Tangier disease. *Orphanet J Rare Dis.* 2014;**9**: 143.

# 5.3.e Organic Acid Disorders

Cristina Tiu, Vlad Eugen Tiu, Elena Oana
Terecoasă

## Case Presentation

An 8-month-old male infant was brought to the ER by his parents because they had noticed that despite the fact he ate enough he had not gained weight in the past month and in the last 24 hours he had vomited several times. The laboratory work-up revealed metabolic acidosis, and thrombocytopenia, so he was admitted to hospital and scheduled for a more extensive work-up over the next few days.

The next day the patient became drowsy, developed hypotonia and blood analysis showed a mild hyperammonemia. A metabolic disorder was suspected and a dried blood spot exam was performed for acylcarnitine, followed by a mass spectrometry analysis to search for an enzymatic defect. A deficiency of glutaryl-coenzyme A (CoA)- dehydrogenase (GCDH) helped to establish the diagnosis of glutaric aciduria type I.

The patient received an intravenous dextrose in saline solution infusion and parenteral solutions containing lipids, with a quick improvement in his general status and lab analysis.

He was discharged with the recommendation of protein restriction (maximum 0.8 g/kg body weight). The parents were instructed to avoid giving their child food that contain the amino acids that were deficiently metabolized (lysine, hydroxylysine, tryptophan) such as whole milk, red meat, parmesan or soy beans, and to ask for medical advice for any new symptom or fever. Doctors also recommended adding dietary supplements of L-carnitine (100 mg/kg body weight). The patient was scheduled for a monitoring visit after six months.

The evolution was good, the patient gained weight and had normal development. At the age of three, he caught a cold, started to cough and developed a fever of 39 °C. He was promptly brought to the hospital. At the ER, he vomited and had a seizure. Postictal he remained lethargic, and in the following hours developed dystonic movements in his right limbs. The brain MRI revealed a hyperintense signal in the left basal ganglia on diffusion-weighted imaging (DWI) and fluid-attenuated inversion recovery (FLAIR) sequences and a right temporal arachnoid cyst. Metabolic stroke was diagnosed. He received antibiotics for the infection, natural protein intake was ceased for several days, he received dextrose and the daily intake of L-carnitine was doubled.

After this episode he developed a dystonic posture and spasticity, which were partially ameliorated by baclofen. He did not have another episode. He was more closely monitored for serum levels of L-carnitine, every three months, and for complete blood count, ferritin, transaminases, calcium phosphate, alkaline phosphatase (for bone status) every six months.

1. Newborn baby: usually acute/subacute onset (screening may depict OAD in asymptomatic phase)
2. Childhood: slowly progressive, more rare

**General**

**Failure to thrive, vomiting** poor feeding, developmental delay

**Neurological**

**Encephalopathy, seizures,** ataxia, choreoathetosis, dystonia, dyskinesia, hypotonia, lethargy, coma

**Other**

Osteoporosis, osteomalacia, liver diseases

**Laboratory:** Metabolic acidosis, elevated anion gap, hyperammonemia, neutropenia, thrombocytopenia

**Acylcarnitines in dried blood spot**

**Organic acids in blood and urine**

**Enzyme activity analysis**

**GA1**- GCDH
**PA**- PCC
**MMA**- MCM, AdoCbl, MCE

**Genetic analysis**

**GA1**- GCDH mutations (cz. 19p13.2)
**PA**- PCC *A* mutations (cz. 13), PCC *B* cz. 3)
**MMA**- MUT mutations Cz. 6p21, AdoCbl mutations cz. 1p34.1(cblC), cz. 4q31(cblA), cz. 12q24.1 (cblB), MCE mutations cz. 2p13.3

**Acute metabolic stroke**
**T2, FLAIR:** hyperintense signal in BG (globus pallidus more affected in GA1 and MMA)
**DWI (BG):** DWI ↑, ADC ↓
**MRS:** NAA ↓, Lactate ↑, Glutamate ↑, Choline ↑

*Subdural hematoma* in GA1

**Chronic metabolic stroke**
**Structural MRI:** Necrosis of BG, macrocephaly, temporal arachnoid cysts, enlarged sylvian fissure (GA1), brainstemand corpuscallosum atrophy (MMA)
**DTI:** FA ↓ in frontal, temporal and occipital white matter

**Prevention of acute decompensation**
**Protein allowance 0.8 g/kg b.w.**
Prefer natural sources to special AAdf supplements of L-carnitine
Supplements of B12 in vitB12-responsive MMA
**Do not give aspirin** in isovaleric aciduria
**Monitor closely** in case of acute infectious illnesses, surgery, immunization or other events which accelerate catabolism

**Acute decompensation**

Should be suspected in the presence of fever, vomiting or diarrhea
**Infections – antibiotics** promptly
**Sufficient caloric intake**
IV dextrose in saline solution
Correction of electrolytes
Parenteral solutions containing lipids
**Ammonia scavengers**
(N-carbamyl glutamate, sodium phenylacetate-sodium glutamate)

**Chronic monitoring**
**Routine lab analysis**
(every six months)
**ECG, ETT** once/year (PA)
Ophtalmological+ renal evaluation (PA, MMA)
DXA after the age of five years
**Neurologic monitoring** for
- spasticity
- movement disorders
- epilepsy, cognition

*Liver or kidney transplant –* can stabilize the patient but cannot always prevent stroke

OAD- organic acid disorders, BG- basal ganglia, IV- intravenous, MRI- magnetic resonance imaging, DWI- diffusion weighted imaging, DTI- diffusion tensor imaging, FA- fractional anisotpy, MRS- magnetic resonance spectroscopy, kg b.w.- kilograms body weight, AAdf- aminoacids deficient formulas. ECG- electrocardiogram, ETT- transthoracic echocardiography, DXA- osteo-densitometry

# Discussion

Organic acid disorders belong to the group inborn errors of metabolism (IEM) caused by enzymatic or transport protein defects in the metabolic pathways of amino acids, lipids or carbohydrates. These disorders lead to an energetic failure due to insufficient "fuel" for the Krebs cycle and an accumulation of intermediate metabolites with a deleterious effect on different organs, including the nervous system. They are called organic acidemias or acidurias (OAs) and their incidence ranges from 1 in 1,000,000 to 1 in 10,000 live births.[1] All OAs have two main evolutive forms: clinical onset during the neonatal period (most frequent) and forms which progress slowly, and onset in childhood (depending on the residual activity of the affected enzyme). With the extension of newborn screening there is an increasing number of cases diagnosed in an asymptomatic phase. There are several clinical signs that must raise suspicion of OAs (see Table 5.3.1), and also distinctive features of each disease, but the diagnosis ultimately requires a genetic or enzymatic analysis. All OAs are inherited following an autosomal recessive pattern, except 3-methylglutaconic aciduria type 2 (Barth syndrome) and a subtype of methylmalonic aciduria (cblIX), which have X-linked inheritance.[2] The risk of infantile mortality and neurological sequelae is high if acute metabolic decompensations occur, precipitated by infections, prolonged fasting, surgery or other stressful situations.

Stroke related to OAs belongs to the *metabolic stroke* category for glutaric, isovaleric, methylmalonic (MMA) and propionic acidurias (PA) and is *related to clot formation* in the dilated cardiac chambers and *to infections* facilitated by neutropenia, in Barth syndrome.[3]

# Diagnosis

Since early diagnosis and adequate therapy can avoid a severe clinical course, some countries have introduced newborn screening for OAs, especially in high-risk communities, where the percentage of consanguinity is elevated (areas in the USA, Canada, countries in the Middle East). When screening is not available, diagnostic procedures are initiated when clinical suspicion is raised, usually the first step being tandem mass spectrometry on a dried blood spot for detection of acylcarnitines, followed by detection of the organic acids in body fluids (urine preferred) – see Table 5.3.2. An algorithm proposed by a panel of experts,[4] details the diagnostic work-up which is needed to confirm positive newborn screening for GA1: determination of C5DC in a dried blood spot, quantitative analysis of glutaric acid (GA) and 3-OH-GA in blood and urine, mutation analysis and if available, enzyme analysis in cultured fibroblasts, but the methods recommended are different according to the high

**Table 5.3 1** Features that raise suspicion of OA[2]

| General | Neurological | Laboratory | Other |
| --- | --- | --- | --- |
| **Failure to thrive** | **Encephalopathy** | **Metabolic acidosis** | Osteoporosis |
| **Vomiting** | **Seizures** | **Elevated anion gap** | Osteomalacia |
| Poor feeding | Ataxia | Hyperammonemia | Liver disease |
| Developmental delay | Hypotonia | Neutropenia | |
| | Lethargy | Thrombocytopenia | |
| | Coma | | |

**Table 5.3.2** Laboratory and genetic diagnosis of organic acidurias

| OAs and affected metabolism of: | MS/MS of dried blood spot | GC/MS of blood | GS/MS of urine | Enzyme activity analysis | Genetic analysis | Diagnostic confirmation |
|---|---|---|---|---|---|---|
| GA1 / Lysine / HO-lysine / Tryptophan | Acylcarnitines (C5DC) | Glutaric acid / 3-OH- GA / Glutaconic acid | | GCDH | GCDH mutations (cz. 19p13.2) | Enzyme analysis / or / two disease-causing mutations |
| PA / Valine / Odd fatty acids / Methionine / Isoleucine / Threonine | Acylcarnitines | Propionyl-carnitine 2 / Glycine (↑) / Methionine | Propionic acid / 3-OH-propionic acid / Methyl citric acid / Propionyl glycine | PCC | PCC A mutations cz. 13 / PCC B mutations cz. 3 | Detection of mutations in PCCA or PCCB |
| MMA / Valine / Odd fatty acids / Methionine / Isoleucine / Threonine | Acylcarnitines | Methylmalonic acid / Glycine (↑) | Methylmalonic acid / Methylcitrate | MCM / AdoCbl / MCE | MUT mutations Cz. 6p21 (Mut°,Mut⁻) / AdoCbl mutations cz. 1p34.1(cblC) / cz. 4q31(cblA) / cz. 12q24.1 (cblB) / MCE mutations cz. 2p13.3 | Combined detection of high levels of acylcarnitines and organic acids in urine |

MS/MS = tandem mass spectrometry, GC/MS = gas chromatography/mass spectrometry, C5DC = glutarylcarnitine, GCDH = glutaryl-CoA-dehydrogenase, PCC = propionyl-CoA-carboxylase, MCM = methylmalonyl-CoA mutase, AdoCbl = adenosyl cobalamin, MCE = methylmalonil-CoA-epimerase

**Table 5.3.3** Imagistic diagnosis of organic acidurias

| OAs | Structural MRI | DWI (BG) | MR spectroscopy (BG) | DTI |
|---|---|---|---|---|
| Acute | Metabolic stroke: T2, FLAIR hyperintense signal in BG (globus pallidus more affected in GA1 and MMA) Subdural hematoma in GA1 | DWI↑ ADC↓ | NAA↓ Lactate↑ Glutamate↑ Choline↑ | |
| Chronic | Necrosis of BG Macrocephaly, temporal arachnoid cysts, enlarged sylvian fissure (GA1) Brainstem and corpus callosum atrophy (MMA) | | | FA ↓ in frontal, temporal and occipital white matter |

ADC = apparent diffusion coefficient, DT I= diffusion tensor imaging, FA = fractional anisotropy, BG = basal ganglia

(MS/MS methods) or low excretor phenotype (DNA-based methods; as MS/MS methods can give false negative results).

The laboratory work-up must include: full blood count (in order to detect infection or pancytopenia), blood glucose, urea, creatinine, transaminases, lactic acid, pH, bicarbonate and ammonia blood levels, blood culture and urine ketones.

*Brain imaging* is mandatory for the evaluation of patients presenting with acute neurological signs, but should not be used for routine monitoring. Acute changes can be reversible, but more often they are replaced by necrosis and gliosis (Table 5.3.3, Figure 5.3.10).

# Glutaric Aciduria type I (GA1)

## Clinical Presentation

An initial period of normal development, quickly followed by macrocephaly and the onset of neurological signs (the symptom-free interval is on average 12 months, range 6–36 months). The onset is frequently abrupt, and the acute signs and symptoms can be misinterpreted as encephalitis.[5] These encephalopathic crises are expected to occur until the

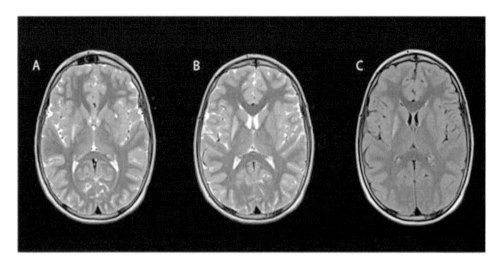

**Figure 5.3.10** Brain MRI. (A,B) Axial T2-weighted image (T2w) at basal ganglia level. (C) Axial FLAIR at basal ganglia level documenting the extent of the basal ganglia abnormalities.
*Reproduced with permission from Demailly D, Vianey-Saban C, Acquaviva C, et al. Atypical Glutaric Aciduria Type I with Hemidystonia and Asymmetric Radiological Findings Misdiagnosed as an Ischemic Stroke. Mov Disord Clin Pract. 2018;5(4):436-438. Published 2018 Jul 19. doi:10.1002/mdc3.12633*

age of six years and are associated with increased mortality and disability. In some patients, the neurological signs can have an insidious onset, without being preceded by an encephalopathic crisis. Macrocephaly is present in 75% of the cases, being highly suggestive for GA1, although it is not pathognomonic. Basal ganglia are always affected and the patients develop dystonia, dyskinesia, hypotonia, choreoathetosis (alone or in combination). Both ischemic and hemorrhagic strokes can occur in these patients, hemorrhages being mainly of venous origin. A particular problem is the presence of a subdural hemorrhage, which can lead to suspicion of shaken baby syndrome, sometimes creating legal issues for the parents.

## Pathophysiology

The mechanism of metabolic stroke in GA1 has been studied using several models, but it is still a matter of debate. According to Zinnanti,[6] if GCDH-deficient mice ($GCDH^{-/-}$) are fed with a diet rich in lysine and proteins, they accumulate high brain levels of glutaric (GA) and hydroxyglutaric acid (OH-GA) and subsequently develop hemorrhagic stroke, symptoms of encephalopathy and basal ganglia dysfunction. The consequences are age dependent, being more severe in younger mice (less than four weeks old) compared with adult mice (over eight weeks old). In this model the steps are as follows: (a) accumulated GA and 3-OH-GA lead to energetic failure of the $Na^+/K^+$ ATPase pump with development of neuronal cytotoxic edema, (b) the swollen neurons compress the neighboring capillaries, inducing hypoxia, which further aggravates the cytotoxic edema, (c) the compression of the capillaries leads to shunting of the blood to the veins, via non-exchange vessels, (d) the increased pressure in the venous drainage system leads to thalamic and striatal hemorrhage and vasogenic edema, (e) blood extravasation is also favored by the altered structure of the blood–brain barrier (BBB), with the loss of occludin in the tight junctions. Subdural hematoma and retinal hemorrhage are frequently seen in GA1. The striatum is particularly vulnerable, due to higher permeability of the BBB and an increased number of N-methyl-D-aspartate (NMDA) receptors. A role also seems to be played by the cortico-striatal glutamatergic projections, which expose the striatum to excitotoxicity. The relationship between cortical and striatal metabolic dysfunction needs further study, as certain experimental models show that cortical involvement precedes the striatal injury.[7]

In another model, consisting of a single direct intracisternal injection of GA in newborn rats, the leading role is given to pericytes and astrocytes, their structural and functional defects being responsible for the altered permeability of the BBB, in the absence of disruption of the tight junctions.[8]

## Methylmalonic Aciduria (MMA)

This organic aciduria can have multiple causes. More than half of patients will have a deficiency of methylmalonyl-CoA-mutase (MCM), a mitochondrial enzyme able to transform methylmalonyl-CoA to succinyl-CoA. MMA can be further classified, according to the residual enzyme activity, into Mut$^-$ (low level) and Mut° (enzyme non-detectable). Another cause of MMA can be deficiency of adenosylcobalamin (an essential cofactor for MCM); there are several subtypes determined by genetic defects on different chromosomes, which are usually responsive to vitamin B12 therapy. The Mut forms of MMA do not respond to vitamin B12 therapy. Apart from the laboratory analysis listed in Table 5.3.2, in MMA it is necessary to determine the blood level of homocysteine, which contributes to further identification of MMA subtypes.[9]

## Clinical Presentation

The onset is usual in the first few days of life, but it can also occur later on, in infancy, childhood or even adolescence [usually Mut$^-$ or cobalamin deficiencies type A (cbl A) or B (cbl B)]. Late onset patients have a median age at diagnosis of seven to nine months and can present with progressive tubular renal dysfunction or progressive neurological signs (tetraparesis, optic atrophy or movement disorders due to basal ganglia dysfunction). Metabolic strokes can be suspected if new abnormal movements occur or the patient develops significant acute changes in mental status and it can occur even in metabolically stable patients (MMA > PA).

## Propionic Aciduria

The clinical presentation does not differ from MMA, at least in the early onset type. In, late-onset PA, patients are more prone to cardiomyopathy due to secondary carnitine deficiency and to arrhythmias due to increased level of components of propionylcarnitine and prolonged QTc interval. PA can also have a purely neurological presentation.

## Principles of Treatment

### Prevention of Acute Decompensation

- Nutrition should be coordinated by a metabolic dietician.
- The primary goal is to reduce the intake of proteins containing the amino acids that cannot be metabolized in each specific OA, while offering enough protein to permit normal growth (daily allowance 0.8 g protein/kg body weight).

- The protein intake should preferably be from natural sources and medical foods, with amino-acid deficient formulas, should be used to a lesser degree.
- Supplements of L-carnitine are required in GA1, MMA and PA, as these patients develop secondary carnitine deficiency.
- B12-responsive MMA (the most common, cblA, should receive 1mg/day hydroxicocobalamin.
- Antibiotics (metronidazole) can reduce propionate production in the gut.
- Aspirin is contraindicated in isovaleric aciduria as it can impede the activity of glycine-N-acylase, an endogenous detoxifying mechanism.

## Acute Decompensation

- Acute decompensations can be caused by acute infectious illnesses, surgery, immunization or other events which accelerate catabolism, and should be suspected in the presence of fever, vomiting or diarrhea. Treatment should be prompt, preferably before the onset of severe neurological symptoms.
- In acute decompensation, sufficient caloric intake must be supplied (intravenous dextrose in saline solution, correction of electrolytes and even parenteral solutions containing lipids); ammonia scavengers (N-carbamylglutamate, sodium phenylacetate-sodium glutamate) can be used to reduce hyperammonemia.
- Neurosurgery in case of subdural hematoma.

## Chronic Monitoring

- Intermediate metabolite level is not recommended for routine monitoring in GA1.
- Electrocardiography (ECG) and echocardiography yearly, especially for PA (less for MMA).
- Ophthalmological examination and renal function evaluation (especially for MMA).
- DXA scan evaluation for osteopenia and osteoporosis starting at the age of five in both PA and MMA; surveillance for fractures including the vertebrae, vertebral fusion anomalies or compressions.
- Neurological monitoring for the management of movement disorders, spasticity, cognition and epilepsy.

*Organ transplantation* has emerged as a solution to stabilize patients with PA (liver transplant) or MMA (liver, kidney, or liver and kidney transplant), but there are patients who still suffer a metabolic stroke or optic atrophy post transplantation.

## References

1. Villani GR, Gallo G, Scolamiero E, Salvatore F, Ruoppolo M. Classical organic acidurias: Diagnosis and pathogenesis. *Clin Exp Med*. 2017;**17**(3): 305–323.

2. Manoli I, Venditti CP. Disorders of branched chain amino acid metabolism. *Transl Sci Rare Dis*. 2016;**1**(2): 91–110.

3. Clarke SL, Bowron A, Gonzalez IL, et al. Barth syndrome. *Orphanet J Rare Dis*. 2013;**8**: 23.

4. Kolker S, Christensen E, Leonard JV, et al. Diagnosis and management of glutaric aciduria type I–revised recommendations. *J Inherit Metab Dis*. 2011;**34**(3): 677–694.

5. Hoffmann GF, Trefz FK, Barth PG, et al. Macrocephaly: an important indication for organic acid analysis. *J Inherit Metab Dis.* 1991;**14**(3): 329–332.

6. Zinnanti WJ, Lazovic J, Housman C, et al. Mechanism of metabolic stroke and spontaneous cerebral hemorrhage in glutaric aciduria type I. *Acta Neuropathol Commun.* 2014;**2**: 13.

7. Nishino H, Czurko A, Fukuda A, et al. Pathophysiological process after transient ischemia of the middle cerebral artery in the rat. *Brain Res Bull.* 1994;**35**(1): 51–56.

8. Isasi E, Barbeito L, Olivera-Bravo S. Increased blood-brain barrier permeability and alterations in perivascular astrocytes and pericytes induced by intracisternal glutaric acid. *Fluids Barriers CNS.* 2014;**11**: 15.

9. Keyfi F, Talebi S, Varasteh AR. Methylmalonic acidemia diagnosis by laboratory methods. *Rep Biochem Mol Biol.* 2016;**5**(1): 1–14.

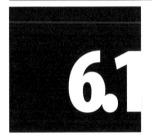

# Paradoxical Embolism: Patent Foramen Ovale

Hrvoje Budinčević, Petra Črnac Žuna, Edvard Galić, Vida Demarin

## Case Presentation

A 62 year-old female was admitted to the emergency department with acute-onset right-sided weakness and speech difficulties.

On arrival she was quantitatively conscious, she presented with sensorimotor aphasia, right-sided supranuclear facial palsy and ipsilateral hemiplegia with weakened myotatic reflexes on the right side, and no pathologic reflexes. The NIHSS score was 12. Her blood pressure was 135/70 mmHg.

The physical examination was unremarkable. The patient's past medical history revealed depression, hysterectomy due to uterine fibroid and arterial hypertension. Her regular medication included alprasolame, risperidone and escitalopram; she didn't use any anti-hypertensive therapy. She was a non-smoker and non-alcoholic.

Brain computed tomography (CT) and CT angiography of the head and neck were performed; the native CT scan of the brain showed no abnormalities, while the CT angiography showed a semiocclusive thrombus in the M1 segment of the left middle cerebral artery (Figure 6.1.1.).

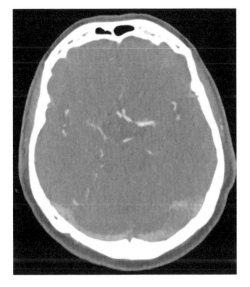

**Figure 6.1.1** CT angiography shows a semiocclusive thrombus in the M1 segment of the left middle cerebral artery.

Considering the appropriate timeframe, she underwent systemic thrombolysis, followed by a mechanical thrombectomy. After the acute stroke treatment, the follow-up neurological examination revealed an NIHSS score reduction (from 12 to 6), with a residual sensorimotor dysphasia, right-side supranuclear facial palsy, a mild ipsilateral hemiparesis with weakened myotatic reflexes. The modified Rankin scale (mRS) score was 2.

The follow-up brain CT scan revealed an acute-subacute ischemia in the left caudate nucleus and the left basal ganglia. Acetylsalicylic acid treatment was started as a secondary prevention of stroke and physical therapy was initiated.

Laboratory studies, including complete blood count, biochemical profile and coagulation tests were normal. Doppler ultrasound imaging of the carotid and vertebral arteries was unremarkable. A transcranial Doppler (TCD) examination revealed normal flow and mean blood flow velocity in the right anterior cerebral artery (ACA), middle cerebral artery (MCA) and posterior cerebral artery (PCA), while no flow was recorded on the left due to inadequate acoustic windows because of ossification of the skull. A transcranial Doppler ultrasound "bubble test" was positive: grade III (Figure 6.1.2).

Subsequently, she underwent a cardiologic examination and diagnostic work-up, to investigate for a possible source for an embolic stroke. A 24-hour Holter monitor revealed sinus rhythm. Cardiac ultrasound was suspicious for a patent foramen ovale (PFO). Transesophageal echocardiography showed a patent foramen ovale with a diameter of 3 mm in the proximal part of the interatrial septum, with a minimal right-to-left shunt. Bubble contrast echocardiography with Valsalva maneuver showed 20–30 bubbles in the left atrium. Doppler ultrasound of the veins of the legs was unremarkable.

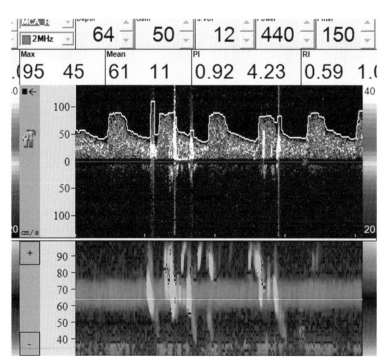

**Figure 6.1.2** Positive transcranial Doppler ultrasound "bubble test."

Antithrombotic treatment was then discontinued, and the patient started with direct oral anticoagulant therapy (dabigatran) 150 mg twice daily. Daily physical therapy was continued.

There was substantial clinical improvement after acute stroke treatment and acute rehabilitation. At hospital discharge, the neurological examination revealed mild right-sided hemiparesis and minor motor dysphasia; the NIHSS score at discharge was 4, while the mRS score was 2.

Four months after hospital discharge, the patient was seen by a neurologist in the outpatient follow-up clinic. Dabigatran was discontinued and acetylsalicylic acid was restarted.

Periodically, she underwent neurological follow-ups. Further laboratory testing revealed hypovitaminosis B12, therefore she started with substitutional therapy with B12. Control TCD "bubble tests" were positive, verifying 10 microembolic signals (MES) during the performance of the Valsalva maneuver, revealing indirect signs of a right-to-left shunt. Acetylsalicylic acid was continued indefinitely. The patient further improved clinically, with a residual mild right-sided supranuclear facial palsy and ipsilateral mild hemiparesis (NIHSS score 3).

## Clinical suspicion of embolic stroke

Clinical manifestations: sudden onset to maximal deficit (<5 min) in 47–74% of cases; decreased level of consciousness at onset in 19–31% of cases; rapid regression of symptoms in 4.7–12% of cases; Wernicke's aphasia or global aphasia without hemiparesis; a Valsalva maneuver at the time of stroke onset; co-occurrence of cerebral and systemic emboli. Cardiac embolism often affects distal arteries in the cerebral cortex while small-vessel occlusion affects subcortical areas, so cardioembolic stroke can be differentiated from lacunar stroke by cortical signs (e.g., aphasia, visual-field deficits). Lacunar clinical presentations make cardioembolic origin unlikely.

Additional signs of *possible paradoxical embolism*: deep-vein thrombosis, with or without pulmonary embolism at time of stroke; abnormal communication between the right and left sides of the circulatory system; clinical, angiographic or pathologic evidence of systemic embolism; presence of a favorable pressure gradient promoting right-to-left shunting.

## Neuroimaging

**Brain CT/brain magnetic resonance imaging (MRI):** confirm stroke size and distribution, assessing for an embolic pattern or a lacunar infarct (typically involving a single deep perforator, <1.5 cm in diameter); simultaneous or sequential strokes in multiple cerebral arterial territories (e.g., bihemispheric combined anterior and posterior circulation, or bilateral or multilevel posterior infarcts); lesions in a cortical territory (e.g., massive, superficial, single large striatocapsular or multiple infarcts in the middle cerebral artery); cardioembolic infarctions predominate in the carotid and middle cerebral artery distribution territories. MRI studies can increase the suspicion of cardioembolism by demonstrating lesions not visible on CT scans. Hemorrhagic transformation of an ischemic infarct and early recanalization of an occluded intracranial vessel are suggestive of a cardiac origin of the stroke.

**CT angiography or MR angiography**: in the acute phase often reveals an abrupt vessel cut-off without significant atherosclerotic narrowing of the upstream vessel. Angiography of the cervical and intracranial vessels are essential to exclude alternative sources of stroke, such as dissection, vasculopathy and atherosclerosis.

### Vascular and cardiac evaluation, possible systemic embolism evaluation

**Vascular evaluation** is essential to rule out large artery plaque (carotid color Doppler ultrasound, TCD). TCD with a 'bubble test' (agitated saline contrast) is a relevant screening method to detect extracardiac right-to-left shunts; but this does not obviate the need for transthoracic echocardiogram (TTE) and transesophageal echocardiogram (TEE) to rule out alternative mechanisms of cardioembolism and confirm that right-to-left shunting is intracardiac and transseptal.

**Cardiac evaluation** is important to identify a high-risk source of cardiac embolism: electrocardiography (ECG) and Holter monitoring for the assessment for atrial fibrillation; echocardiography and transesophageal echocardiography (TEE studies should use bubble contrast, with and without Valsalva maneuver, to assess for right-to-left shunt and determine degree of shunting) for the assessment of: mechanical prosthetic valve; left atrial or ventricular thrombus; recent myocardial infarction (within four weeks); dilated cardiomyopathy; infective endocarditis; regional left ventricular akinesis; atrial myxoma; rheumatic heart disease; paradoxical embolism sources: patent foramen ovale with thrombus in situ, pulmonary arteriovenous (AV) fistula, atrial septal defects, ventricular septal defects.[1]

**Systemic embolism evaluation**: performance of hypercoagulable studies that would be considered a plausible high-risk stroke mechanism; venous Doppler ultrasound of the legs; CT pulmonary angiography.

### Diagnosis of paradoxical embolism: integration of neuroimaging, cardiac, vascular and systemic embolism evaluation

- Presence of a typical clinical presentation and neuroimaging profile
- Exclusion of a large artery plaque as a source of stroke
- Positive evidence of a high-risk cardiac source
- Abnormal communication between the right and left sides of the circulatory system
- Evidence of systemic embolism; presence of a pressure gradient promoting right-to-left shunting

### Confirmation of PFO as probable source of cardioembolic stroke

**Treatment**: 1. antiplatelet medication; 2. anticoagulation therapy; 3. PFO closure.

It is important to counsel patients that having a PFO is common; that it occurs in about one in four adults in the general population; that it is difficult to determine with certainty whether their PFO caused their stroke and that PFO closure probably reduces recurrent stroke risk in selected patients.

If PFO closure is considered, clinicians should ensure that an appropriately thorough evaluation has been performed to rule out alternative mechanisms of stroke; in patients with a higher risk, or an alternative mechanism of stroke identified, closure should not be routinely recommended.

In patients younger than 60 years with a PFO and embolic-appearing infarct and no other mechanism of stroke identified, clinicians may recommend closure following a discussion of potential benefits (absolute recurrent stroke risk reduction of 3.4% at five years) and risks (periprocedural complication rate of 3.9% and increased absolute rate of non-periprocedural AF of 0.33% per year).[2]

In patients who opt to receive medical therapy alone without PFO closure, clinicians may recommend an antiplatelet medication or anticoagulation. Current evidence suggests that for patients with cryptogenic stroke and PFO, anticoagulation and antiplatelet medication are

### Confirmation of PFO as probable source of cardioembolic stroke

possibly equally effective at reducing recurrent stroke; specific antithrombotic management for patients with stroke thought to be caused by PFO remains uncertain. Existing randomized studies comparing anticoagulation with antiplatelet therapy do not indicate that either treatment option is superior, although most recent studies suggest that the Risk of Paradoxical Embolism (RoPE) score might help in selecting patients that would benefit from anticoagulation.[3]

# Discussion

A precise definition of the mechanism of stroke is essential for the implementation of the most effective care and therapy. Embolism from the heart to the brain can be a result of several mechanisms: blood stasis and thrombus formation in a dilated (or affected by another structure) left cardiac chamber, release of material from an aberrant valvular surface, atrial fibrillation and abnormal flow from the venous to the arterial circulation (paradoxical embolism). Cardiac emboli can be of any size, but those arising from the cardiac chambers are often large and likely to cause severe stroke.

There is no gold standard for making the diagnosis of cardioembolic stroke. The existence of a potentially significant cardiac source of embolism in the absence of significant arterial disease is decisive in the clinical diagnosis. When cardiac and arterial disease exist side-by-side, the etiology of the ischemic stroke becomes more complex.

Clinical features that support the diagnosis of cardioembolic stroke are: sudden onset to maximal deficit (<5 min), decreased level of consciousness, rapid regression of symptoms (the spectacular shrinking deficit syndrome may be due to distal migration of the embolus followed by recanalization of the occluded vessel), aphasia without hemiparesis, in the posterior circulation, Wallenberg's syndrome, multilevel infarcts, cerebellar infarcts, top-of-the basilar syndrome or posterior-cerebral-artery infarcts. Visual-field abnormalities and neglect are also more common in cardioembolic strokes. A classic cardioembolic stroke presents with onset of symptoms after a Valsalva-provoking activity suggesting paradoxical embolism promoted by a transitory increase in right atrial pressure and the co-occurrence of cerebral and systemic emboli.

Neuroimaging data suggesting cardioembolic stroke include sequential or simultaneous strokes in different arterial territories. Cardiac emboli are often of large size and flow to the intracranial vessels, in most cases causing massive, superficial, single large striatocapsular or multiple infarcts in the irrigation territory of the middle cerebral artery; cardioembolic infarctions predominate in the carotid and middle cerebral artery distribution territories. The CT scan often shows bihemispheric combined anterior and posterior circulation, or bilateral or multilevel posterior infarcts. MRI can increase the suspicion of cardioembolism by showing lesions not visible on CT scans.

Hemorrhagic transformation of an ischemic infarct and early recanalization of an occluded intracranial vessel are suggestive of a cardioembolic stroke. Hemorrhagic transformation occurs in up to approximately 70% of cardioembolic strokes. About 95% of hemorrhagic infarcts are caused by cardioembolism.[4]

Paradoxical embolism (PDE) is a diagnosis of exclusion. In most patients, the integration of history, physical examination and several diagnostic tests for cardiac and vascular assessment, as well as systemic embolism assessment are necessary to make the diagnosis of presumed paradoxical embolism as a source of stroke. Paradoxical embolism should be included in the differential diagnosis for arterial embolism for which there is no obvious source, particularly when there is also evidence of venous thrombosis or pulmonary embolism. In all patients with arterial embolism without an obvious source, a complete work-up should include a lung scan, whether or not there are overt symptoms and signs of pulmonary embolism, a peripheral venogram to detect phlebothrombosis, whether or not the patient has symptoms and signs of thrombophlebitis, and complete right and left cardiac catheterization and angiography. The latter should be performed to rule out atrial myxoma, cardiomyopathy with mural thrombosis, myocardial infarction with mural thrombosis, mitral stenosis and an intracardiac septal defect.

The role of a PFO as a risk factor for ischemic stroke has been established in recent years, particularly for strokes that lack an apparent cause (cryptogenic). Approximately 25% of the general population has a PFO, and it has not been shown to increase the risk of ischemic stroke. On the other hand, the prevalence of PFO is significantly higher in patients with cryptogenic stroke; up to 40% of ischemic cryptogenic strokes have a PFO, suggesting that paradoxical embolism through a PFO may be associated with a number of cryptogenic strokes.[5]

Treatment strategies have been developed to decrease the risk of recurrent events in patients with PFO, but whether antithrombotic treatment or closure of the PFO should be preferred remains uncertain. Considering the high prevalence of PFO in the general population, the identification of patients at higher risk of stroke before the stroke occurs would be essential.

A PFO is usually identified by transthoracic echocardiography (TTE) with injection of contrast material, usually aerated saline solution. Transesophageal echocardiography (TEE), a semi-invasive test that requires conscious sedation, is used when additional assessment is necessary. TEE is the most sensitive technique for PFO detection, and mostly allows direct visualization of the separation between the two septal components, using its measurement as an indication of shunting potential. The use of Valsalva maneuver to increase the right atrial pressure, making a right-to-left shunt visible increases the sensitivity of both TTE and TEE. The risk of stroke related to a PFO appears rather low in the general population. Other associated factors may come into play that enhance the risk of events associated with PFO in stroke patients: anatomical variants of the PFO (size, prominent Eustachian valve) and the right atrium, and the coexistence of thrombotic or prethrombotic conditions (deep venous thrombosis and hypercoagulable states).[6]

# References

1. Kamel H, Healey JS. Cardioembolic Stroke. *Circ Res.* 2017;**120**(3): 514-526.

2. Messé SR, Gronseth GS, Kent DM, et al. Practice advisory update summary: Patent foramen ovale and secondary stroke prevention. Report of the Guideline Subcommittee of the American Academy of Neurology. *Neurology.* 2020;**94**(20): 876–885.

3. Romoli M, Giannandrea D, Eusebi P, et al. Aspirin or anticoagulation after cryptogenic stroke with patent foramen ovale: Systematic review and meta-analysis of randomized controlled trials. *Neurol Sci.* 2020;**41**(10): 2819–2824.

4. Arboix A, Alió J. Cardioembolic stroke: Clinical features, specific cardiac disorders and prognosis. *Curr Cardiol Rev.* 2010;**6**(3): 150-161.

5. Collado FMS, Poulin MF, Murphy JJ, Jneid H, Kavinsky CJ. Patent foramen ovale closure for stroke prevention and other disorders. *J Am Heart Assoc.* 2018;**7**(12): e007146.

6. Di Tullio MR, Homma S. Patent foramen ovale and stroke: What should be done? *Curr Opin Hematol.* 2009;**16**(5): 391-396.

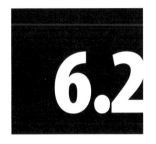

# Infective Endocarditis

Filipa Dourado Sotero, Diana
Aguiar de Sousa

**6.2**

## Case Presentation

A 41-year-old man was admitted to the emergency department with sudden onset of left-sided hemiparesis one hour before. He also reported diffuse holocranial headache and fever in the previous two days. He had history of heroin and cocaine use and chronic liver disease (alcoholic and hepatitis C virus).

At admission he was drowsy, with an arterial blood pressure of 148/84 mmHg, heart rate 67bpm, respiratory rate 22 breaths/min, oxygen saturation 99%, tympanic temperature 38°C. On physical examination, there were multiple skin tracks and needle puncture marks, suggestive of past and recent drug injection. Neurological examination revealed drowsiness, right homonymous hemianopia, left central facial palsy and left-sided hemiplegia and hemihypoesthesia. A brain CT showed a fronto-parietal hemorrhage with moderate perilesional edema and slight midline shift (Fig.6.2.1).

The patient underwent cranial MRI that confirmed the right intracranial hematoma and also showed multiple acute ischemic lesions in several other arterial territories (Figure 6.2.2).

Laboratory studies disclosed an elevated C reactive protein (11 mg/dl). A urine drug screen test was positive for cocaine. Blood cultures were drawn.

The patient was admitted at the stroke unit. A new regurgitant heart murmur was noted. The transthoracic and transesophageal echocardiograms showed a small and

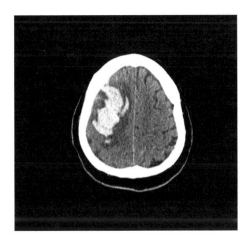

**Figure 6.2.1** Cranial CT (axial) showing an intracranial hemorrhage within the right frontal and parietal lobes, with moderate perilesional edema and slight midline shift.

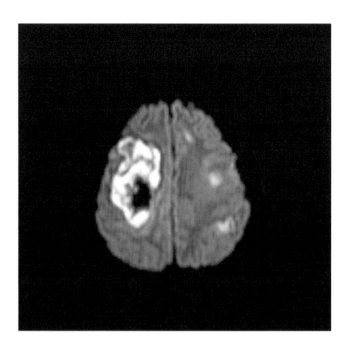

**Figure 6.2.2** Brain MRI (axial) showing multiple acute ischemic lesions in multiple vascular territories in diffusion-weighted imaging (DWI), contralateral to the subacute frontal and parietal hematoma.

mobile mass compatible with a vegetation on the mitral valve and another on the aortic valve with resultant moderate regurgitation, suggestive of native valve infective endocarditis. He started empirical antimicrobial therapy with vancomycin 60 mg/kg/day plus gentamicin 3 mg/kg/day. Serial blood cultures identified a methicillin-susceptible *Staphylococcus aureus*. A diagnosis of definitive infective endocarditis was made, according with modified Duke criteria. He also underwent digital subtraction angiography but no intracranial aneurysm was detected. The next day, the patient developed hemodynamic instability and was admitted to the intensive care unit. Echocardiographic evaluation was repeated with similar findings. A multidisciplinary team including cardiology and cardiothoracic surgery evaluated the patient and conservative treatment and monitoring was suggested. Antibiotic treatment was maintained for six weeks with favorable clinical evolution.

## Clinical suspicion of infective endocarditis in patients with stroke

### Clinical Factors

Young age without vascular risk factors

Cardiac risk factors: native valve abnormalities, prosthesis or indwelling cardiac devices

Non-cardiac risk factors: intravenous drug use, immunosuppression or recent dental procedure

Preceding non-specific systemic symptoms and fever

Clinical stigmata of embolism

Janeway's lesion; Osler's node; splinter hemorrhage; purpura and petechial hemorrhages in the skin

Cardiac murmurs

Immune complex formation or very high inflammatory markers

### Neuroimaging Findings

**Cranial CT/MRI:** Multiple ischemic lesions (symptomatic or asymptomatic), often at different ages; hemorrhagic lesions; combination of hemorrhagic and ischemic lesions; cranial abscesses; subarachnoid hemorrhage. MRI has better sensitivity for ischemic lesions and can also show microbleeds on T2*-weighted gradient-echo (GRE) or susceptibility-weighted imaging (SWI), which typically have cortical distribution

## Work-up

**Routine Laboratory Tests:** Peripheral blood count, hemogram, erythrocyte sedimentation rate, C-reactive protein, urea, creatinine, homocysteine, antiphospholipid antibody, lupus anticoagulant, anticardiolipin antibody, anti-beta-2-glycoprotein-1 antibody, prothrombin time, activated partial thromboplastin time, antinuclear antibodies, rheumatoid factor, cryoglobulins, complement levels C4, C5, CH50, urinalysis, urine drug screening.

**Microbiology:** 24h serial blood cultures (buffered charcoal and yeast agar for *Legionella;* blood, bone marrow or liver cultures up to six weeks for *Brucella* spp.). If culture-negative IE: *Coxiellaburnetii* and *Bartonella* spp.serology; PCR for *Coxiella Burnetti, Bartonella* spp., *T. whipplei* and broad range fungi; serology for *Mycoplasma pneumoniae, Legionella pneumophila, Brucellamelitensis* and *Bartonella* multi-species Western Blot If culture-negative and serology-negative IE, especially with previous antibiotic therapy: Blood PCR for streptococci and staphylococci.

**Transthoracic Echocardiogram (TTE) and Transesophageal Echocardiogram (TEE):** TTE is the first diagnostic test but in certain circumstances it is reasonable to undergo immediate TEE, especially in patients with mechanical prosthetic valves (higher sensitivity, detection of abscess, leaflet perforation and pseudoaneurysm).

**F-FDG-PET/CT, Cardiac CT, MRI or Leucocyte-labeled SPECT/CT:** Consider for diagnostic or management questions that remain after echocardiographic imaging. These new imaging modalities improve the sensitivity of the modified Duke criteria and have been incorporated as part of the diagnostic algorithm for prosthetic valve endocarditis in the 2015 European Society of Cardiology guidelines (9).

**Electrocardiography:** New or evolving conduction disease (atrioventricular block, bundle branch block, or complete heart block), reflecting paravalvular or myocardial extension of infection.

**Conventional Angiography:** If there is suspicion of infectious intracranial aneurysms, which are typically fusiform shaped, thin walled, with a distal location, and usually change in size on follow-up angiography.

## Diagnosis according to the modified Duke Criteria[9]

## Management and Treatment

### Antibiotherapy

### Aniplateletst

Initiation is not recommended

Continuation of long-term antiplatelet may be considered, except for the presence of major bleeding.

### Anticoagulants

Should be avoided in the acute phase.

Intracardiac thrombus, atrial fibrillation and mechanical prosthetic valves: the risk should be weighted.

Ischemic stroke: discontinuation for at least two weeks or switch from oral anticoagulant to unfractionated or low-molecular-weight heparin for one to two weeks should be considered under close monitoring.

Intracranial hemorrhage: interruption of all anticoagulation, in mechanical valves the risk must be weighted.

### Intravenous Thrombolysis

Intravenous thrombolysis is not recommended.

### Mechanical Thrombectomy

Only case series of mechanical thrombectomy in IE: recanalization rates and neurological outcomes similar to other stroke patients.

### Surgical Valve Treatment (preventing further embolization)

Silent embolism or transient ischaemic attack: if cardiac surgery is indicated, it is recommended without delay.

Major ischemic stroke or intracranial haemorrhage: delay surgery for at least four weeks.

Small cerebral lesions and decline in cardiac function or recurrent embolism or antibiotic failure: a delay of fewer than four weeks may be reasonable.

Infective endocarditis (IE) is a disease of the endocardial surface of the heart, native or prosthetic heart valves or intracardiac cardiac devices with an estimated annual incidence ranging from 3 to 14 per 100,000 person-years.[1-3] The causes and epidemiology have changed in recent decades due to the growing number of health-related procedures and lower incidence of rheumatic heart disease.[4]

Although IE is a rare cause of stroke, this is the most common neurological complication of IE, affecting up to 35% of all patients.[5] Risk factors for brain embolization include vegetation size and mobility,[6] left-side vegetation and a *Staphylococcus aureus* infection.

There are several predisposing risk factors for IE, including patient features such as male sex, older age, injectable drug use, dental condition or infection, and comorbid conditions, namely, acquired or congenital structural or valvular heart disease, prosthetic heart valves, intracardiac or intravascular devices or catheter, chronic hemodialysis or HIV infection.[7,8]

The diagnosis of IE is based on clinical, echocardiographic and microbiologic findings, assessed by the updated Duke criteria.[9] When IE is suspected, transthoracic echocardiography (TTE) should be performed first, as it can reveal vegetations in up to 90% of cases.[10] Transesophageal echocardiogram is superior to TTE and especially important when mechanical prosthetic valves are present, to detect right-sided lesions, to visualize myocardial abscesses and in all cases of uncertainty or negative results when there is high clinical suspicion.[9] The identification of the causative agent to guide the antimicrobial treatment is another important step.[11] *Staphylococcus aureus* is the most common causative organism, being isolated in up to 30% of IE.[12]

In the acute stroke setting, intravenous (IV) thrombolysis is not recommended, as it has been associated with a high rate of hemorrhage.[13] Thus, a clinical challenge is recognizing the possibility of IE in the setting of an acute ischemic stroke. Careful consideration of the typical clinical features of IE is crucial. Regarding mechanical thrombectomy in IE, only few case series have been reported, with similar recanalization rates and neurological outcomes to general stroke patients.[14-18] However, more studies are needed and caution is necessary.

Acute ischemic lesions are usually multiple cortical and subcortical infarcts, disseminated in multiple vascular territories, often with various ages. Intracerebral hemorrhage accounts for nearly 20% of cerebrovascular complications of IE, with 15% being hemorrhagic transformations.[6] The underling mechanisms are rupture of infectious intracranial aneurysms (Figure 6.2.3), septic necrotic arteritis with vessel rupture or hemorrhagic transformation of ischemic lesions. In suspected cases, digital subtraction angiography should be considered for aneurysm detection. Ruptured aneurysms should be immediately secured by surgical or endovascular procedures as this situation bears a poor outcome and high mortality rate.[19]

Infectious intracranial aneurysms are thin-walled and fusiform-shaped, within a distal location, and often have a wide or absent neck. Therefore, treatment may be laborious due to the wide aneurysm neck and vascular fragility. For unruptured aneurysms, a conservative approach with antibiotic therapy guided by blood cultures and serial angiography follow-up may be a reasonable option.[9]

Antimicrobial therapy is the mainstay of treatment for patients with IE and guidelines for appropriate case management have been published by several professional societies.[9,20,21] Initiation of targeted antibiotic therapy has been shown to lower the embolic

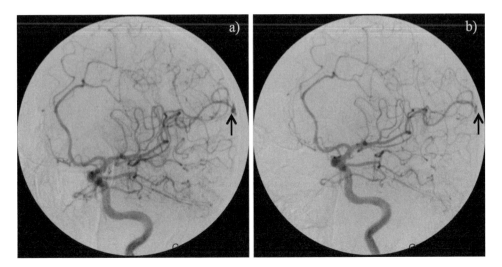

**Figure 6.2.3** Digital subtraction angiography showing an asymptomatic fusiform shaped aneurism on distal branches of the medial cerebral artery in a patient with diagnosis of infective endocarditis: (a) angiography at admission, (b)follow-up cerebral angiogram after four months showing resolution of the aneurysm.

risk of IE from 10–50% to 6–21%, with most events occurring in the first two weeks of treatment.[22]

Regarding antithrombotic treatment, initiation of antiplatelets is not recommended. The continuation of previous long-term antiplatelet therapy may be considered, except in cases of bleeding.[20] There is no evidence to support use of anticoagulants in acute stroke due to IE. If, due to another condition, there is a formal indication, the risk of hemorrhage should be carefully weighed.

The timing and indications for valvular surgery to prevent systemic embolism remains controversial. In cases of major ischemic stroke or intracranial hemorrhage, it is reasonable to delay surgery.[20] In cases of small brain lesions in patients with a decline in cardiac function, recurrent embolism or failure of antibiotic therapy, shorter delays may be considered.[21]

Despite the advances in diagnostic tools, antimicrobials and valve surgery, morbidity and mortality remain high in stroke patients.[6] Independent predictors of mortality include older age, cerebrovascular events, *Staphylococcus aureus* infection and healthcare-associated IE.[4]

# References

1. Dayer MJ, Jones S, Prendergast B, et al. Incidence of infective endocarditis in England, 2000–13: A secular trend, interrupted time-series analysis. *Lancet*. 2015;**385**(9974): 1219–1228.

2. Duval X, Delahaye F, Alla F, et al. Temporal trends in infective endocarditis in the context of prophylaxis guideline modifications: Three successive population-based surveys. *J Am Coll Cardiol*. 2012;**59**(22): 1968–1976.

3. Pant S, Patel NJ, Deshmukh A, et al. Trends in infective endocarditis incidence, microbiology, and valve replacement in the

United States from 2000 to 2011. *J Am Coll Cardiol.* 2015;**65**(19): 2070–2076.

4. Pericart L, Fauchier L, Bourguignon T, et al. Long-term outcome and valve surgery for infective endocarditis in the systematic analysis of a community study. *Ann Thorac Surg.* 2016;**102**(2): 496–504.

5. Jiad E, Gill SK, Krutikov M, et al. When the heart rules the head: Ischaemic stroke and intracerebral haemorrhage complicating infective endocarditis. *Pract Neurol.* 2017;**17**(1): 28–34.

6. García-Cabrera E, Fernández-Hidalgo N, Almirante B, et al. Neurological complications of infective endocarditis risk factors, outcome, and impact of cardiac surgery: A multicenter observational study. *Circulation.* 2013;**127**(23): 2272–2284.

7. Holland TL, Baddour LM, Bayer AS, et al. Infective endocarditis. *Nat Rev Dis Prim.* 2016;**2**(16059): 1–23.

8. Hill EE, Herijgers P, Claus P, et al. Infective endocarditis: Changing epidemiology and predictors of 6-month mortality. A prospective cohort study. *Eur Heart J.* 2007;**28**: 196–203.

9. Habib G, Lancellotti P, Antunes MJ, et al. 2015 ESC guidelines for the management of infective endocarditis. *Eur Heart J.* 2015;**36**(44): 3075–3123.

10. Murdoch DR, Corey GR, Hoen B, et al. Clinical presentation, etiology and outcome of infective endocarditis in the 21st century: The International Collaboration on Endocarditis-Prospective Cohort Study. *Arch Intern Med.* 2009;**169**(5): 463–473.

11. Thuny F, Grisoli D, Collart F, Habib G, Raoult D. Management of infective endocarditis: Challenges and perspectives. *Lancet.* 2012;**379**(9819): 965–975.

12. Hoen B, Duval X. Infective endocarditis. *N Engl J Med.* 2013; 300–313.

13. Asaithambi G, Adil MM, Qureshi AI. Thrombolysis for ischemic stroke associated with infective endocarditis: Results from the nationwide inpatient sample. *Stroke.* 2013;**44**(10): 2917–2919.

14. Ambrosioni J, Urra X, Hernández-Meneses M, et al. Mechanical thrombectomy for acute ischemic stroke secondary to infective endocarditis. *Clin Infect Dis.* 2018;**66**(8): 1286–1289.

15. Scharf EL, Chakraborty T, Rabinstein A, Miranpuri AS. Endovascular management of cerebral septic embolism: Three recent cases and review of the literature. *J Neurointerv Surg.* 2017;**9**(5): 463–465.

16. Sveinsson O, Herrman L, Holmin S. Intra-arterial mechanical thrombectomy: An effective treatment for ischemic stroke caused by endocarditis. *Case Rep Neurol.* 2016;**8**(3): 229–233.

17. Madeira M, Martins C, Koukoulis G, et al. Mechanical thrombectomy for stroke after cardiac surgery. *J Card Surg.* 2016;**31**(8): 517–520.

18. Bolognese M, von Hessling A, Müller M. Successful thrombectomy in endocarditis-related stroke: Case report and review of the literature. *Interv Neuroradiol.* 2018;**24**(5): 529–532.

19. Cahill TJ, Baddour LM, Habib G, et al. Challenges in infective endocarditis. *J Am Coll Cardiol.* 2017;**69**(3): 325–344.

20. Baddour LM, Wilson WR, Bayer AS, et al. Infective endocarditis in adults: Diagnosis, antimicrobial therapy, and management of complications. A scientific statement for healthcare professionals from the American Heart Association. *Circulation.* 2015;**132**(15): 1435–1486.

21. Byrne JG, Rezai K, Sanchez JA, et al. Surgical management of endocarditis: The society of thoracic surgeons clinical practice guideline. *Ann Thorac Surg.* 2011;**91**(6): 2012–2019.

22. Vilacosta I, Graupner C, Roma AS, et al. Risk of embolization after institution of antibiotic therapy for infective endocarditis. *J Am Coll Cardiol.* 2002;**39**(9): 1489–1495.

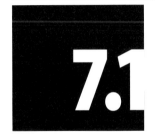
# 7.1 Reversible Cerebral Vasoconstriction Syndrome

Dejana R. Jovanović, Predrag Stanarčević

## Case Presentation

A previously healthy 41-year-old woman presented to the emergency department with bilateral loss of vision and an occipital headache. The patient reported diffuse headache with sudden onset two weeks ago as severe occipital pain "like a thunder strike," intensity 10/10 on the analog pain scale, associated with nausea and vomiting. Ten days later, in addition to a continual occipital throbbing headache, she noticed blurred vision with an unsteady gait. An ophthalmological examination was performed, which revealed bilateral amblyopia (VOU 0.2–0.3; FOU, TOU, eyeball motility normal) and cranial computerized tomography (CT) showed hypodense zones in the left parietal subcortical and left occipital regions (Figure 7.1.1A). Three days later an outpatient cranial magnetic resonance imaging (MRI) showed bilateral occipital and parietal parasagittal hyperintense zones on T2-weighted (T2 W)/T2 fluid attenuated inversion recovery (FLAIR) images, with a clear pathological diffuse restriction and without postcontrast signal enhancement (Figure 7.1.1B). On arrival, the physical examination and vital functions were normal. Initial neurological examination showed that she was conscious, disoriented in time, fulfilled only simple orders after repeated asking, with spatial and body neglect. Bilateral amblyopia was registered, recognizing only light and dark, and the pupils were about 5 mm in diameter, reactive to light. She demonstrated discrete sinking of the right extremities with symmetrical muscle reflexes and an atypical right plantar response. The gait was insecure due to amblyopia, without other pathological characteristics. The day after admission, the typical signs of cortical blindness and Anton's syndrome, with confusion, occasional psychomotor agitation and visual hallucinations were confirmed by examination.

The head CT at admission showed bilateral occipital hypodense zones with some signs of diffuse edema (Figure 7.1.1C). CT venography showed no signs of venous sinus thrombosis and CT angiography (CTA) showed left vertebral artery spasm in the V4 segment with slow and discrete basilar and posterior cerebral artery filling (Figure 7.1.1D). A few days later color Doppler sonography (CDS) of the neck vessels was normal, but a transcranial Doppler (TCD) showed a significant flow acceleration in both middle cerebral arteries (MCA) along their entire course, with maximal peak systolic velocity (PSV) values of 170 cm/s, and slight flow acceleration in the right anterior cerebral artery (ACA) with maximum PSV of 70cm/s. Vertebral and basilar arteries showed moderate hemodynamic acceleration without indirect signs of stenosis. Electroencephalography (EEG) showed the presence of moderate electrocortical dysfunction, predominantly on the left side.

On the 20th day from disease onset, repeated MRI showed bilateral multiple focal parietal and occipital confluent hyperintense zones in T2 W/FLAIR images with restrictive

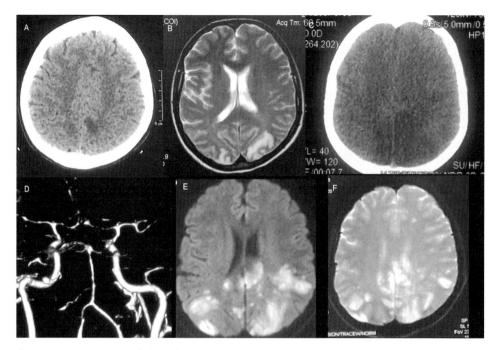

**Figure 7.1.1** Neuroimaging findings: head CT, head MRI and CT angiography (described in the text).

diffusion, and discrete zones of the same characteristics in the frontal left and insular left regions (Figure 7.1.1E,F).

After application of a contrast agent, several zones of spotted and gyral enhancement were observed. TCD repeated three weeks after disease onset showed normal hemodynamic flow parameters in both ACMs, as well as in the left ACA. CTA on the 30th day from disease onset showed only a narrowing of the ophthalmic segment of the left internal carotid artery of about 60% with a normal finding on other blood vessels. Digital subtraction angiography, six weeks after onset, was completely normal with no signs of any vessel stenosis. On the computerized perimetry, four weeks from the start of the disease, bilateral lower altitudinal hemianopia, predominantly right lower homonymous quadrantanopia was recorded.

To determine the etiology of multifocal cerebral artery vasospasm, laboratory studies were performed: complete blood count, erythrocyte sedimentation rate, biochemical screen of hepatic and renal functions, C reactive protein, thyroid function, vitamin B12 and folic acid were normal. Routine and extended coagulation tests (antithrombin III, protein C, protein S, lupus anticoagulant, plasminogen inhibitor activator PAI-1, D-dimer, activated protein C resistance, factor VIII and factor XII levels, homocysteine) were normal. Tumor markers (α-fetoprotein (AFP), CA 125, CA 19–9, CEA 15–3, CA 72–4, Cyfra 3) were negative. Immunoserological analyses (antinuclear antibodies, antineutrophilic cytoplasmic autoantibodies, anticardiolipin antibodies, anti-β-2-glycoprotein antibodies) were negative. The cytochemical cerebrospinal fluid (CSF) examination and isoelectric focusing were normal. Serum and CSF *Treponema pallidum* hemagglutination assay (TPHA) and virologic tests (CMV, HSV1, HSV2, HIV, HCV, HBs Ag) were negative. Lung X-ray, abdominal echo and transthoracic echocardiography were normal.

As all the findings were compatible with a diagnosis of reversible cerebral vasospasm syndrome (RCVS), the patient was treated with an intravenous infusion of nimodipine for five days, then continued with tablets for another 10 days until vasospasm was resolved according to TCD. In addition, she received aspirin 100 mg daily. The patient was discharged home after about six weeks from the onset of the disease with signs of lower right homonymous hemianopia and signs of spatial disorientation. In the follow-up examination four months later, she had no visual disturbances and repeat cranial MRI showed left parietal subcortical infarction in the level of supramarginal gyrus.

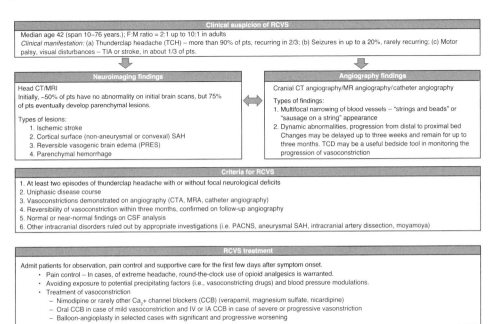

**Clinical suspicion of RCVS**

Median age 42 (span 10–76 years.); F:M ratio = 2:1 up to 10:1 in adults
*Clinical manifestation:* (a) Thunderclap headache (TCH) – more than 90% of pts, recurring in 2/3; (b) Seizures in up to a 20%, rarely recurring; (c) Motor palsy, visual disturbances – TIA or stroke, in about 1/3 of pts.

**Neuroimaging findings**

Head CT/MRI
Initially, ~50% of pts have no abnormality on initial brain scans, but 75% of pts eventually develop parenchymal lesions.

Types of lesions:
1. Ischemic stroke
2. Cortical surface (non-aneurysmal or convexal) SAH
3. Reversible vasogenic brain edema (PRES)
4. Parenchymal hemorrhage

**Angiography findings**

Cranial CT angiography/MR angiography/catheter angiography

Types of findings:
1. Multifocal narrowing of blood vessels – "strings and beads" or "sausage on a string" appearance
2. Dynamic abnormalities, progression from distal to proximal bed
   Changes may be delayed up to three weeks and remain for up to three months. TCD may be a useful bedside tool in monitoring the progression of vasoconstriction

**Criteria for RCVS**

1. At least two episodes of thunderclap headache with or without focal neurological deficits
2. Uniphasic disease course
3. Vasoconstrictions demonstrated on angiography (CTA, MRA, catheter angiography)
4. Reversibility of vasoconstriction within three months, confirmed on follow-up angiography
5. Normal or near-normal findings on CSF analysis
6. Other intracranial disorders ruled out by appropriate investigations (i.e. PACNS, aneurysmal SAH, intracranial artery dissection, moyamoya)

**RCVS treatment**

Admit patients for observation, pain control and supportive care for the first few days after symptom onset.
- Pain control – In cases, of extreme headache, round-the-clock use of opioid analgesics is warranted.
- Avoiding exposure to potential precipitating factors (i.e., vasoconstricting drugs) and blood pressure modulations.
- Treatment of vasoconstriction
  - Nimodipine or rarely other $Ca_2+$ channel blockers (CCB) (verapamil, magnesium sulfate, nicardipine)
  - Oral CCB in case of mild vasoconstriction and IV or IA CCB in case of severe or progressive vasoconstriction
  - Balloon-angioplasty in selected cases with significant and progressive worsening

# Discussion

RCVS is a clinical radiological syndrome that typically presents with severe headache, with or without other neurological symptoms, and is associated with diffuse multifocal vasoconstriction of the cerebral arteries that resolves spontaneously within three months.[1,2] This is known as Call–Fleming syndrome, as it was first described by Call and associates in 1988.[3] Other names for this syndrome that can be found in the literature include isolated benign cerebral vasculitis, acute benign cerebral angiopathy, benign CNS angiopathy, migraine angiitis, primary thunderclap headache, postpartum benign angiopathy, among others.[4] The term RCVS was proposed by Calabrese and colleagues in 2007 as a way to recognize the similarities among these entities and to unify this group of related conditions.[5]

The pathophysiology of RCVS is still unknown. The proposed mechanism is that cerebral vasoconstriction, due to sympathetic overactivity, leads to breakdown of the blood–brain barrier (BBB) and transitory cerebrovascular autoregulation dysfunction.[5,6]

It has been suggested that the vasoconstriction observed in RCVS starts in small distal arteries and progresses centrally toward medium- and large-sized arteries.[1] This may be an explanation for normal findings in early angiography. As cerebral blood vessels are densely innervated with sensory afferents from the trigeminal nerve, the vasoconstriction of small distal arteries may be responsible for recurrent thunderclap headaches that resolve with progression of vasospasm to medium- and large-sized arteries.[1,4] Potential triggers of RCVS are numerous exogenous or endogenous factors. Most of the RCVS cases are associated with vasoactive medications (sympathomimetic drugs, bromocriptine, ergotamine, pseudoephedrine, selective serotonin uptake inhibitors, interferon, tacrolimus, cyclophosphamide, fingolimod, triptans, diet pills, non-steroidal anti-inflammatory drugs, indomethacin, erythropoietin, oral contraceptive pills, nicotine patches, blood transfusions, intravenous immunoglobulins, etc.) or recreational drugs (binge alcohol drinking, amphetamines, cannabis, cocaine, ecstasy, nicotine).[2,4] About 10% of RCVS appears during pregnancy and postpartum and up to 40% with migraine headaches.[4] Other conditions associated with RCVS are catecholamine-secreting tumors, head trauma, antiphospholipid antibody syndrome, thrombotic thrombocytopenic purpura, carotid dissection, unruptured cerebral aneurysm, and head and neck surgery.[2,4] The delay in exposure to an exogenous trigger and the development of RCVS can be anything between a few days and several months. In the absence of any of the precipitating factors, RCVS is marked as idiopathic or primary, which makes up less than a third of patients.[7]

RCVS typically involves adults aged 20–50 years with women more commonly affected than men.[2] Men with RCVS are a decade younger than female patients.[8] It usually begins with an acute, extremely severe thunderclap headache, that reaches peak intensity within 60 seconds of onset, similar to the headache in a subarachnoid hemorrhage (SAH).[2,4,8] The headache is typically bilateral, begins in the posterior parts of the head with subsequent involvement of the entire head, and is often accompanied by nausea, vomiting, photophobia and phonophobia. The headache gradually subsides after one to three hours and recurs several times in the next one to three weeks.[8] Most patients report that even between attacks of these thunderclap headaches, there may be a mild, continuous headache. The onset of headache is mainly provoked by some kind of stress (e.g., sexual activity, sudden emotions, straining, coughing, sneezing, urinating, defecation, bending forward, etc.).[2] Epileptic seizures have been reported in up to 20% of patients with RCVS.[1] The incidence of focal neurological deficit ranges from 8–43% and may present as a transient ischemic attack (TIA) or with visual disturbances similar to a migraine aura.[2,8] Transient or permanent focal neurologic deficits encountered with RCVS include visual deficits, hemiplegia, dysarthria, aphasia, numbness, cortical blindness or ataxia.

In more than 90% of patients, complete withdrawal of symptoms occur, but RCVS may be complicated with cerebral infarction, intracerebral hemorrhage (ICH), SAH or posterior reversible encephalopathy syndrome (PRES).[8,9] Rarely, these complications lead to death, which has been reported in about 5–10% of these patients.[2,6,9] Some factors, such as glucocorticoid therapy, intra-arterial vasodilator therapy and infarction on baseline imaging are associated with a poor outcome.[6]

The typical radiological presentation of RCVS includes vasoconstriction of medium and large-sized arteries, with at least two narrowings in the same artery, on two different cerebral arteries, which commonly disappear within three months.[6] Catheter angiography, MR angiography (MRA) or CT angiography (CTA) may disclose diffuse or focal vasoconstriction and vasodilation, or a "string-of-beads" and "sausage-string" appearance.[2,6] Arterial involvement is usually bilateral, with diffuse involvement of the anterior and posterior circulations. However, cerebral vasoconstriction may not be visualized in patients with RCVS during the first week and may be delayed up to three weeks after the initial thunderclap headache.[2,10] Transcranial Doppler sonography is a good, bedside, non-invasive way of monitoring cerebral vasospasm.

Initial CT or MRI brain imaging may be normal in 30–70% of RCVS patients and if the diagnosis is suspected, repeat imaging should be performed.[2,10] In one-third to a half of cases, brain imaging reveals cortical surface SAH(cSAH), PRES, ICH, subdural hemorrhage, and ischemic stroke.[2,10] cSAH is usually seen in the first week after onset of symptoms and is generally minor, restricted to a few hemispheric sulci, and most commonly located over the frontal and parietal lobes.[2] In a minority of patients, ischemic strokes may occur generally at the end of the second week, often after the resolution of the headache. They are typically bilateral in arterial watershed areas.[2,4,6] Rarely, isolated deep ICH may occur. PRES is reported in 10–38% of RCVS, but the edema is typically asymmetric.[2,6]

The main differential diagnosis of RCVS includes an aneurysmal SAH and primary angiitis of CNS (PACNS). In an aneurysmal SAH, typical findings are the presence of blood in a basal cistern and subsequent vasospasm of long segments of the proximal arteries, contrary to focal cSAH, with a disproportionate, beaded peripheral vasoconstriction seen in RCVS.[4] It is important to differentiate RCVS from PACNS because prescribing glucocorticoids to patients with RCVS is associated with clinical worsening and delaying it in PACNS patients means a poor prognosis.[4] The deep brainstem infarcts and abnormal CSF findings typically seen in PACNS patients are rare in RCVS.[2,4] Rocha and colleagues developed an RCVS2 score to distinguish between these two entities.[11] Other conditions that should be differentiated from RCVS are cervical artery dissection, cerebral venous thrombosis, acute stroke, unruptured aneurysm, third ventricular colloid cyst, spontaneous intracranial hypotension and primary headache disorders.[2]

Treatment of RCVS is currently based on expert opinion and reported case series. The majority of RCVS patients have a self-limited course and only require an early withdrawal of precipitating vasoactive agents, avoidance of any stress and headache triggers, use of sedatives, analgesia and bed rest.[2,7] Paracetamol and opioids are recommended for pain control of headache and indomethacin and triptans should be avoided.[1,2] In cases of seizure, an antiepileptic drug should be given for a short period. It is important to maintain optimal blood pressure values, avoiding hypotension, which may lead to watershed infarctions. In the treatment of cerebral vasospasm, the use of calcium channel blockers for about four to eight weeks may be considered, although there is no evidence that they bring faster resolution of vasospasm or prevent complications.[1] Oral nimodipine is most commonly prescribed in a dose of 30–60 mg every four hours and in cases of severe vasospasm a nimodipine infusion may be considered.[1,2,7,9] The use of verapamil hydrochloride, magnesium sulfate or nicardipine is also possible. One should be cautious in the use of these drugs due to their hypotensive effects, which may contribute to the development of ischemic lesions. The use of glucocorticoids is not recommended due to the observed clinical deterioration with their use.[2,7] Invasive neurointerventional techniques of intra-arterial nimodipine and balloon angioplasty should be reserved for RCVS patients with clinical deterioration and severe refractory vasoconstriction.[2]

# References

1. Ducros A. Reversible cerebral vasoconstriction syndrome. *Lancet Neurol.* 2012;**11**: 906–917.

2. Cappelen-Smith C, Calic Z, Cordato D. Reversible cerebral vasoconstriction syndrome: Recognition and treatment. *Curr Treat Options Neurol.* 2017;**19**: 21.

3. Call GK, Fleming MC, Sealfon S, et al. Reversible cerebral segmental vasoconstriction. *Stroke.* 1988;**19**: 1159–1170.

4. Levitt A, Zampolin R, Burns J, Bello JA, Slasky SE. Posterior reversible encephalopathy syndrome and reversible cerebral vasoconstriction syndrome: Distinct clinical entities with overlapping pathophysiology. *Radiol Clin N Am.* 2019;**57**: 1133–1146.

5. Calabrese LH, Dodick DW, Schwedt TJ, Singhal AB. Narrative review: Reversible cerebral vasoconstriction syndromes. *Ann Intern Med.* 2007;**146**: 34–44.

6. Pilato F, Distefano M, Calandrelli R. Posterior reversible encephalopathy syndrome and reversible cerebral vasoconstriction syndrome: Clinical and radiological considerations. *Front Neurol.* 2020;**11**: 34.

7. Chen SP, Fuh JL, Wang SJ. Reversible cerebral vasoconstriction syndrome: Current and future perspectives. *Expert Rev Neurother.* 2011;**11**: 1265–1276.

8. Miller TR, Shivashankar R, Mossa-Basha M, Gandhi D. Reversible cerebral vasoconstriction syndrome, part 1: Epidemiology, pathogenesis, and clinical course. *Am J Neuroradiol.* 2015;**36**: 1392–1399.

9. Velez A, McKinney JS. Reversible cerebral vasoconstriction syndrome: A review of recent research. *Curr Neurol Neurosci Rep.* 2013;**13**: 319.

10. Miller TR, Shivashankar R, Mossa-Basha M, Gandhi D. Reversible cerebral vasoconstriction syndrome, part 2: Diagnostic work-up, imaging evaluation, and differential diagnosis. *Am J Neuroradiol.* 2015;**36**: 1580–1588.

11. Rocha EA, Topcuoglu MA, Silva GS, Singhal AB. RCVS2 score and diagnostic approach for reversible cerebral vasoconstriction syndrome. *Neurology.* 2019;**92**: e639–e647.

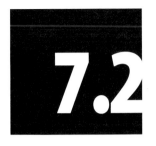

# 7.2 Eclampsia and Strokes during Pregnancy and Postpartum

Dejana R. Jovanović

## Case Presentation

A 36-year-old woman was admitted to the emergency neurological department due to three convulsive seizures with the development of drowsiness after a cesarean section. She was a pregestationally healthy person and this was her first pregnancy after treated infertility. During the VIII lunar month of pregnancy, pretibial edema became profound and edema of the hands and face appeared. In the 34th week of gestation, the patient complained about general malaise, vomiting, diarrhea and headache, and elevated blood pressure values were recorded. The gynecologist confirmed severe pre-eclampsia and threatening eclampsia with signs of fetal distress, and an emergency delivery by cesarean section was performed. The patient developed a series of three generalized seizures 2, 10 and 21 hours after delivery, between which she was drowsy and complained of a headache. In laboratory analyses, signs of HELLP (Hemolysis, Elevated Liver enzymes, Low Platelets) syndrome were suspected. At admission, the patient was somnolent, easily wakened upon call and adequately oriented. The somatic examination revealed tachycardia 98 beats/min, blood pressure 160/90 mmHg, obesity, pallor, moderate pretibial and edema of the hands, and mild periorbital edema. The neurological examination disclosed partial right-sided homonymous hemianopia, right central facial palsy and discrete right-sided pyramidal deficit with positive Babinski sign. Initial head computerized tomography (CT), 24 hours after delivery, showed signs of diffuse edema with bilateral circular hypodense zones, predominantly in the occipital and parietal regions, in both thalamus and bilaterally in the basal ganglia, consistent with posterior reversible encephalopathy syndrome (PRES) (Figure 7.2.1A). CT angiography was without pathological findings. Electroencephalography (EEG) recorded persistent pseudorhythmic

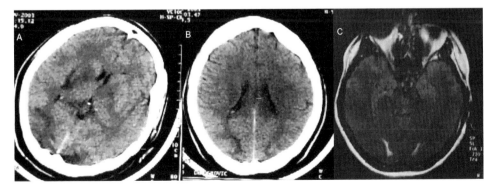

**Figure 7.2.1** Neuroimaging findings: head CT and head MRI in patient with eclampsia (described in the text).

theta activity over both frontotemporal regions. In the complete blood count, hemoglobin (Hb) was 91 g/l, leukocytes $20 \times 10^3/mm^3$ (91% neutrophils), platelets $37 \times 10^3/mm^3$, and the presence of schistocytes in the peripheral blood smear. An elevated sedimentation rate (55 mm/h) and fibrinogen (4.3 g/l) with normal activated partial thromboplastin time (aPTT) and prothrombin time (PT) were recorded. The biochemical analysis showed slightly elevated transaminases (aspartate transaminase (AST) 60 IU/l, alanine transaminase (ALT) 87 IU/l), elevated lactate dehydrogenase (LDH) 1605 IU/l, and creatine kinase 827 IU/l. Glycemia, urea, creatinine, bilirubin, electrolytes and serum proteins were normal. In the routine urine analysis, proteinuria 3+ was detected. A lung X-ray and abdominal ultrasound examination were normal. Repeated gynecological examination on three occasions showed a regular postoperative finding and involution of the uterus. The patient was treated with a continuous IV infusion of magnesium sulfate for five days, antihypertensives, fresh frozen plasma for the first three days, continuous infusion of oxytocin, antibiotics, preventive doses of low-molecular-weight heparin (LMWH), and other symptomatic and rehydration therapies. On the second day after admission, variations in blood pressure were still registered, and in the neurological finding only symmetrically enhanced muscle reflexes. An anemia (Hb 91–99 g/l) was maintained in laboratory analyses with gradual normalization of platelet count, transaminases, LDH and creatine kinase values. The repeat EEG still showed bilateral theta activity on the third day, and a normal finding was registered on the eighth day. Head CT on the seventh day showed significant regression of multifocal zones of PRES edema and on day 9, magnetic resonance imaging (MRI) showed small zones of occipital edema bilaterally (Figure 7.2.1B and Figure 7.2.1C).

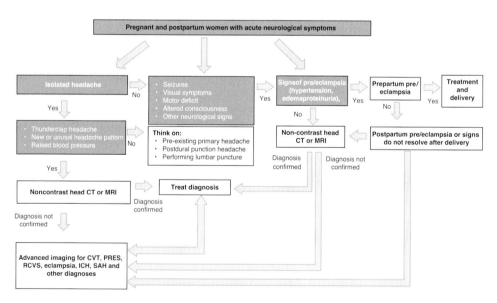

## Discussion

In developed countries, two of the most common causes of maternal death are eclampsia and stroke, although their occurrence in the peripartum period is rare.[1,2] The incidence rate of gestational stroke is three to nine times higher compared to non-pregnant women.[3]

During pregnancy, there is a significant increase in hormonal activity, significant cardiovascular, hemodynamic and coagulation changes.[4] All these physiological gestational adjustments can predispose pregnant women to the appearance of cerebrovascular disorders.

# Pre-Eclampsia/Eclampsia

Pre-eclampsia is a multisystem disorder diagnosed by the presence of de novo hypertension after the 20th week of pregnancy, and no later than 48 hours after birth, accompanied by proteinuria or evidence of maternal acute kidney injury, liver dysfunction, neurologic changes (encephalopathy, seizures), hemolysis or thrombocytopenia, or fetal growth restriction.[5] Eclampsia means the occurrence of convulsions or coma, which are not caused by a coincidental neurological disease, in the setting of pre-eclampsia. In developed countries, pre-eclampsia occurs in about 6–8% and eclampsia in 0.1% of all pregnancies.[2,5]

In pre-eclampsia, high arterial pressure causes cerebral vasospasm, and due to the loss of the cerebral autoregulation mechanism, subsequent focal vasodilation develops, leading to breakdown of the blood–brain barrier with extravasation of serum proteins and water.[5,6] Due to the persistence of focal vasoconstriction, microinfarcts, hypoxic-ischemic lesions and cytotoxic edema develop, and due to endothelial damage and coagulopathy, pericapillary, petechial or even small parenchymal hemorrhages appear.

In more severe forms of pre-eclampsia, typical neurological symptoms are headaches and various visual disturbances in the form of scotoma, blurred vision, amblyopia, cortical blindness and visual hallucinations.[6,7] In addition, patients may be confused, disoriented and drowsy, and rarely have a discrete focal neurological deficit. Eclampsia is the most severe clinical form of the disease and is characterized by the appearance of convulsions.[4,5,7] HELLP syndrome occurs in 0.5–0.9% of all pregnancies, mostly in those with severe pre-eclampsia or eclampsia.[8] It usually begins with malaise, nausea, vomiting, epigastric or pain in the right hypochondrium, and approximately 30–60% of patients have headaches and about 20%, visual symptoms.[8] Other symptoms and complications such as jaundice, subcutaneous edema, mucosal hemorrhages, hematuria, convulsions and disturbances of consciousness, acute renal failure, disseminated intravascular coagulation (DIC), pulmonary edema and acute liver necrosis may occur.[8]

Head CT in patients with severe pre-eclampsia and eclampsia shows transient focal hypodensities, particularly in the occipital-parietal regions, less often temporally, frontally or in the basal ganglia.[9] Cranial MRI shows hypointense or isointense changes in the T1 sequence and hyperintense changes in the T2 and FLAIR sequences that are rarely contrast-enhanced-localized at typical sites.[7,9] These neuroimaging changes are reversible, resolve within 10–20 days, and represent a recognizable clinical entity of PRES.[10] In eclamptic forms of PRES, the thalamus, mesencephalon and pons are rarely affected and severe forms of vasogenic edema, cytotoxic edema and contrast enhancement are less common.[9,11] PRES develops more often in postpartum eclampsia than in that occurring during pregnancy.[11] The occurrence of PRES in the gestational period is not only associated with pre-eclampsia/eclampsia, but also with reversible cerebral vasoconstriction syndrome (RCVS) or with the use of some drugs in the peripartum period.[7] Besides the signs of edema, unifocal or multifocal intracerebral hemorrhages (ICH) can be visualized, mostly in the occipital-parietal regions, and less often cerebral infarctions or cerebral venous thrombosis.[9,12]

In patients with pre-eclampsia/eclampsia, angiographic scans often show diffuse or focal beaded arterial vasoconstriction, mostly in the proximal portions of the large arteries, but also in their extracranial segments and variably distal arteries are affected.[7,9,11,12] Such angiographic findings are consistent with RCVS and confirm the role of vasospasm in the pathogenesis of preeclampsia and delayed postpartum eclampsia. These patients with eclampsia and RCVS are more likely to develop craniocervical arterial dissections.[7] Vasospasm gradually subsides in eclampsia, but focal spasms of individual arteries can be seen even after several weeks.[7,9,11]

# Stroke

The rate of gestational stroke in developed countries is ~ 30 per 100,000 pregnancies, mostly the ischemic type.[4,5] Arterial infarctions mainly occur in the second and third trimesters of pregnancy and the first week of puerperium, and cerebral venous thrombosis in the first two weeks of puerperium, while the occurrence of hemorrhagic forms is more common pre-partum, except those caused by eclampsia.[2,4]

### Ischemic Stroke

The etiology of ischemic stroke in pregnancy and puerperium are similar to the etiology of stroke among young people in general. Some of the causes may be more common in pregnant women, due to physiological cardiovascular, hormonal and hematological changes. In addition, stroke can appear as a complication of pregnancy-specific conditions, such as eclampsia, peripartum cardiomyopathy and postpartum benign angiopathy, or very rarely amniotic fluid embolization and choriocarcinoma.

*Eclampsia* carries a high risk for stroke, both hemorrhagic and ischemic. It is blamed for the occurrence of 16–23% of ischemic and up to 50% of hemorrhagic strokes during gestation.[4,6] The existence of endothelial damage, cerebral vasospasm and activation of coagulation mechanisms predisposes to an arterial or venous cerebral infarction.

*Postpartum benign angiopathy* means the appearance of RCVS in the postpartum period and, apart from headaches, generally does not lead to neurological deficits. However, cases of less favorable outcomes with arterial infarctions or ICH have also been reported.[4]

*Peripartum cardiomyopathy* is a dilated cardiomyopathy of unknown etiology that occurs during the last month of pregnancy or within five months after birth in the absence of previous heart disease and accounts for less than 1% of all cardiac gestational complications.[13] About 5% of patients with peripartum cardiomyopathy develop cerebral infarction.

*Pregnancy non-specific causes.* Among these causes of ischemic stroke during pregnancy and puerperium, the most common are cardioembolic causes.[14] The gestational period favors the occurrence of paradoxical embolization due to hypercoagulability associated with the presence of a foramen ovale apertum.[2] Hormonal changes may affect arterial walls and provoke spontaneous arterial dissections or stroke in moyamoya disease. Strokes in migraine patients are significantly more common during pregnancy.[2,14] Risk factors for stroke in pregnancy/puerperium are age >35 years, multi-parity, twin pregnancy, hyperemesis, pre-eclampsia, cesarean section, then the presence of antiphospholipid antibodies, sickle cell anemia, thrombotic thrombocytopenic purpura and blood transfusion.[14,15]

## Cerebral Venous Thrombosis

The incidence of CVT in the gestational period is similar to arterial infarctions, but the greatest risk is during the puerperium.[2,4] This risk for CVT is increased in older women, cesarean delivery or epidural anesthesia, in the presence of hypertension, infection, antiphospholipid antibodies or congenital thrombophilia, dehydration or obesity.[9] Venous infarctions are typically associated with hemorrhagic transformation and mass effect, ICH is typically cortically localized, while subarachnoid hemorrhages (SAHs) are smaller in size and localized on convexities.[9,16]

## Hemorrhagic Stroke

Pregnancy and puerperium carry an increased risk of hemorrhagic stroke, but it is rare.[6] Risk factors for hemorrhagic stroke during gestation are older age, pregestational and gestational hypertension, pre-eclampsia/eclampsia, coagulopathies and smoking.[16] The main causes of hemorrhagic stroke during the gestational period are eclampsia, rupture of aneurysms and vascular malformations, or hemorrhage in cerebral venous thrombosis.

Pre-eclampsia and especially eclampsia increase the risk of developing ICH by about eight to ten times.[4,6,16] Malignant hypertension in a setting of coagulation disorders (DIC, HELLP) may cause the appearance of visible ICH and SAH. Intracerebral hemorrhages are often multifocal and less often associated with a mass effect, and SAHs are small, cortical and usually absent in basal cisterns.[9] Unlike hemorrhages that occur as a result of vascular anomalies, these hemorrhages mostly present in the postpartum period.[2,4,16]

# References

1. Chang J, Elam-Evans LD, Berg CJ, et al. Pregnancy-related mortality surveillance: United States 1991–1999. *MMWR Surveill Summ.* 2003;**52**: 1–8.

2. Miller EC, Leffert L. Stroke in pregnancy: A focused update. *Anesth Analg.* 2020;**130**: 1085–1096.

3. Ban L, Sprigg N, Abdul Sultan A, et al. Incidence of first stroke in pregnant and nonpregnant women of childbearing age: A population-based cohort study from England. *J Am Heart Assoc.* 2017;**6**: e004601.

4. Feske SK, Singhal AB. Cerebrovascular disorders complicating pregnancy. *Continuum (Minneap Minn).* 2014;**20**(1 Neurology of Pregnancy): 80–99.

5. Camargo EC, Feske SK, Singhal AB. Stroke in pregnancy: An update. *Neurol Clin.* 2019;**37**: 131–148.

6. Crovetto F, Somigliana E, Peguero A, Figueras F. Stroke during pregnancy and pre-eclampsia. *Curr Opin Obstet Gynecol.* 2013; **25**: 425–32.

7. Edlow JA, Caplan LR, O'Brien K, Tibbles CD. Diagnosis of acute neurological emergencies in pregnant and post-partum women. *Lancet Neurol.* 2013;**12**: 175–185.

8. Dusse LM, Alpoim PN, Silva JT, et al. Revisiting HELLP syndrome. *Clin Chim Acta.* 2015;**451**(Pt B): 117–120.

9. Mortimer AM, Bradley MD, Likeman M, Stoodley NG, Renowden SA. Cranial neuroimaging in pregnancy and the post-partum period. *Clin Radiol.* 2013;**68**: 500–508.

10. Levitt A, Zampolin R, Burns J, Bello JA, Slasky SE. Posterior reversible encephalopathy syndrome and reversible cerebral vasoconstriction syndrome distinct clinical entities with overlapping pathophysiology. *Radiol Clin N Am.* 2019;**57**: 1133–1146.

11. Liman TG, Bohner G, Heuschmann PU, et al. Clinical and radiological differences in posterior reversible encephalopathy syndrome between patients with preeclampsia/eclampsia and other predisposing diseases. *Eur J Neurol.* 2012;**19**: 935–943.

12. Hugonneta E, Da Inesa D, Bobyb H, et al. Posterior reversible encephalopathy syndrome (PRES): Features on CT and MR imaging. *Diag Interv Imaging.* 2013;**94**: 45–52.

13. Biteker M, Kayatas K, Duman D, Turkmen M, Bozkurt B. Peripartum cardiomyopathy: Current state of knowledge, new developments, and future directions. *Curr Cardiol Rev.* 2014;**10**: 317–326.

14. Del Zotto E, Giossi A, Volonghi I, et al. Ischemic stroke during pregnancy and puerperium. *Stroke Res Treat.* 2011; 606780.

15. Cauldwell M, Rudd A, Nelson-Piercy C. Management of stroke and pregnancy. *Eur Stroke J.* 2018;**3**: 227–236.

16. Khan M, Wasay M. Haemorrhagic strokes in pregnancy and puerperium. *Int J Stroke.* 2013;**8**: 265–272.

# 7.3 Migraines and Migraine-Like Conditions

Yagmur Turkoglu Comert, Peter J. Goadsby

## Case Presentation

A 41 year-old male with a history of chronic migraine without aura was admitted to the emergency department with a severe left-sided persistent headache. The headache had been present for two days, and was associated with nausea and dizziness. On the morning of admission his wife noticed a droopy left eyelid and he complained of right-arm numbness. He had no other notable medical history, part from an eight packet a year history of cigarette smoking. He was on candesartan 8 mg as a migraine preventive. A neurological exam demonstrated mild left ptosis, right-side subjective hemi-hypoesthesia and no other pathological findings. He underwent a brain computed tomography (CT) scan and lumbar puncture at the emergency department, which were reported to be normal. His admission diagnosis was status migrainosus.

## Additional history

Taking a more detailed history, he began to have periodic left frontal headache nine years earlier. Initially, the pain was in the bifrontal area and pressure-like, with occasional vertex pain. He noted the pain was throbbing as it moved to the forehead. There could be a tingling sensation. The headache was consistently associated with photophobia, lasting some hours, and less often with nausea and phonophobia. At first, his headaches occurred two to three times per month. He reported an average severity of 6–7/10 as a verbal pain rating. He was not on any medication in that period.

The headache became problematic in 2016 when he developed pain involving the parietal regions as well, and increased frequency to 20 days per month. He had worsening lasting 45 minutes on average, and occurring three to four times per week, which he reported as pain up to 8/10 in severity. There was no circadian variation. As associated symptoms, he had nausea without vomiting, bilateral photophobia, both allodynic and photosensitivity, phonophobia, aggravation of pain with movement and internal vertigo. Cranial autonomic symptoms sometimes included left-sided lacrimation, left tinnitus and he could have bilateral ptosis. As premonitory-like symptoms, during the headache he had neck discomfort, concentration impairment and tiredness. He had a postdrome including fatigue lasting up to 36 hours. Triggers to worsening included alcohol, undersleeping, skipping meals and dehydration.

## Progress

On day two after admission he developed dysphagia to solids and liquids. His weight was 75 kg, blood pressure 130/80 mmHg and pulse 72 beats/minute. On examination of the cranial nerves, fundi were normal, and pupils were equal and reactive to light. He had left ptosis, visual fields were normal and eye movements full with horizontal nystagmus on leftward gaze. He had a swollen tongue base with bilateral depressed gag reflex and diminished soft palate elevation, as well as left-sided ataxia. Given the findings, a vertebral artery dissection was considered. Cranial magnetic resonance imaging (MRI) and diffusion-weighted magnetic resonance imaging (DWI) were performed. Both T2/fluid-attenuated inversion recovery (FLAIR) (Figure 7.3.1) and DWI (Figure 7.3.2) showed a clear hyperintensity in the left medullar area consistent with the clinical findings. Anticoagulant therapy was commenced with warfarin and low-molecular-weight heparin. Digital subtraction angiography (DSA) demonstrated thrombotic stenosis and left vertebral artery dissection, which was effectively treated with coil embolization. At discharge, on day 11, his swallowing was normal. He continued to have some residual right-sided numbness. He was discharged on clopidogrel. He had continued low-level (3/10) daily headaches.

## Discussion

Our case is a young healthy male who had troublesome chronic migraine without aura for nearly ten years. The patient had no recent history of any head or neck trauma. From time to time, he had migraine attacks that could come along with posterior circulation symptoms, specifically nausea, vomiting and vertigo. On admission day he had non-diagnostic symptoms and examination findings. Initial radiological imaging was unremarkable. Persistent headache, relative refractoriness to analgesics, paracetamol/caffeine and naproxen, and subtle neurological signs led a diagnosis of status migrainosus. Cervical artery dissection

(a)                                            (b)

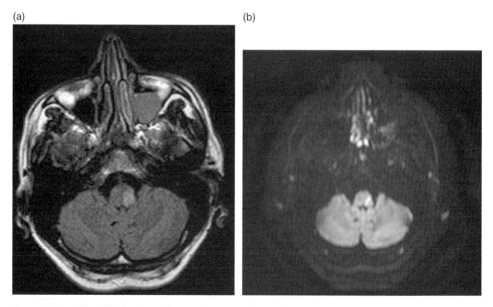

**Figure 7.3.1** (a)T2A /FLAIR MRI and (b) DWI showing nodular infarction measuring about 1 cm in left medulla.

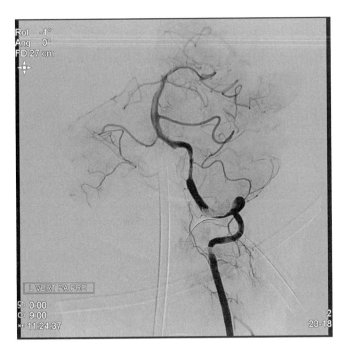

Rot -1°
Ang 0°
FD 27 cm

L VERT PA PRE

0:00
9:00
11:24:37

2
23-18

**Figure 7.3.2** Thrombotic stenosis and luminal irregularities of left VA are seen in DSA.

(CAD) was diagnosed when he developed findings of brainstem ischemia. Headache is commonly seen in patients with CAD, and the characteristics of a CAD headache might be easily confused with migraine. Initial notable manifestations of CAD are posterior headache or neck pain. In our case the persistent pain was localized on entire left side of the head. Migrainous features in the presentation included: unilateral pain, throbbing quality, accompanying nausea and photophobia. Given the history of chronic migraine without aura and a duration of nearly 72 hours, the diagnosis of status migrainosus was made. Migraine is associated with a higher risk of CAD than of non-CAD ischemic stroke, and this risk is especially evident for migraine without aura.[1] Our patient had a history of chronic migraine without aura and newly-emerging findings, such as persistence of severe headache, posterior circulation symptoms, led to further investigation. Migraine without aura is more common among CAD stroke patients compared to non-CAD ischemic stroke patients.[2] In addition, in a meta-analysis, migraine was found to be associated with a twofold increased risk of CAD.[3] The pathophysiology causing the increased risk of ischemic stroke among patients with migraine is not understood.

### Possible mechanisms behind the association between migraine and CAD

1. Endothelial dysfunction, which may be partially genetically determined by an insertion/deletion polymorphism in the angiotensin-converting enzyme gene, has been reported in migraineurs and may account for the altered systemic vascular reactivity among migraine patients; such vessel wall pathologies are also among the most important risk factors for CAD

(cont.)

### Possible mechanisms behind the association between migraine and CAD

2. Biological evidence is provided by studies suggesting that migraine and CAD share common genetic susceptibility factors, such as the 677C>T variant in the gene coding for methylenetetrahydrofolate reductase

3. The activity of serum elastase, a metalloendopeptidase involved in extracellular matrix degradation, is increased among migraineurs, providing a physiological explanation for the increased risk of CAD

### Diagnosis of CAD associated with migraine

- Clinical and laboratory investigations (complete blood cell count, biochemical profile, urinalysis, 12-lead electrocardiogram, chest radiography, Doppler ultrasonography, with frequency spectral analysis and B-mode echotomography of the cervical arteries, transcranial Doppler ultrasonography and CT and/or MR angiography, to investigate extracranial and intracranial vessels)

- Coagulation testing, included prothrombin and activated partial thromboplastin times, lupus anticoagulant, circulating antiphospholipid antibodies (anticardiolipin antibodies and anti–$\beta_2$-glycoprotein I antibodies), fibrinogen, protein C, protein S, activated protein C resistance, antithrombin III and genotyping to detect factor V Leiden and the G20210A mutation in the prothrombin gene

- Transthoracic and/or transesophageal echocardiography to rule out cardiac sources of emboli

- Neuroimaging methods (four-vessel conventional angiography, MRI with MR angiography (three-dimensional time of flight), and/or CT angiography of the brain and neck. The presence of the double-lumen sign (a false lumen or an intimal flap), luminal narrowing with the "string sign" and gradual tapering ending in total occlusion of the lumen (flame-like occlusion) are considered reliable angiographic findings in CAD, whereas a narrowed lumen surrounded by a semilunar-shaped intramural hematoma on axial T1-weighted images is considered the pathognomonic MRI sign

Our case is consistent with chronic migraine without aura as a marker for increased risk of cerebral infarction in young people, caused by CAD. The relationship between migraine without aura and stroke, compared to migraine with aura, remains an important area for research.

# References

1. DeGiuli V, Grassi M, Lodigiani C, et al. Association between migraine and cervical artery dissection: The Italian project on stroke in young adults. *JAMA Neurol.* 2017;**74**: 512.

2. Metso TM, Tatlisumak T, Debette S, et al. Migraine in cervical artery dissection and ischemic stroke patients. *Neurology.* 2012;**78**: 1221–1228.

3. Rist PM, Diener H-C, Kurth T, Schürks M. Migraine, migraine aura, and cervical artery dissection: A systematic review and meta-analysis. *Cephalalgia.* 2011;**31**: 886–896

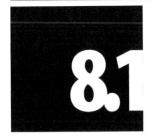

# Moyamoya Disease

Bojana Žvan, Marjan Zaletel

## Case Presentation

A 26-year-old student was examined in the outpatient clinic because of headaches. For eight months, she had been admitted daily into the emergency hospital due to acute, unbearable headaches, which woke her up from sleep. It was the worst headache she had ever had and often depicted it as 10/10 on a numeric scale. She described the pain as a tense and stabbing. She experienced nausea and vomiting and had the perception of tingling, and a pins and needles feeling in both upper extremities, exchanging between the right and left sides, in the temples and occiput. She had no photo- or sonophobia. Previous headaches were of the same intensity and were associated with sleep, waking her up one to two hours after she fell asleep. She complained of a vigorously distressed condition, which she connected with symptomatology. She had been taking oral contraceptives. No abnormalities were revealed during a neurologic examination. Because of the unusual pattern of the headaches, we were suspicious of a secondary condition and decided to do magnetic resonance imaging (MRI) of the head. The MRI showed striped hyperintense changes in sulci along both convexities in all parts of the brain on the fluid-attenuated inversion recovery (FLAIR)-weighted sequence (Figure 8.1.1A), because of a slow flow through the leptomeningeal collateral vessels (white arrows). Six non-specific hyperintense, round-to-oval lesions of the deep white cerebellum, were arranged bilaterally at the border between the anterior cerebral artery (ACA) and middle cerebral artery (MCA) lobes, most likely chronic ischemic changes. On the T2 sequence of the MRI (Figure 8.1.1B), the leptomeningeal vessels at the base are visible in the suprasellar cistern, in the cistern ambience (white arrow).

After we recognised abnormalities in the MRI we suspected moyamoya disease and continued with angiography (Figure 8.1.2A). We found occlusion of the intracranial portion of the internal carotids, which were normal up to the ophthalmic portion, and occluded distally with a moyamoya vessel pattern. Angiographic changes in the patient were consistent with grade 3 involvement. Digital subtraction angiography of the vertebrobasilar region (Figure 8.1.2B) showed that the posterior region was filled via a distinctly well-developed vertebral artery on both sides. From the vertebrobasilar system, the anterior region was filled distally from the occlusion of the internal carotid arteries via well-developed posterior communicating arteries.

To exclude other vasculopathies, we performed ultrasound of the abdomen, kidney and heart; blood was collected to conduct rheumatology and thrombophilia tests, thyroid hormones, and serology on borreliosis and lues. All results were within normal limits but elevated protein values stood out in the cerebrospinal fluid.

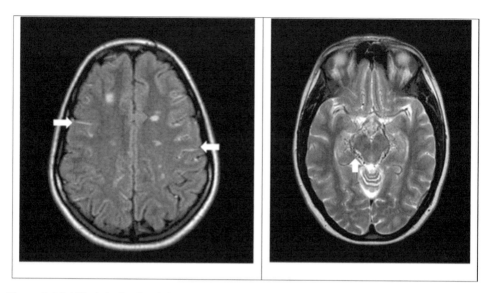

**Figure 8.1.1** MRI of the head with (A) FLAIR and (B) T2-weighted sequences, with changes consistent with moyamoya disease.

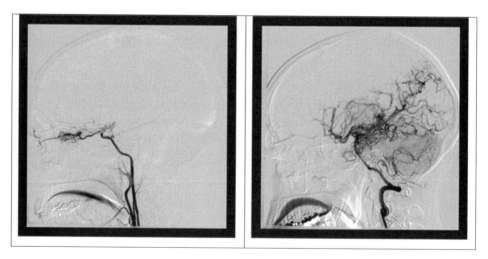

**Figure 8.1.2** Digital subtraction angiography of (A) the carotid and (B) vertebrobasilar territories.

Clinical suspicion of moyamoya
Stroke in young adults and children, unusual headache, asian, female, CT scan findings in basal brain regions including basal ganglia, deep white matter, temporal lobes and border zone territories infarctions and hemmorrages)

MRI scan
Absence of flow voids in the distal ICA and MCA, multiple signal voids in the basal ganglia, and dilated leptomeningeal and cortical collateral vessels

Non-invasive angiographic techniques (MRA, CTA)
Detection of steno-occlusion of the distal ICA, MCA and ACA

Invasive angiography (DSA) (when MR angiography clearly demonstrates all the subsequently described findings, conventional cerebral angiography is not mandatory) [follow on] demonstrating basal moyamoya vessels, small saccular aneurysms, status of the external carotid artery circulation, findings should present bilaterally

Histopathological features
Analysis of the surgical specimens: fibrocelular thickening of the intima, irregular undulation of the internal elastic laminae, medial thinness at stenotic arterial segments

Treatment
Surgical revascularization; recommended for MMD patients presenting with cerebral ischemic symptoms[4] direct revascualrization and/or combined direct/indirect procedures are recommended for adult MMD patients. Antiagregation in ischemic events, no antiagragation in haemorraghe

Clinical conditions that should be excluded:

1. Arteriosclerosis
2. Autoimmune disease
3. Meningitis
4. Brain neoplasm
5. Down syndrome
6. Recklinghausen disease
7. Head trauma
8. Irradiation to the head
9. Others (sickle cell disease, tuberous sclerosis, etc.)

# Discussion

Moyamoya disease (MMD) is a cerebrovascular disorder characterized by progressive stenosis of the terminal portion of the internal carotid artery (ICA). The perforating arteries in the basal ganglia and thalamus markedly dilate and serve as an important collateral circulation, known as "moyamoya" vessels. MMD is found predominantly in East Asian populations and can be overlooked in other patient populations. In Japan, the annual prevalence has been estimated to be 3.16 to 10.5 per 100,000. The female to male ratio was shown to be 1.8.[1] This strongly suggests that the female gender may be highly susceptible. MMD remains rare outside the Far East, but the condition has been described on every continent and in all ethnic groups. Studies involving non-Asian populations are rare. In the states of Washington and California, the annual incidence of MMD is 0.086 per 100,000.[2] The incidence among all patients with MMD in Europe appears to be about 1/10th of that observed in Japan. The onset of the disease has been suggested to have two peaks: one at five years of age and one lower peak at about 40 years of age.[1]

The clinical presentations of MMD include TIA, ischemic strokes, hemorrhagic strokes, seizures, headaches and cognitive impairments. An ischemic event is the most-important clinical manifestation. The infarct topography in MMD often extends beyond the classical vascular territories. Approximately 30% of MMD patients present with intracerebral hemorrhage or, less commonly, subarachnoid hemorrhage. The cause of headaches in MMD remains unclear, but it is possible that dilatation of meningeal and leptomeningeal collateral vessels may stimulate dural nociceptors. Patients may also have seizures, visual deficits, syncope or personality changes that can be mistaken for a psychiatric illness.

In spite of this, the specific mechanism has not been elucidated and the pathogenesis of MMD is still unclear. It has been suggested that the clinical presentation of affected patients may be the result of underlying genetic and environmental causes. The main pathological changes induced by MMD in the stenotic segment are fibro cellular thickening of the intima, irregular undulation of the internal elastic laminae, medial thinness (weakening of the media), and a decrease in the outer diameter.[3]They suggest that MMD is primarily a proliferative disease of the intima. Cortical micro vascularisation is considered specific for MMD. Associated collaterals are generally dilated perforating arteries.

The exact etiologic process of MMD is unknown, although myriad environmental, genetic, and infectious causes have been proposed. Approximately 10% of individuals with MMD exhibit a familial occurrence. Most familial cases appear to be polygenic or inherited in an autosomal dominant fashion. Several genetic loci have been identified in familial MMD, including 3p24-26, 6q25, 8q23, 10q23.31, 12p12 and 17q25.[5] Levels of many growth factors, enzymes and other peptides have been reported to be increased. For example, fibroblast growth factor, transforming growth factor β-1, hepatocyte growth factor, vascular endothelial growth, matrix metalloproteinases, intracellular adhesion molecules, and hypoxia-inducing factor 1α are elevated in the dura of patients with MMD. It appears that in susceptible persons, when particular environmental triggers, such as radiation, are present, it results in the moyamoya phenotype.

The diagnostic criteria for MMD, stated by the Research Committee on Spontaneous Occlusion of the Circle of Willis in Japan, is well established and generally accepted around the world as the definition of this disease.[4] Most patients first have computed tomography (CT) of the head, which can show ischemic changes in the borderline territories, basal nuclei and deep white matter, bleeding in the basal nuclei, ventricular system and temporal lobe, and in the thalamus. MRI can reveal the following features, which should lead clinicians to suspect MMD. These are the absence of flow voids in the distal ICA and middle cerebral artery (MCA), multiple signal voids in the basal ganglia, and dilated leptomeningeal and cortical collateral vessels. Diminished cortical blood flow due to moyamoya can be suspected from FLAIR sequences showing high linear signals that follow a sulcal pattern, which is called the "ivy sign." On cerebral angiography, bilateral carotid forks were involved in the majority of asymptomatic patients with MMD. Between 15 and 44% of adult patients with MMD have silent microbleeds in the basal ganglia, thalamus and periventricular white matter. CT angiography (CTA) and MR angiography (MRA) are important to non-invasively detect steno-occlusion of the distal ICA, MCA and anterior cerebral artery (ACA). Catheter angiography is usually used for demonstrating basal moyamoya vessels with a typical pattern (smoke-like) and small saccular aneurysms, and for assessing the status of the external carotid artery circulation. Based on various angiographic findings, six stages of angiographic evolution have been proposed. In the last stages, there is an increase in collateral circulation from the external carotid artery (stage 5) with the final disappearance of the moyamoya pattern with cerebral circulation maintained only by the external carotid artery or the vertebral artery (stage 6).

Surgical revascularisation is the mainstay of MMD treatment. It prevents ischemic attacks by improving the cerebral blood flow. The surgery includes both microsurgical reconstruction, using an extracranial–intracranial bypass, and consolidation for future vasculogenesis by indirect pialsynangiosis. Surgical treatment of MMD is also indicated for hemorrhagic-onset patients, but not for asymptomatic patients with MMD. There is no specific treatment to prevent ischemic events in MMD. Administration of antiplatelets can be considered for patients with ischemic symptoms, but there is only weak evidence supporting this approach. Antiplatelet agents are not recommended for hemorrhagic-onset or asymptomatic patients. Headaches persist in up to 63% of patients, even after successful surgical revascularisation. Calcium-channel blockers may be useful in ameliorating intractable headaches.

# References

1. Kuroda S, Houkin K. Moyamoya disease: Current concepts and future perspectives. *Lancet Neurol.* 2008;7(11): 1056–1066.

2. Uchino K, Johnston SC, Becker KJ, Tirschwell DL. Moyamoya disease in Washington state and California. *Neurology.* 2005;**65**(6): 956–958.

3. Scott RM, Smith ER. Moyamoya disease and moyamoya syndrome. *N Engl J Med.* 2009;**360**(12): 1226–1237.

4. Research Committee on the Pathology and Treatment of Spontaneous Occlusion of the Circle of Willis: Health Labour Sciences Research Grant for Research on Measures for Intractable Diseases. Guidelines for diagnosis and treatment of moyamoya disease (spontaneous occlusion of the circle of Willis). *Neurol Med Chir (Tokyo).* 2012;**52**(5): 245–266.

5. Bang OY, Fujimura M, Kim SK. The pathophysiology of moyamoya disease: An update. *J Stroke.* 2016;**18**(1): 12–20.

# Cerebral Amyloid Angiopathy

Matija Zupan

## Case Presentation

An 82-year-old gentleman was admitted to the neurology department due to six repetitive stereotyped episodes over the last three days, each lasting approximately 30 minutes, consisting of clonic convulsions associated with paraesthesia of his left upper limb and left facial muscula-ture. He had no headache, nausea or vomiting. His medical history was otherwise remarkable for cognitive impairment, depression, arterial hypertension and benign prostatic hyperplasia. He was regularly taking an antidepressant, an antidementive, antihypertensives and a hypolipemic. An anticonvulsant, lacosamide, prescribed during a previous hospitalization had been stopped 11 months prior to admission. Two years earlier, we had treated him due to repetitive intermittent paraesthesia of his right limbs followed by transient clumsiness of the right hand. At that time, a non-contrast computed tomography (CT) head scan had revealed a convexity subarachnoid hemorrhage (cSAH) in the left central sulcus. CT angiography of cervical and intracranial arteries, as well as intracranial veins and venous sinuses had been unremarkable. A magnetic resonance imaging (MRI) head scan had additionally shown signs of cortical superficial siderosis (cSS) emphasized over both frontoparietal cortices and chronic partly confluent ischemic lesions of cerebral white matter predominantly parietally. After the introduction of an anticonvulsant, the presenting symptoms had subsided completely. It had been concluded that the patient had suffered a convexity subarachnoid hemorrhage of unknown cause.

On present admission, he was alert, attentive and oriented to space but not time. Speech was unremarkable. After five minutes he recalled two to three objects only after prompting. Examination of cranial nerves was unremarkable, with the exception of a previously known dilated and unreactive right pupil after prior ocular trauma. He had no sensorimotor deficits in his limbs. Gait and stance were adequate for his age. Temperature was 36.6 °C and no meningeal signs were present. Blood pressure was 150/90 mmHg and respiratory rate was 15 breaths/min with an oxygen saturation of 96% on room air. The physical examination was otherwise unremarkable.

A non-contrast CT head scan showed fresh blood in the right central sulcus and a chronic ischemic lesion in the right frontal lobe. CT angiography of intracranial arteries showed no signs of aneurisms, vasospasm or vascular malformations. CT angiography of intracranial veins and venous sinuses showed no signs of thrombosis. An MRI head scan revealed hyperdensity in the right central sulcus on fluid-attenuated inversion recovery (FLAIR) sequence consistent with cSAH. Chronic (cSS) was seen over both cerebral hemispheres, especially frontally and parietally, estimated to be more pronounced than at the time of the first presentation in 2017. Two novel microhemorrhages were seen in the cerebellar hemispheres on

314

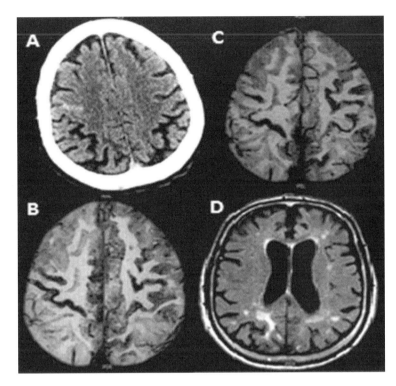

**Figure 8.2.1** (A) Non-contrast CT head scan showing a hyperdense signal of fresh blood in the right central sulcus. (B) SWI MRI showing hypointense signal in sulci over both cerebral hemispheres, reflecting cSS. (C) SWI MRI showing comparatively less advanced cSS in 2017. (D) FLAIR MRI showing partly confluent hyperintense ischemic lesions, pronounced in the parietal regions.

susceptibility-weighted imaging (SWI). Chronic partly confluent ischemic lesions of cerebral white matter were found, especially in the parietal lobes (Fazekas scale 2). Generalized cerebral atrophy was estimated to be more pronounced than previously (Figure 8.2.1). Ultrasound examination of cervical vessels showed signs of non-obstructive atherosclerosis of moderate degree in extracranial parts of the carotid arteries. A subcortical cognitive impairment most consistent with a predominantly vascular etiology was evident during the hospital stay.

Extensive laboratory work-up (biochemistry, complete blood count and differential, C-reactive protein, sedimentation rate and coagulation tests) did not yield any significant aberrations. The patient suffered an additional three episodes that were interpreted as transient focal neurological symptoms (TNFS) that ceased to repeat after the reinstitution of an anticonvulsant. We concluded that thus far the patient had suffered two clinically apparent episodes of cSAH. We did not opt for cerebral biopsy due to its invasive nature in an otherwise elderly patient with vascular cognitive impairment because the results would not have changed the management of the patient. According to the Modified Boston Criteria the patient fulfilled the criteria for probable cerebral amyloid angiopathy (CAA). We introduced no additional pharmacotherapy and advised tight blood pressure control and a consultation with a vascular neurologist if antithrombotics were contemplated in future.

| Clinical presentations of CAA | Radiological findings |
|---|---|
| Headache, focal neurological deficits, focal seizures, nausea and vomiting, and decreased consciousness | Multiple or single lobar/cortico-subcortical/ cerebellar hemorrhage(s), predominantly lobar CMBs on SWI MRI |
| | May have concomitant WMI/lobar lacunae, pronounced in occipitoparietal lobes or CMIs, CSO-DPVS, predominantly posterior cortical atrophy |
| TFNS (amyloid spells): aura-like (positive) and/or TIA-like (negative) symptoms | cSAH ± cSS, predominantly lobar CMBs on SWI MRI |
| Cognitive impairment: predominantly subcortical (vascular) type (up to 25% diagnosed with AD), gradually progressive; repetitive intracranial hemorrhage (ICH) associated with stepwise cognitive decline | Any of the above findings (in the absence of ICH especially WMI, CMI, lobar lacunae, cortical, atrophy, CMBs) |
| Subacute or rapidly progressive cognitive decline, headache, hallucinations, behavioral changes, decreased consciousness; less often focal neurological signs and focal seizures | **Distinct entity CAA-ri/ABRA**: WMH on T2 and FLAIR MRI sequences reflecting vasogenic edema, contrast enhancement, sometimes mass effect, highly frequent lobar CMBs |

| Modified Boston Criteria | Description |
|---|---|
| Definite CAA | *Full post-mortem examination demonstrating*: lobar, cortical, or cortical–subcortical hemorrhage, severe CAA with vasculopathy, absence of other diagnostic lesions |
| Probable CAA with supporting pathology | *Clinical data and pathological tissue (evacuated hematoma or cortical biopsy) demonstrating*: lobar, cortical, or cortical– subcortical hemorrhage (including ICH, CMB, or cSS), some degree of CAA in specimen, absence of other diagnostic lesion |
| Probable CAA | *Clinical data and MRI or CT demonstrating*: multiple hemorrhages (ICH, CMB) restricted to lobar, cortical or cortical–subcortical regions (cerebellar hemorrhage allowed), or single lobar, cortical or cortical–subcortical hemorrhage and cSS (focal or disseminated), age ≥55 years, absence of other cause of hemorrhage* |
| Possible CAA | *Clinical data and MRI or CT demonstrating*: single lobar, cortical or cortical–subcortical ICH, CMB, or cSS (focal or disseminated), age ≥55 years, absence of other cause of hemorrhage* |

* Other causes of hemorrhage (differential diagnosis of lobar hemorrhages): antecedent head trauma, hemor- rhagic transformation of an ischemic infarction, arteriovenous malformation, hemorrhagic tumour, warfarin therapy with international normalized ratio >3, and vasculitis.

| Additional investigations | Findings |
| --- | --- |
| CTA/CTV, MRA/MRV, DSA | Normal except for CAA-ri/ABRA: typical findings of vasculitis (beading) may be found on DSA |
| CSF diagnostics | Increased protein and decreased soluble Aβ or APOE in non-inflammatory forms of CAA; CAA-ri: increased anti-Aβ autoantibodies and tau/phosphotau proteins, even lower Aβ42 than in CAA |
| Routine blood tests | No specific abnormalities, at first ICH presentation imperative to rule out hemorrhagic diatheses (e.g., anticoagulation) |
| Genetic tests | Younger onset/family history suspicious of hereditary forms (e.g., Dutch, Icelandic), APOE genotyping useful in suspicious CAA-ri (>75% homozygosity for APOE ε4) |
| PET brain scan | In doubtful cases; if CSF unobtainable: cortical retention of PIB is an *in vivo* marker of CAA |
| Brain and leptomeningeal biopsy | Mandatory for (1) definite CAA, (2) probable CAA with supporting pathology and (3) to confirm the diagnosis of CAA-ri |

| Treatment | Aims and Description |
| --- | --- |
| Standard treatment for ICH | To lower intracranial pressure (ICP) and prevent herniation |
| | Non-surgical: head elevation, osmotic diuretics, hyperventilation (+intensive neurological care) |
| | Neurosurgical: ICH evacuation (+histopathology!), ICP electrode, placing EVD in intraventricular extension of ICH |
| Hemostasis | To correct any significant hemorrhagic diathesis (e.g., low platelet count; immediate withdrawal of antithrombotics; to revert anticoagulant effects of medications) according to standard care |
| TFNS | To halt amyloid spells: anticonvulsants may be of help |
| Cognitive impairment | To slow down worsening: antidementives may be of help, especially in concomitant AD |
| CAA-ri | To suppress the autoimmune response: initially high-dose corticosteroids, later on cyclophosphamide, duration not well established; individualized approach |
| Prevention of recurrent ICH | Strict blood pressure control |
| | Caution when (re)instituting statins |

| Treatment | Aims and Description |
|---|---|
| | (Re)instituting anticoagulation in particular only after prudent consideration of multiple factors; not earlier than one month after ICH, consider non-pharmacologic treatment (e.g., LAA closure in patients with concomitant AF) |
| | Avoiding even trivial head trauma |

Aβ: amyloid beta; ABRA: amyloid beta-related angiitis; AD: Alzheimer disease; AF: atrial fibrillation; APOE: apolipoprotein E; CAA: cerebral amyloid angiopathy; CAA-ri: cerebral amyloid angiopathy-related inflammation; CMI: cortical microinfarct, CMB: cerebral microbleed; cSAH: convexity subarachnoid hemorrhage; CSF: cerebrospinal fluid; CSO-DPVS: centrum semiovale dilated perivascular space; cSS: cortical superficial siderosis; CT: computerized tomography; CTA: computerized tomography arteriography; CTV: computerized tomography venography; DSA: digital subtraction angiography; EVD: external ventricular drainage; FLAIR: fluid attenuated inversion recovery; ICH: intracerebral hemorrhage; ICP: intracranial pressure; LAA: left atrial appendage; MRA: magnetic resonance imaging arteriography; MRV: magnetic resonance venography; MRI: magnetic resonance imaging; PET: positron emission tomography; PIB: Pittsburgh compound B; SWI: susceptibility-weighted imaging; TIA: transient ischemic attack; TFNS: transient focal neurological symptoms; WMH: white matter hyperintensity; WMI: white matter ischemia.

CAA is characterized by the deposition of Aβ proteins in the media and adventitia of small and mid-sized cortical and leptomeningeal arteries (and, less frequently, veins). It is a component of any disorder in which amyloid is deposited in the brain, and it is not associated with systemic amyloidosis. The prevalence of CAA increases with advancing age. Some autopsy series have found CAA in 5% of individuals in the seventh decade but in 50% of those older than 90 years. While often asymptomatic, CAA is being increasingly recognized as an important cause of ICH in the elderly, accounting for up to one-fifth of all spontaneous ICH in this group.

Most cases of CAA are sporadic. Hereditary types represent only a minor proportion and are associated with ICH at younger ages. The Aβ in CAA is predominantly a soluble 40 amino-acid-long form. This is in contrast to the parenchymal Aβ in senile plaques of AD, which is predominantly a longer and less soluble 42-amino-acid-long form. These amyloid proteins are derived from a larger amyloid precursor protein (APP), encoded by the APP gene on chromosome 21. APP is expressed and metabolized into Aβ in especially high levels by neurons in the brain. CAA is thought to result from a defect in the central nervous system clearance mechanism of interstitial fluid (ISF), and thus, also the Aβ. In the initial stages, Aβ deposition is limited to the tunica adventitia, resulting in thickening of the vessel. With progression, the tunica adventitia becomes saturated, resulting in further Aβ deposition in the smooth muscle of the tunica media and further thickening of the vessel wall. Due to the cytotoxic effects of Aβ, there is subsequent degeneration and eventual loss of the smooth muscle, resulting in thinning and fragility of the vessel wall. CAA affects vessels in a characteristic patchy manner with a predilection for the occipital lobe. Sporadic CAA has known genetic risk factors in APOE alleles, as APOE is an important lipoprotein involved in ISF drainage pathways. The two alleles thought to be implicated in increasing risk of developing sporadic CAA are APOE ε2 and APOE ε4, where APOE ε2 induces vessel fragility, while APOE ε4 promotes Aβ intravascular deposition. Another common genetic risk factor is Down syndrome (trisomy 21), presumably because there is increased expression of APP. Importantly, CAA is considered to be a distinct entity from, yet highly associated with, AD, with up to 90% of those with AD having pathologically determined CAA, but only 25% of patients with advanced CAA having AD.

The diagnosis of CAA is based on the Modified Boston Criteria. The key diagnostic category for clinical practice is probable CAA, the highest level of diagnostic certainty currently achievable without obtaining brain tissue. Spontaneous ICH is the most disabling manifestation of CAA and occurs in peripheral cortical and subcortical lobar locations. This is a key differentiating factor from causes of ICH in deep locations (e.g., basal ganglia, pons), such as chronic hypertensive arteriopathy. Clinical manifestations of lobar ICH include headache, focal neurological deficits, focal seizures, nausea and vomiting, and depressed consciousness. In CT scanning, the finding of a single or even multiple lobar ICHs with superficial location and cortical involvement is suggestive of a CAA-related hemorrhage. CAA-related lobar ICH is recurrent in up to 30% of patients per year.

The diagnosis of CAA before ICH manifests is paramount, especially in light of the high prevalence of antithrombotics, especially anticoagulants, in elderly patients that can increase the risk of ICH. Clinically, patients can develop TFNS (amyloid spells) from cSAH, a form of a non-aneurysmal SAH, characterized by bleeding localized to one or more adjacent cortical sulci at the convexity of the brain. CAA should never be assumed to be the cause of an isolated SAH unless all other causes, particularly aneurysmal, have been excluded. The vast majority of cSAH in CAA occurs due to rupture of fragile Aβ-laden convexity leptomeningeal vessels. Amyloid spells, thought to be due to cortical spreading depression triggered by breakdown products of cSAH, are characteristically described as recurrent, stereotyped, spreading paresthesias lasting several minutes, but a range of both positive (e.g., scintillating scotoma) and negative (e.g., paresis, dysphagia) transient symptoms have been described. TFNS should not be mistaken for sensory TIAs. The headache in cSAH tends to either be very mild or absent.

SWI MRI sequences can be used to detect lobar CMBs and cSS associated with CAA. CMBs refer to small 2–10 millimeter, round or ovoid, low-signal areas evident on SWI. Histologically, they represent small areas of blood extravasation into the perivascular space. Subacutely and chronically, SWI MRI sequences can be used to detect the low-signal hemosiderin residues that are left after cSAH resolution, known as cSS. However, cSS should not be confused with infratentorial superficial siderosis of unknown etiology. CMBs and cSS have been incorporated into the Modified Boston Criteria, which allows for reliable diagnosis of CAA without the need for histopathology. Chronic periventricular posteriorly located WMI sparing the U fibres, CMI and lobar lacunae, cortical atrophy of the posterolateral cortices and increased CSO-DPVS have each been recently described as promising MRI biomarkers of moderate to severe stage CAA. PVSs are the major route for the drainage of ISF, including Aβ, from the brain. It has been proposed that as vessel walls become saturated with Aβ, this results in retrograde dilation of these PVSs, and actually causes further impairment to perivascular drainage. This leads to further Aβ deposition resulting in a vicious cycle.

Increasing evidence speaks in favor of chronic WMI, CMBs, CMI and lobar lacunae to significantly contribute to cognitive and functional decline independent of AD in CAA. These lesions cause gradual cognitive impairment by either disrupting neuronal circuits or occurring in strategic locations. In addition to gradual chronic cognitive decline, patients with CAA can also experience acute stepwise decline in cognitive function after lobar ICH, or may present with a rapidly progressing cognitive decline caused by CAA-ri.

An autoimmune response to Aβ, termed CAA-ri or ABRA, is another important albeit uncommon autoimmune response to vascular Aβ. Histopathologically, there is perivascular inflammation and inflammation confined to the Aβ-laden vessel wall itself. Similar findings have been observed in studies of Aβ immunotherapy in AD with resultant amyloid-related imaging abnormalities (ARIA) seen on MRI. Pathologically, ARIA is characterized by a shift of Aβ into the vasculature. Clinically, CAA-ri can present with subacute or rapidly progressive cognitive decline, headache, hallucinations, focal neurological signs, focal seizures or decreased consciousness. Angiographic findings can be typical of vasculitis (beading of vessels on DSA). MRI may show more extensive WMH due to vasogenic edema, sometimes causing a mass effect resembling a tumor, with concomitant abundant lobar CMBs. Brain biopsy is usually needed to confirm the diagnosis of CAA-ri.

No specific laboratory findings are diagnostic of CAA. However, there is an emerging role of CSF abnormalities that may serve as biomarkers of CAA; specifically, increased protein and decreased soluble Aβ or APOE in non-inflammatory CAA. In contrast, in CAA-ri, decreased levels of Aβ (especially the less soluble form, 1–42), and additionally increased levels of Aβ autoantibodies and markers of axonal injury, such as tau and phosphotau, may be found. Genetic evaluation can be considered, especially in patients with a family history of CAA. In cases of CAA-related ICH, laboratory studies should rule out other possible etiologies (e.g., anticoagulation). PET brain scanning with [18]F-labeled Pittsburgh compound B (PIB) derivative may be useful in some patients where the diagnosis is doubtful (e.g., unobtainable CSF), where cortical retention of PIB may serve as an *in vivo* marker of CAA.

Currently, CAA is largely untreatable. The management of CAA-related ICH is identical to the standard management of ICH. Special attention should be paid to the reversal of anticoagulation, the management of intracranial pressure and the prevention of complications. ICH evacuation should be considered in patients with intermediate-sized ICHs (20-60 ml) who have a progressive deterioration in their level of consciousness. It is imperative for a neurosurgeon to send a specimen for histopathological study. Some patients with CAA-ri improve clinically when given corticosteroids or cyclophosphamide (duration is not well established, treatment should be individualized). TFNS can be successfully suppressed with anticonvulsants. There is evidence supporting the treatment of arterial hypertension to prevent hemorrhage recurrence in CAA. CAA increases the risk of antithrombotic-associated ICH. Reinstitution of anticoagulation after CAA-related ICH should be considered after carefully weighing the risks and benefits in a given individual. In patients with coronary artery disease, cardiac stents and/or ischemic stroke, the benefit of antithrombotic therapy is clear and withdrawal of antiplatelets requires prudent consideration of multiple factors. The use of statins after a lobar ICH may increase the risk for a clinically manifest recurrent ICH, so they should be prescribed with caution. Patients should avoid any degree of head trauma. In future, development of methods for imaging perivascular drainage would be a key step towards identifying treatments for enhancing Aβ clearance and reducing vascular and parenchymal deposition, which may possibly decelerate the clinical progression of CAA.

# References

1. Greenberg SM, Bacskai BJ, Hernandez-Guillamon M, et al. Cerebral amyloid angiopathy and Alzheimer disease: One peptide, two pathways. *Nat Rev Neurol.* 2020;**16**(1): 30–42.

2. Sharma R, Dearaugo S, Infeld B, O'Sullivan R, Gerraty RP. Cerebral amyloid angiopathy: Review of clinico-radiological features and mimics. *J Med Imaging Radiat Oncol.* 2018. doi: 10.1111/1754–9485.12726. Online ahead of print.

3. Banerjee G, Carare R, Cordonnier C, et al. The increasing impact of cerebral amyloid angiopathy: essential new insights for clinical practice. *J Neurol Neurosurg Psychiatry.* 2017;**88**(11): 982–994.

4. Greenberg SM, Charidimou A. Diagnosis of cerebral amyloid angiopathy: Evolution of the Boston criteria. *Stroke.* 2018;**49**: 491–497.

# Dolichoectasia and Fusiform Aneurysms

Jernej Avsenik, Bojana Žvan

## Case Presentation

59-year-old male presented to the neurological emergency department with acute vertigo, drowsiness, nausea and sudden worsening of bilateral hearing loss. He initially presented with vertigo five years earlier when he was diagnosed with vertebrobasilar fusiform aneurysm (Figure 8.3.1).

Despite receiving dual antiplatelet therapy, the patient had recurrent episodes of acute vertigo and hearing loss in the following years. During that period he was also diagnosed with ischemic infarct in the right cerebellar hemisphere (Figure 8.3.2).

Neurological examination revealed somnolence, bilateral hearing loss, horizontal nystagmus and mild lower limb ataxia. Non-contrast computed tomography (CT) showed no acute lesion in the brain parenchyma. On the other hand, significant enlargement of the fusiform aneurysm involving basilar and left vertebral artery was evident on CT angiography (CTA) (Figure 8.3.3).

Laboratory results showed hyperlipidemia and mildly elevated sedimentation rate, but were otherwise normal. Paroxismal atrial fibrillation was noted on electrocardiography

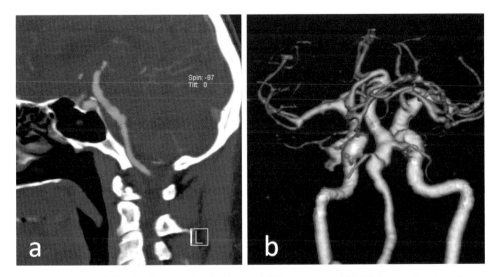

**Figure 8.3.1** Sagittal (a) and volume-rendered technique (VRT) reconstructed (b) CTA images show irregular dilatation of basilar artery, extending to distal segment of the left vertebral artery. Right vertebral artery is occluded. Findings are consistent with fusiform vertebrobasilar aneurysm.

321

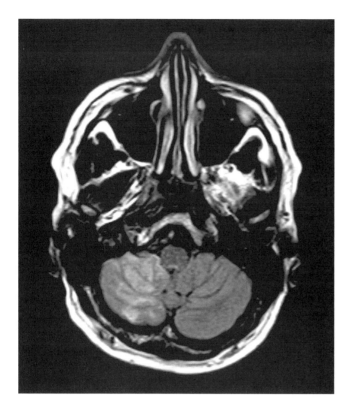

**Figure 8.3.2** Fluid attenuated inversion recovery (FLAIR) MRI image shows high intensity signal in the caudal part of the right cerebellar hemisphere, consistent with acute ischemic lesion in the right posterior inferior cerebellar artery (PICA) vascular territory.

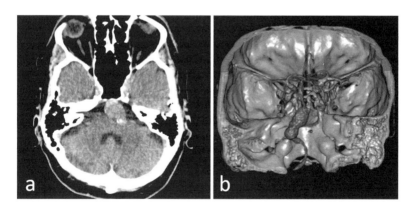

**Figure 8.3.3** Computed tomography (a) shows oval heterogeneously hyperdense lesion in the course of the basilar artery, compressing the pons, representing a partially thrombosed fusiform aneurysm. Surface rendered CTA imaging (b) shows significant enlargement of the aneurysm in comparison to Figure 8.3.1.

(ECG). Magnetic resonance imaging (MRI) showed an area of chronic postischemic encephalomalacia in the right cerebellum; however, no acute ischemic lesion could be seen. A vertebrobasilar aneurysm with mural thrombus and turbulent blood flow was

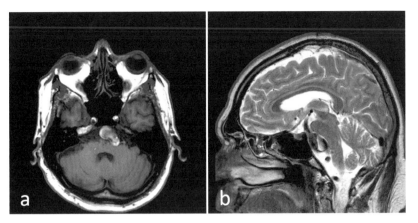

**Figure 8.3.4** Axial T1-weighted (a) and sagittal T2-weighted (b) MRI images show heterogeneous signal intensity of the vertebrobasilar fusiform aneurysm due to irregular blood flow and complex thrombus structure. There is significant indentation of brainstem due to mass effect of the aneurysm (b).

identified, compressing the pons and lower mesencephalon (Figure 8.3.4). There was no hydrocephalus and no edema was present in the adjacent brain parenchyma.

Due to the enlargement of the vertebrobasilar fusiform aneurysm and severe clinical deterioration, a multidisciplinary board decided to treat the patient endovascularly, using a combination of flow diverter and stents.

**Population**
- Middle-aged and older patients with systemic atherosclerosis, predominantly in posterior circulation
- Non-atherosclerotic types more often in younger patients with systemic inflammatory connective tissue disorders, acquired immunodeficiency or viral disease; posterior and anterior circulation equally affected

**Presentation**
- TIA or ischemic stroke, more common in posterior circulation
- Compressive symptoms due to brainstem compression, hydrocephalus or cranial neuropathies
- Hemorrhage due to aneurysm rupture

Wide clinical differential diagnosis, depending on presentation: other causes of stroke, cranial neuropathy, brain compression or subarachnoid hemorrhage

**Computed tomography (CT) and magnetic resonance (MRI) imaging**
- Evidence of ischemic stroke, mass effect, edema or bleeding
- Signs of generalized atherosclerosis may be present
- Mural calcification and partial thrombosis of the aneurysm are common
- Complex MR signal due to layered thrombus structure and slow or turbulent residual flow

**Angiographic techniques (CTA, MRA, DSA)**
- Focal fusiform or ovoid luminal dilatation
- Commonly superimposed on ectatic parent vessel
- May show evidence of generalized vasculopathy

Imaging differential diagnosis included olichoectasia (generalized non-focal elongation) and dissecting aneurysm

**Treatment**
- Medical: antiplatelat, anticoagulant
- Endovascular: parent vessel occlusion, stenting, stent-assisted coiling, deployment of flow diverter
- Surgical: flow reduction or bypass/trapping, flow reversal, trapping with aneurysm decompression

**Follow-up**
- Clinical follow-up at 1 month, 3–6 months, 12–18 months, later at 1–3 year intervals
- Radio logical follow-up: post perative control, then at 3–6 months, 12–18 months, then at 1–3 year intervals
- Convention angiography is the gold standard in first 12 months, MRA may be acceptable alternative

## Discussion

The term dolichoectasia refers to generalized non-focal vessel elongation and tortuosity, and is a frequent manifestation of advanced atherosclerosis. It most commonly occurs in the posterior circulation (vertebrobasilar dolichoectasia), followed by the supraclinoid internal cerebral artery. However, any part of the intracranial circulation may be involved. Elderly and middle-aged patients are most commonly affected. Ectatic vessels are usually asymptomatic and present as incidental findings on imaging or at autopsy.[1]

On the other hand, fusiform aneurysms (FA) are true focal arterial enlargements, commonly associated with underlying dolichoectasia. These aneurysms are rare, representing 3–13% of all intracranial aneurysms. They are usually atherosclerotic in origin and present in the vertebrobasilary circulation of elderly patients. Significant male predominance for posterior circulation fusiform aneurysms has been found. Incidence is also higher in patients with hypertension, diabetes, hyperlipidemia, coronary artery disease and smoking. However, non-atherosclerotic types occurring in younger patients have also been described, mostly in association with systemic vascular disorders, such as systemic lupus, Marfan syndrome, Ehlers–Danlos syndrome, Fabry disease, autosomal-dominant polycystic kidney disease and neurofibromatosis, as well as with viral infections such as varicella zoster or human immunodeficiency virus (HIV). Interestingly, in the non-atherosclerotic form, anterior and posterior intracranial circulations are equally affected.[2]

Patients with vertebrobasilar fusiform aneurysms may present with symptoms related to mass effect, ischemia or hemorrhage. Compression of the brainstem may result in headache due to hydrocephalus.[3] However, patients may also present with trigeminal neuralgia, hemifacial spasm or abducens palsy due to cranial nerve compression. Cranial nerves (CN) V to VIII are most commonly affected by fusiform aneurysms, followed by CN IX, X and XII. On the other hand, clinical syndromes due to ischemic events are even more common and range from mild transient ischemic attacks (TIAs) to locked-in syndrome secondary to large pontine infarcts. Areas most commonly affected by ischemia include the pons, thalamus, lateral medulla, cerebellum, and occipital and temporal lobes.[4] The third and the least common clinical presentation is with a sudden headache due to aneurysmal rupture and subsequent subarachnoid hemorrhage. The natural history is unfavorable, with especially poor prognosis for those symptomatic patients with untreated aneurysms who initially present with compressive symptoms or ischemia. Nevertheless, rebleeding rate and mortality for untreated ruptured aneurysms is also very high.

Histologically, irregular or hyperplastic intima with extensive fragmentation of internal elastic lamina and loss of reticular fibers in tunica media have been described. Commonly, the residual vessel lumen is surrounded by layers of organized thrombus. This may be appreciated as heterogeneously hyperdense areas on non-contrast CT. On MRI, signal intensity is often extremely heterogeneous due to the combination of complex thrombus structure and slow or turbulent blood flow. However, a prominent flow void surrounded by heterogeneous thrombus may frequently be appreciated. Furthermore, by employing vessel wall imaging techniques, inflammatory processes inside the vessel wall may be evaluated by short-segment patchy enhancement following intravenous administration of gadolinium contrast agent. CTA and digital subtraction angiography (DSA) confirm fusiform or ovoid luminal dilatation, commonly superimposed on an ectatic parent vessel.

Recently, endovascular techniques, including parent vessel occlusion, stenting, stent-assisted coiling and deployment of flow diverters have become the primary treatment modality for most patients, reserving traditional microsurgical management for patients who cannot be treated endovascularly.

# References

1. Awad AJ, Mascitelli JR, Haroun RR, et al. Endovascular management of fusiform aneurysms in the posterior circulation: The era of flow diversion. *Neurosurg Focus.* 2017;**42** (6): E14.

2. Barletta EA, Gaspar RHML, Araújo JFM, et al. Nonsaccular aneurysms: A wide comparison between the four main types. *Surg Neurol Int.* 2019;**10**: 30.

3. Osborn AG, Hedlund GL, Salzman KL. *Osborn's Brain: Imaging, Pathology, and Anatomy, 2nd Edn.* Philadelphia, PA: Elsevier; 2017. 1300.

4. Serrone JC, Gozal YM, Grossman AW, et al. Vertebrobasilar fusiform aneurysms. *Neurosurg Clin N Am.* 2014;**25**: 471–484.

# Carotid Artery Dissection

Füsun Mayda Domaç, Mustafa Ülker

## Case Presentation

A 17-year-old male was admitted to the emergency department with a headache. Two days ago he had a sudden hypoesthesia and weakness in his left arm that has lasted for one to two hours. After these symptoms had disappeared, he had a sudden onset of a throbbing headache located on the right frontal region with a visual analog scale (VAS) score of 5–6/10 that he claimed he had not experienced before. Over a duration of approximately two hours, the severity of the headache increased with a VAS score of 9/10 and spread throughout his head. He did not have nausea or vomiting. Neither photophobia nor phonophobia accompanied the headache. After left-sided weakness and hypoesthesia had been supervened by a headache two days later, lasting for an hour, he was admitted to the emergency department. Except for a febrile convulsion at the age of three, his medical history was totally normal. He did not have a history of trauma or a recent infection. His elder brother had a history of epilepsy and his aunt had a history of ischemic cerebrovascular disease.

On physical examination, his temperature was 36.7 °C, heart rate 82 beats/min and blood pressure 110/75 mmHg. On neurological exam, he was cooperative and oriented. Cranial nerves were intact. Motor strength and sensory examination were normal. Deep tendon reflexes and plantar reflexes were normal with flexor response bilaterally. Because of having experienced similar complaints two days ago, brain computed tomography (CT) and magnetic resonance imaging (MRI) were performed and neither hemorrhage nor ischemia were seen (Figure 8.4.1).

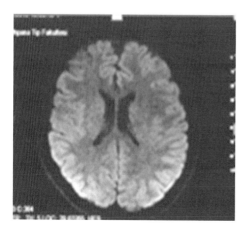

**Figure 8.4.1** Cranial diffusion MRI is normal.

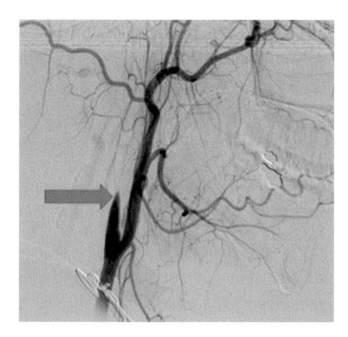

**Figure 8.4.2** Digital subtraction conventional angiography; right internal carotid artery thins out and disappears 2–3 cm proximal to the origin of the bulbar segment, which is compatible with dissection.

A bilateral carotid ultrasound with color Doppler was suspicious of right carotid artery dissection at the cervical segment, so digital subtraction angiography was performed to verify the dissection. On digital subtraction angiography, the right internal carotid artery was found to thin out and disappear at 2–3 cm proximal to the bulbar segment, which was compatible with dissection (Figure 8.4.2).

As the patient did not have a history of trauma and had a family history of ischemic stroke, he was examined for diseases that may predispose spontaneous carotid artery dissection. Routine biochemical and microbiological studies, including total peripheral blood count, fasting glucose, HbA1c, low-density lipoprotein (LDL), very-low-density lipoprotein (VLDL), high-density lipoprotein (HDL) and triglyceride, thyroid, hepatic and renal functions, vitamin B12, folic acid, homocysteine, erythrocyte sedimentation rate and C-reactive protein were all normal. Examinations for lupus anticoagulant, rheumatoid factor, serum angiotensin-converting enzyme, antineutrophilic cytoplasmic autoantibodies, human leukocyte antigen (HLA) B27, antithrombin-III, protein S, protein C, antiphospholipid antibodies and genetic tests for factor V Leiden mutation and activated protein C resistance were negative. Only the antinuclear antibody (ANA) test was slightly positive. Abdominal CT did not show any evidence of renal or hepatic disease. He also did not have any signs of connective tissue disease.

The patient was diagnosed with spontaneous carotid artery dissection (sCAD) presenting with headache and transient ischemic attacks. He was hospitalized and treated with subcutaneous low-molecular-weight heparin, followed by transition to therapeutic oral warfarin. The headache was treated with paracetamol and during his short hospital stay his headache diminished. On follow-up warfarin was ceased at the third month and replaced with acetylsalicylic acid. At one-year follow-up the patient remained symptom-free.

---

**Clinical Suspicion of CAD**

**Age**: 30–45 years

**Gender:** slight gender predisposition favoring males

**Type of onset:** especially sudden onset

**Clinical manifestations:** (a) sudden onset, unilateral, constant, and throbbing headache,

(b) neckpain (with headache >90%), (c) transient ischemic attack or stroke symptoms (50–90%)

---

- **Magnetic resonance angiography (MRA):** along with a T1 axial cervical MRI with fat saturation: high sensitivity and specificity, and ability to visualize an intramural hematoma

- **Computeed tomographic angiography (CTA):** can show the double lumen sign (true and false lumen), but is associated with radiation exposure and potential technical challenges

- **Carotid ultrasound with color Doppler:** this non-invasive technique is operator dependent and is of poor diagnostic value in patients with intracranial carotid dissection

- **Conventional angiography:** an invasive test that may potentially cause an iatrogenic dissection, especially in a patient population with underlying vessel wall weakness

---

**Etiological Investigations**

Spontaneous or traumatic

**Traumatic dissection:** blunt or penetrating trauma

**Spontaneous caroti dissections:** family history of

- Marfan syndrome

- Ehlers–Danlos Syndrome

- Fibromuscular dysplasia

- Autosomal dominant polycystic renal disease

- Other connective tissue disorders

- Eagle syndrome (elongated styloid process)

---

**Treatment of CADs**

- The main purpose of treating CAD is to prevent stroke

- **Antithrombotic treatment** for at least three to six months is reasonable

- **Anticoagulation therapy** is still often used in practice as a stroke prevention

- No difference shown between stroke recurrence and bleeding complications between antitrombotic and anticoagulation treatments

---

# Discussion

Carotid artery dissection (CAD) occurs in young people. In population-based studies, the mean age of occurrence of is approximately 45 years. Dissection is found to be as high as 20% in stroke patients younger than 30 years of age. There is a variation in the presenting signs and symptoms of this disease, which makes it extremely difficult to diagnose on initial presentation. The incidence of bilateral carotid dissections is considered rare and is not exactly known, but may be as high as 22% of sCADs.[1]

The presentation can range from an asymptomatic patient one that presents with an acute stroke. The most common presenting symptom (80–90%) is unilateral headache at the same side as the arterial dissection. The headache has no specific features and can resemble migraine or cluster headaches. In 20% of the patients a severe and sudden thunderclap headache may be the initial symptom. Classically the patient describes a headache, facial or eye pain and neck pain. Focal neurological symptoms as a result of cerebral or retinal ischemia may be transient or persistent. Partial Horner's syndrome with miosis and ptosis but without anhidrosis may be present in a quarter of the patients and this may be due to compression of the adjacent sympathetic nerves by a hematoma of the cervical artery. Pulsatile tinnitus may be seen in 15–20% of patients. Intracranial CADs are complicated by pseudoaneurysm formation; cranial nerves IX, X and XII are the closest in proximity to the carotid artery and are most commonly involved in CAD. Rupture of a pseudoaneurysm can cause subarachnoid hemorrhage.[2]

Patients with CAD are more likely to have hypertension. Migraine, particularly with aura, hyperhomocysteinemia, hypertension, smoking, family history of arterial dissection and recent infection have been identified as the risk factors for the development of CAD. A family history of carotid dissection or connective tissue disorders may heighten suspicion. Certain genetic connective tissue conditions such as Ehlers–Danlos syndrome, Marfan's syndrome, osteogenesis imperfecta and fibromuscular dysplasia increase the risk of CAD. One of the well-known risk factors that has been identified is a recent history of minor cervical trauma. In traumatic dissection the presence of blunt or penetrating trauma is helpful in making the diagnosis.[3]

CAD is suspected clinically and confirmed by neuroimaging techniques including MRI, CT angiography (CTA) and conventional angiography. The preferred method of diagnosis is magnetic resonance angiography (MRA) along with T1 axial cervical MRI with fat saturation due to its high sensitivity and specificity, and ability to visualize an intramural hematoma. CTA be used, but is associated with radiation exposure. In patients with CAD, a CTA can show the double lumen sign (true and false lumen) or a flame-like taper of the lumen. Carotid ultrasound with color Doppler is another screening test that can be used. In patients with only local symptoms, the dissection rarely causes luminal narrowing and thus may be missed on color Doppler. Catheter angiography is not routinely used to diagnose, being an invasive test that may potentially cause an iatrogenic dissection, especially in a patient population with underlying vessel-wall weakness.[4]

The main purpose of treating CAD is to prevent stroke. Several retrospective studies and a meta-analysis did not show any difference between stroke recurrence and bleeding complications between the two treatments. The guidelines also recommend intravenous thrombolysis for eligible patients with acute ischemic stroke, including those with isolated extracranial or intracranial carotid artery dissection, provided that treatment is initiated within 3–4.5 hours of symptom onset. Mechanical thrombectomy has proven effective for selected patients with acute ischemic stroke caused by a proximal intracranial arterial occlusion in the anterior circulation.[5] Headache can be treated with paracetamol, NSAIDs (naproxen sodium) or ibuprofen.

# References

1. Lee VH, Brown RD, Mandrekar JN, et al. Incidence and outcome of cervical artery dissection: A population-based study. *Neurology.* 2006;**67**: 1809–1812.

2. Blum CA, Yaghi S. Cervical artery dissection: A review of the epidemiology, pathophysiology, treatment, and outcome. *Arch Neurosci.* 2015;**2**(4): e26670.

3. Hassan AE, Zacharatos H, Mohammad YM, et al. Comparison of single versus multiple spontaneous extra- and/or intracranial arterial dissection. *J Stroke Cerebrovasc Dis.* 2013;**22**(1): 42–48.

4. Debette S, Leys D. Cervical-artery dissections: Predisposing factors, diagnosis, and outcome. *Lancet Neurol.* 2009;**8**: 668–678.

5. Cervical Artery Dissection in Stroke Study (CADISS) Investigators, Markus HS, Levi C, King A, et al. Antiplatelet therapy vs anticoagulation therapy in cervical artery dissection: The Cervical Artery Dissection in Stroke Study (CADISS) randomized clinical trial final results. *JAMA Neurol.* 2019;**76** (6): 657.

# Cerebral Venous Sinus Thrombosis

Taşkın Duman, Derya Uludüz

## Case Presentation

A 24 year-old female, primigravida, was admitted to the emergency department with a generalized tonic-clonic seizure two weeks after normal vaginal delivery. In addition to the seizure, she had left-sided weakness. The seizure lasted for about three minutes and she was unconscious for 20 minutes afterwards. She reported a severe headache in the previous three days. The headache was in the occipital region extending to the neck and vertex. It was throbbing and associated with nausea and vomiting.

On arrival she was drowsy with fluctuating consciousness. Temperature was 36.6 °C, heart rate 70 beats/min, blood pressure 110/60mHg and respiratory rate 22 breaths/min with an oxygen saturation of 99% on room air. A physical examination revealed no abnormalities in the head, neck, chest, abdomen or lymph nodes. On neurological exam, she demonstrated slightly decreased motor strength in her left side, predominantly upper extremity. Fundoscopic examination was normal. Her medical and family history, including occurrence of thromboembolism, were unremarkable. She had no history of use any drug or hormone therapy.

Considering the patient's age and lack of past medical history, brain computed tomography (CT) and magnetic resonance imaging (MRI) were performed, followed by MR angiography and venography to rule out vascular abnormalities such as aneurysm, arteriovenous malformation or sinus thrombosis. Cortico-subcortical areas of higher signal intensity in bilateral parietal and left frontal regions with no arterial distribution were observed in the brain MRI, which was best seen in fluid-attenuated inversion recovery (FLAIR) and diffusion-weighted images (Figure 9.1.1).

Cranial MR venography revealed venous thrombosis in the anterior two-thirds of the superior sagittal sinus. This was compatible with superior sagittal sinus thrombosis explaining venous infarctions (Figure 9.1.2).

Laboratory studies, including total peripheral blood count, biochemical screen, Fe, ferritin, HbA1c, vitamin B12, folic acid, erythrocyte sedimentation rate, C-reactive protein, thyroid functions, and renal and hepatic functions were normal. Inflammatory and coagulopathy panel, antinuclear antibody, rheumatoid factor, antineutrophilic cytoplasmic autoantibody, human leukocyte antigen (HLA) B27, serum angiotensin-converting enzyme (ACE), lupus anticoagulant, antithrombin, protein S, protein C, factor VIII levels, homocysteine levels, antiphospholipid antibodies, factor V Leiden mutation and activated protein C resistance were negative. The patient was diagnosed with cerebral venous sinus thrombosis due to puerperium and treated with heparin, transitioning to therapeutic oral warfarin. On the fourth day of their hospital stay, she had another generalized tonic-clonic

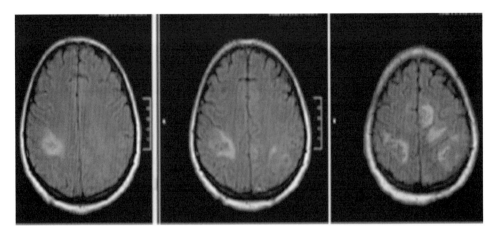

**Figure 9.1.1** FLAIR-weighted axial MR images, cortico-subcortical areas of high signal intensity in bilateral parietal and left frontal regions.

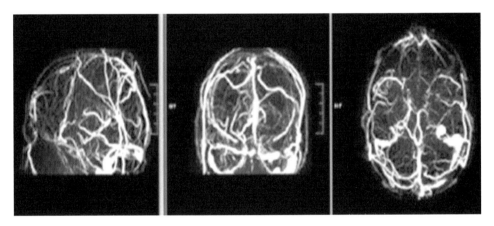

**Figure 9.1.2** Lateral maximum intensity projection (MIP) images of MR venography, showing signal loss in the anterior half of the superior sagittal sinus.

seizure lasting two minutes. Levetiracetam was initiated with an optimal dose of 1000 mg/ daily. She was discharged with full recovery.

**Clinical suspicion of CVST**

Age = 20–50 years; Gender = F/M:3/1; Type of onset = acute (47.1%), subacute (34%) or chronic (18.9%); Clinical manifestations: (a) isolated intracranial hypertension: headache (60–70%), papilledema, (b) focal neurological deficit, (c) seizures (30–40%), (d) diffuse encephalopathy, (e) cavernous sinus syndrome: orbital pain, ophthalmoplegia

Non-specific neurological manifestations

**Cranial CT** = Direct signs; increased attenuation of thrombosed sinus (dense triangle sign, cord sign), contrast enhancement of wall of occluded sinus owing to collateral circulation (empty delta sign). Indirect signs, brain edema, intracerebral hemorrhage (juxtacortical etc.) orbilateral parencyhmal infarction

**Cranial MRI** = Infarction or hemorrhage, often across arterial boundaries, and brain swelling. Lack of signal void from the sinus, abnormal signals from intraluminal clot, depending its age, evidence of collateral formation. SWI: exaggerated magnetic susceptibility effect, intraluminal hypointense thrombus. T2GRE: clots within sinus isorcortical veins. DWI: hyperintensities with decreased apparent diffusion coefficient (ADC).

**Cranial CT Venography/MR Venography** = Lack of high flow signal in venous sinuses, formation of collaterals

**Cerebral Angiogaphy** = Lack of filling of the sinuses, delayed emptying, sudden termination of a cortical vein surrounded by dilated and tortuous collateral veins

**Confirmed CVST–etiological investigations**

| Prothrombotic states | Sex related | Infections | Infections | Hematological Disease | Others |
|---|---|---|---|---|---|
| Antithrombin III deficiency, protein C deficiency, protein S deficiency, antiphospholipid antibodies, factor V Leiden mutation, activated protein C resistance, hyperhomocysteinemia | Pregnancy and puerperium, oral contraceptives/ hormone-replacement therapy | Otitis, mastoiditis, sinusitis, meningitis, systemic infections | Systemic lupus erythematosis, Behçet disease, inflammatory bowel disease, thyroid disease, sarcoidosis | Paroxysmal nocturnal hemoglobinuria, iron deficiency, nephrotic syndrome, polycythemia, thrombocythemia | Lumbar puncture, spinal anesthesia, cancer-related, drugs, dehydration none identified |

Peripheral blood count, hemogram, iron, ferritin, urea, creatinine, free T3, free T4, TSH, calcium, liver enzymes, ACE, thyroid antibodies, sedimentation, CRP, HCG test, antithrombin III, protein C, protein S, factor V Leiden, G20210A prothrombin, homocysteine, antiphospholipid antibody, lupus anticoagulant, anticardiolipin, antibeta 2 glycoprotein-1 antibody, ANCA, activated protein C, prothrombin time, activated partial thromboplastin time, HLAB27, pathergy test

**Treatment of CVST**

| | | |
|---|---|---|
| **Antithrombotic: IV or SC anticoagulation (except*)**<br>**(1) Neurological improvement or stable:** continue with oral anticoagulation for 3–12 months (transient or low-risk etiology) or lifelong (high-risk thrombophilia)<br>**(2) Neurological deterioration despite medical treatment:** consider endovascular therapy. If severe mass effect*; consider decompressive hemicraniectomy | **Intracranial hypertension:** hyperventilation, head elevation (30°), osmotic diuretics, shunt or stenting<br>**Epilepctic seizures:** antiepileptic in first seizure<br>**Herniation:** decompressive hemicraniectomy<br>**Hidrocephalus:** ventriculoperitoneal shunt | **Prothrombotic states**<br>Inflammatory diseases and Behçet disease: steroids<br>Infections: antibiotics |

CVST: Cerebral venous sinus thrombosis; F: Female; M: Male; CT: Computerized tomography; MRI: Magnetic Resonance imaging; SWI: susceptibility weighted imaging; DWI: Difusion weighted imaging; GRE: Gradient echo; ADC: Apparent diffusion coefficient; CRP: C-reactive protein; ACE: angiotension-converting enzyme; HCG: human chorionic gonadotropin; ANCA: Antineutrophil cytoplasmic antibodies

# Case Discussion

Cerebral venous sinus thrombosis (CVST) is thrombosis of the dural sinuses and deep and/ or superficial cerebral venous system. CVST is presumed to be less frequent than ischemic infarction and intracerebral hemorrhage and it accounts for 0.5–3% of all stroke types. As opposed to arterial strokes, CVST has significantly higher incidence before the age of 50 years and is three times more common in women. Sex-specific risk factors in women such as oral contraceptive use, pregnancy and hormone therapy seem to be associated with an increased risk of CVST.[1]

Symptoms and signs of cerebral vein thrombosis can be presented, with two different mechanisms. One of the mechanisms is parenchymal damage due to venous obstruction, increased venous and capillary pressure, and decreased cerebral perfusion. An increase in venous and capillary pressure leads to disruption of the blood–brain barrier, vasogenic edema and blood leakage into the interstitial space. Another mechanism is that increased venous pressure as a result of thrombosis disrupts cerebrospinal fluid absorption and causes increased intracranial pressure.

Clinical symptomatology in CVST cases is quite wide ranging from headache to coma and this may cause difficulties in diagnosis and a delay in treatment. Clinical presentation may vary according to age, etiology, mode of onset, lesion localization and presence of parenchymal involvement. Clinical symptomatology can be classified into five groups, as intracranial hypertension (headache, diplopia, papillary edema, sixth cranial nerve paresis), focal neurological deficit, epileptic seizures, encephalopathy and cavernous sinus syndrome. Headache is the most common symptom in 70–90% of CVST cases and may be accompanied by papilledema (41–82%), nausea and vomiting (27.7%), changes in consciousness or neck stiffness. Clinical features of CVST can also vary according to the localization of thrombosis. Motor deficits and seizures might be presented in superior sagittal sinus thrombosis (SSS), aphasia and headache in left transverse sinus thrombosis (TS), and orbital pain, chemosis and oculomotor paralysis may occur in cavernous sinus thrombosis.[2]

Diagnosis in CVST is based on clinical suspicion and radiological evaluation. It is essential to demonstrate thrombus in sinus or vein. Cerebral CT is the first method in the evaluation of patients with suspected CVST or solely headache symptoms. CT findings can be classified directly and indirectly. Direct findings are: increased attenuation of thrombosed sinus (dense triangle sign, cord sign) or contrast enhancement of the wall of the occluded sinus owing to collateral circulation (empty delta sign). Indirect signs are: brain edema, intracerebral hemorrhage (juxtacortical, etc.) or orbilateral parenchymal infarction. Cranial MRI reveals infarction or hemorrhage, often across arterial boundaries, and brain swelling, lack of signal void from a sinus, abnormal signals from intraluminal clot depending its age and evidence of collateral formation. MRI gradient echo (GRE) and susceptibility-weighted imaging (SWI) sequences may be more useful in diagnosis. SWI demonstrates exaggerated magnetic susceptibility effects and intraluminal hypointense thrombus. GRET2 and diffusion-weighted imaging show clots within sinuses or cortical veins and hyperintensity with decreased apparent diffusion coefficient. Parenchymal lesions can be detected in 40% of cases, hemorrhagic transformation in 16.3% and hemorrhagic stroke in 3.8%. Vascular work-up can be performed in clinical suspicion of CVST. Either CT venography or MR venography are acceptable for evaluation, depending on the patient's clinical status. CT/MR venography may reveal lack of high flow signal in venous sinuses or formation of collaterals. The most commonly involved sinuses are SSS and TS. MR venography is also useful for three to six months follow-up of the patients. Conventional angiography is rarely necessary when clinical diagnosis of CVST is highly suspected, but diagnosis cannot be made. Lack of partial or complete ventricular filling, delayed emptying, sudden ending of cortical veins surrounded by dilated collaterals and dilated tortuous collaterals are clues to the diagnosis. Plasma D-dimer levels are also sensitive for ruling out CVST except in the early stages.

At least one risk factor is present, causing CVST, in 85% of the cases. Risk factors are divided into two groups, temporary or permanent. Up to 50% of common transient risk factors are pregnancy, puerperium and oral contraceptive use. Infections such as otitis, mastoiditis, sinusitis or meningitis contribute 10% risk, particularly in developing countries. Spinal anesthesia, neurosurgical intervention, dehydration, anemia and thyroid diseases are other rare risk factors. Persistent risk factors include genetic or acquired prothrombotic disorders such as prothrombin gene mutation, factor V Leiden mutation, proteins C and S or antithrombin 3 deficiency, hyperhomocysteinemia, inflammatory bowel disease or Behçet's disease.[3]

The first-line treatment in CVST is antithrombotics to ensure recanalization of the occluded veins, prevent pulmonary embolism and spread of the thrombus, and to treat underlying prothrombotic conditions. The guidelines recommend oral warfarin treatment, starting with heparin in the acute phase, even with intracranial hemorrhage (ICH) or hemorrhagic transformation in CVST cases. Novel oral anticoagulants (NOACs) or direct oral anticoagulants (DOACs)(rivaroxaban and dabigatran) might also be used for treatment of CVST, according to the latest studies. Studies also suggest endovascular treatment in the presence of progressive neurological deterioration, despite medical treatment.[4] Mechanical thrombectomy has been found to be effective in CVST cases, but large randomized studies are needed. Decompressive hemicraniectomy or hematoma evacuation should be preferred in patients with malignant hemispheric stroke and progressive neurological deterioration. Anticoagulant therapy is recommended for three to six months in patients with transient risk factors. In cases with idiopathic CVST or "mild" thrombophilia (factor V Leiden heterozygous mutation, hyperhomocysteinemia), warfarin can be given for up to six to twelve months. In cases with severe risk of thrombophilia or recurrent venous thrombosis, an indefinite period of anticoagulant therapy is recommended. It is essential to keep the international normalized ratio between 2 and 2.5 during treatment. In the presence of intracranial hypertension, mannitol, hyperventilation and sedation are recommended. Although there is no controlled data, acetozalamide or furosemide diuretics may be considered in patients with persistent papillary edema. Lumboperitoneal shunt, stenting and optic nerve fenestration may be considered in worsening cases. Antiepileptic treatment should be initiated especially in patients with epileptic seizures with supratentorial lesions. Prophylactic antiepileptic therapy is not recommended in patients without seizures.

# References

1. ISCVT Investigators, Ferro JM, Canhão P, Stam J, et al. Prognosis of cerebral vein and dural sinus thrombosis: Results of the International Study on Cerebral Vein and Dural Sinus Thrombosis (ISCVT). *Stroke.* 2004;**35**: 664–670.

2. VENOST Study Group, Duman T, Uluduz D, Midi I, et al. A multicenter study of 1144 patients with cerebral venous thrombosis: The VENOST Study. *J Stroke Cerebrovasc Dis.* 2017;**26**: 1848–1857.

3. Wasay M, Bakshi R, Bobustuc G, et al. Cerebral venous thrombosis: Analysis of a multicenter cohort from the United States. *J Stroke Cerebrovasc Dis.* 2008;**17**: 49–54.

4. Ferro JM, Dentali F, Coutinho JM, et al. Rationale, design, and protocol of a randomized controlled trial of the safety and efficacy of dabigatranetexilate versus dose-adjusted warfarin in patients with cerebral venous thrombosis. *Int J Stroke.* 2018;**13**: 766–770.

# Bone Disorders

Milija Mijajlovic, Vuk Aleksic, Natasa Stojanovski, Natan M. Bornstein

## Case Presentation

A 19-year-old Caucasian female patient was admitted to the emergency department with episodic piercing-type headaches of moderate intensity not relieved by painkillers. For the last two days before admission, the headache was associated with right-side weakness, which evolved into speech difficulty and finally faintness. There was no associated high fever, loss of consciousness, ataxia, vomiting, photo- or phonophobia, vision problems, hearing difficulty, neck stiffness or other symptoms. Her family history was significant for hypertension. Also, her father had several skeletal deformities, such as deformity of the ankle and short stature, as well as several tumors (probably osteochondromas) on the lower extremities, but he had never undergone any detailed investigation regarding this condition.

On admission, vital signs included a heart rate of 99/min, blood pressure 170/80 mmHg, body temperature 36.7 °C, respiratory rate 23 breaths/min, with 98% oxygen saturation on room air. A general physical examination showed an obese patient (BMI 36 kg/m$^2$) with several tumor changes in the lower extremities. Positive family history, clinical appearance and X-ray findings (Figure 10.1.1) raised the suspicion that the patient had multiple osteochondromatosis (e.g., Hereditary multiple exostoses).

Neurological examination showed mild dysphasia and moderate right-sided hemiparesis. A non-contrast brain computed tomography (CT) scan showed left middle cerebral artery territory cortical and subcortical ischemic stroke. Laboratory biochemical investigations, complete blood count, inflammatory markers, immunological panel, syphilis serology, cerebrospinal fluid findings, electroencephalogram, thrombophilia screening and transthoracic echocardiogram were all normal. Digital subtraction angiography of cerebral blood vessels revealed supraclinoid occlusion of the left internal carotid artery, and filiform middle cerebral artery with proliferation of collateral vessels emerging from the left ophthalmic artery, as well as collaterals bridging the stenosis, reminiscent of a puff of smoke (Figure 10.1.2). These findings are compatible with a progressive vascular occlusive process seen in moyamoya disease (MMD).

The patient was diagnosed with acute ischemic stroke due to MMD, and, although genetic testing was not performed, there was high suspicion of hereditary multiple exostoses, based on clinical presentation, X-ray findings and positive family history.

After discussing the treatment options with the patient, she refused MMD surgery and was treated symptomatically and conservatively during the acute phase of the stroke. Therapy was continued with physical treatment, and antihypertensive and antiplatelet agents. The patient was further followed in the outpatient setting by a neurologist and an orthopedic surgeon. She is stable and stroke-free, without signs of de novo exostosis formation.

MMD is a chronic cerebrovascular occlusion disease. Major symptoms are transient ischemic attacks, and ischemic or hemorrhagic stroke. No evidence suggests that drug treatment is

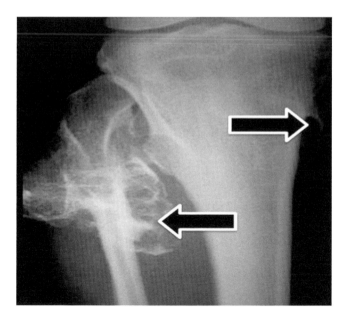

**Figure 10.1.1** X-ray of the lower extremity showing sessile (left arrow) and pedunculated (right arrow) tumor changes in the metaphyseal region, projecting away from the epiphysis, representing a typical finding of osteochondroma.

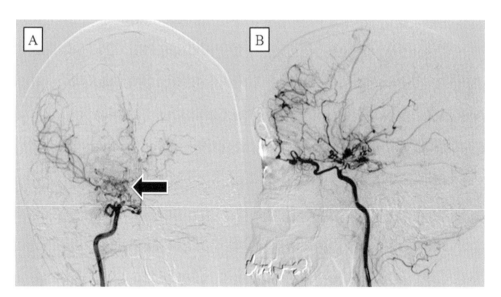

**Figure 10.1.2** Digital subtraction angiography (DSA) showing characteristic findings for moyamoya disease. (A) The arrow shows characteristic sign "puff of smoke". (B) Collateral vessels emerging from the left ophthalmic artery

able to delay disease progression. The current drug treatment targets only clinical symptoms, by exerting anticoagulant or hemostatic effects. Recent guidelines recommend the use of anti-platelet drugs for the treatment of the ischemic form, but the bleeding risk remains. On the other hand, current studies show that MMD patients with any type of stroke should receive surgical (direct, indirect or combined) revascularization. The most common type is direct middle cerebral artery–superficial temporal artery anastomosis.

A definitive connection between moyamoya disease and multiple osteochondromatosis has not been established, but related complex pathophysiological mechanisms and genetic causes may underlie vasculopathy and osteochondroma development. In cases of suspected association between stroke and bone disorders, the following diagnostic work-up should be followed.

| SUSPICION OF BONE-DISORDER-RELATED (CAUSED) STROKE |
|---|
| • Clinical symptoms and signs of TIA/stroke and |
| • Previously diagnosed bone disorder or |
|    o   Clinical suspicion of bone disorder |
|    o   Positive family history of bone disorder |
|    o   Recent orthopedic procedure |

| TIA/STROKE CONFIRMATION | BONE DISORDER CONFIRMATION |
|---|---|
| • Clinical presentation<br>• Cranial CT/MRI | • Osteoporosis<br>• Skull disorders<br>   o  Osteopetrosis<br>   o  Paget's disease<br>   o  Craniosynostosis<br>• Skeletal abnormalities<br>   o  Spondyloepiphyseal dysplasia and Schimke syndrome<br>   o  Camurati–Engelmann disease<br>• Bone tumors<br>   o  Osteochondromas<br>   o  Osteosarcoma |
| | • Fibrocartilaginous (nucleus pulposus) embolism<br>• Fat embolism syndrome<br>• Orthopedic procedures |

| RULE OUT |
|---|
| • **Common causes of stroke** |
| • **Rare causes of stroke** |
|   o **Non-atherosclerotic angiopathies** |
|     (cervicocephalic arterial dissection, cerebral amyoid angiopathy, moyamoya disease, fibromuscular dysplasia, reversible cerebral vasoconstriction syndrome, Susac's syndrome, Sneddon's syndrome, migraine-induced stroke) |
|   o **Hematologic conditions** |
|     (*Hypercoagulable state* due to deficiencies of protein S, protein C or antithrombin; factor V Leiden mutation, prothrombin gene G20210A mutation; acquired *hypercoagulable state* (e.g., cancer, pregnancy, hormonal contraceptive use, exposure to hormonal treatments such as anabolic steroids and erythropoietin, nephrotic syndrome); antiphospholipid syndrome, hyperhomocysteinemia, sickle cell disease, myeloproliferative disorders (e.g., leukemia, lymphoma) |
|   o **Genetic** |
|     (Fabry disease; MELAS; CADASIL; Marfan syndrome; neurofibromatosis; Sturge–Weber disease) |
| • **Stroke mimics** |
|   o SAH |
|   o ICH |
|   o Intracranial mass (tumor, abscess) |

| BONE DISORDER RELATED (CAUSED) STROKE<br>HIGHLY PLAUSIBLE |
|---|

Bone disorders are an extremely rare cause of stroke, but they should be considered when other causes are excluded by a thorough diagnostic work-up. The connection between stroke and bone status is complex. These two conditions have similar intertwined risk factors, but also represent risk factors for each other. However, the current facts show a more pronounced effect of stroke on bone health. Several bone disorders have been shown to be associated with stroke: body bone pathology (osteoporosis), skull disorders (osteopetrosis, Paget's disease and craniosynostosis), skeletal abnormalities (spondyloepiphyseal dysplasia, Schimke syndrome and Camurati–Engelmann disease) and bone tumors (osteochondromas and osteosarcoma). Fibrocartilaginous and fat emboli, as well as orthopedic procedures are among bone pathologies that have to be considered as a possible cause of stroke in specific clinical scenarios.[1]

## Body Bone Pathology: Osteoporosis

Bone mineral density (BMD) and stroke are both related to deficiency of estrogen, high blood pressure, diabetes and reduced physical activity. It has not been fully elucidated whether there is a causal relationship between low BMD and high risk of stroke, or whether low BMD simply represents a sign of poor general health and aging. However, some recent studies show that BMD is an independent risk factor for stroke in the female population.

On the other hand, osteoporosis represents a well-known stroke complication. Hemiparesis/hemiplegia in stroke patients predisposes impaired bone physiology due to increased bone resorption, which, with loss of function, leads to early reduction in BMD. Such a state combined with a higher incidence of falling due to instability in stroke patients, leads to an increase in hip fractures after stroke. This is most likely the most serious stroke complication, since more than 30% of such patients die within the first year after stroke. However, survivors face chronic pain and loss of independence, making this complication a major cause of morbidity in stroke patients. Since half of all strokes occur in older age, the population at high risk of stroke is already at risk of fracture and osteoporosis.[1,2]

## Skull Disorders

*Osteopetrosis* (previously called "marble bone" disease) is a rare hereditary disease characterized by an abnormal accumulation of bone tissue. Diminished bone resorption is the probable cause due to metabolic imbalance. Different neurological conditions are found in patients with osteopetrosis; however, stroke involvement is very rare, and probably due to mechanical compression of blood vessels by osteopetrotic bones.

*Paget's disease* (osteitis deformans) represents a chronic osteodystrophy of unknown etiology. The risk of Paget's disease increases with age and it is usually found in patients over 50 years of age. It is characterized by the extensive replacement of normal bone with bone tissue that is irregular in structure and architecture, causing affected bones to become misshapen and fragile. Different neurological conditions are found in patients with Paget's disease, most often due to vascular steal syndromes. Cerebrovascular disorders of these patients have a mainly mechanical, compressive origin.[3]

*Craniosynostosis* (prevalence 1 in 2500 births) is a clinically and genetically heterogeneous developmental craniofacial anomaly, resulting in an abnormally shaped skull and sometimes impairment of brain development. It may be associated with decreased cerebral blood flow or vessel occlusion caused by compression.[4]

# Skeletal Abnormalities

*Spondyloepiphyseal dysplasia congenita* is a rare genetic (autosomal dominant) disorder characterized by diminished bone growth, resulting in dwarfism and other skeletal abnormalities, sometimes accompanied by vision and hearing problems. It is caused by defects in the gene COL2A1 on the long arm of chromosome 12, whose coding protein is an essential part of normal type II collagen. Spondyloepiphyseal dysplasia tarda is different form of X-linked recessive hereditary skeletal disorder that affects only male patients. In 1971, Schimke defined a genetic autosomal recessive multisystem disorder (*Schimke syndrome*) consisting of short stature due to spondyloepiphyseal dysplasia, facial dysmorphisms, renal failure, immunodeficiency due to lymphopenia and accelerated atherosclerosis leading to stroke in young patients. It is caused by mutations of the SMARCAL1 gene, which encodes the protein of found in chromatin. Renal disease complications of Schimke syndrome, such as hypertension and hyperlipidemia are well-known risk factors for stroke. However, the increasing number of patients with Schimke syndrome and stroke, leads to a suspicion that stroke is one of the standard features of the syndrome and not just a complication.[5]

*Camurati–Engelmann disease* (progressive diaphyseal dysplasia) is a rare autosomal dominant skeletal disease, caused by mutations in the transforming growth factor-β1 (TGFβ1) gene, an important mediator of bone remodeling. It is characterized by a progressive diaphyseal dysplasia with cortical sclerosis of the long tubular bones and the base of the scull. The patients have diffuse painful bony deformities, exophthalmia, a waddling gait, and muscular weakness. Cranial nerve palsy due to restriction of the skull base foramina caused by hyperostosis are rarely found. Higher then normal incidence of stroke in patients with Camurati–Engelmann disease is explained by blood vessel compression caused by a cranial hyperostotic bone. Also, the affected protein inhibits migration of endothelial and smooth muscle cells, which is also associated with an increase in the extracellular matrix and proteoglycan synthesis, leading to thickening of the vessel walls (premature arteriopathy) as a potential cause of stroke.[6,7]

# Bone Tumors

*Osteochondromas* (hereditary multiple osteochondromas) is an autosomal dominant disorder characterized by the development of multiple benign cartilage-capped bony lesions (called osteochondromas or exostoses) in relation to the metaphyses of long bones. With an incidence of 1 in 50,000 people, they represent the most common benign bone tumors, sometimes causing complications due to compression of blood vessels. The prevalence of such vascular complications secondary to exostosis compression can be as high as 11%. This mechanism can be considered as a potential cause of stroke in all conditions with heterotopic ossification. However, cases of vertebral artery dissection in patients with hereditary multiple osteochondromas without direct compression have also been described. Aberrations in structural proteins common to both blood vessels and bones possibly predispose weakness of the arterial wall, which may lead to dissection and subsequently to stroke. So, there are two possible mechanisms of vascular event occurrence in patients with osteochondromas: ([1]) direct compression of blood vessels and ([2]) dissection and/or formation of an aneurysm due to a genetically predisposed weakness of blood vessel walls.

*Osteosarcoma* is a primary malignant bone tumor mostly affecting the long bones with an incidence of about 3 cases/million population/year and slight predominance in the younger population. Cerebrovascular accidents (either ischemic or hemorrhagic) in relation to osteosarcoma are extremely uncommon, and can be related to brain metastasis, paraneoplastic hypercoagulation state, bleeding diathesis or mechanical cranial blood vessel compression. On the other hand, cancer surgery, chemotherapy and radiotherapy have also been shown to increase stroke risk.[8,9]

## Fibrocartilaginous (Nucleus Pulposus), Fat Embolism and Orthopedics Procedures

*Fibrocartilaginous (nucleus pulposus) embolism* could potentially cause spinal cord infarction by a retrograde embolization to the central artery gaining vascular access throughout blood vessels in the intervertebral space when there is neo-vascularization due to inflammation of a herniated disc, formation of Schmorl's hernia or residual embryonic disc vasculature during adulthood. It has been postulated that the initial trigger is increased intradiscal pressure caused by axial forces such as trauma, falls, heavy lifting or even coughing or sneezing (Valsalva maneuver).

*Fat embolism* syndrome is a common complication of long-bone fractures and orthopedic procedures, when fat droplets released from bone marrow enter the blood stream. There are two main theories about pathophysiology: (1) mechanical: fat particles are released directly from the bone marrow into the blood stream, (2) biochemical: local inflammation causes bone marrow to release fatty acids into the venous circulation, after triglycerides are decomposed due to increased lipoprotein lipase activity. About 5–30% of long bone fractures are associated with fat embolism syndrome, but the mortality rate is approximately 15%. Usually it is asymptomatic, but some patients present with embolic stroke.

Stroke after *orthopedic procedures* is extremely rare, but it is thought that incidence is underappreciated. A cardioembolic source due to atrial fibrillation is the most common cause of stroke in orthopedic patients. It has been shown that general anesthesia is associated with higher stroke risk in comparison with neuraxial anesthesia. Depending on the orthopedic procedure, about 0.08–0.7% of patients undergoing elective orthopedic surgery experience a stroke within the 30 days of the procedure. More than half of strokes occur within 48 hours after an operation, and one quarter occur after hospital release. Presumed risk factors for postoperative stroke in orthopedic surgery are older age, diabetes mellitus, hypertension, chronic obstructive pulmonary disease and long procedure time. However, there is no evidence that they are independently associated with stroke after elective surgery. Paradoxically, history of stroke is not independently associated with increased postoperative stroke rates, probably since patients with previous cerebrovascular accident already receive prophylactic therapy.[10]

# References

1. Moayyeri A, Alrawi YA, Myint PK. The complex mutual connection between stroke and bone health. *Arch Biochem Biophys.* 2010;**503**: 153–159.

2. Poole KE, Reeve J, Warburton EA. Falls, fractures, and osteoporosis after stroke: Time to think about protection? *Stroke.* 2002;**33**(5): 1432–1436.

3. Farre JM, Declambre B. Functional consequences and complications of Paget's disease. *Rev Prat.* 1989;**39**: 1129–1136.

4. David LR, Wilson JA, Watson NE, Argenta LC. Cerebral perfusion defects secondary to simple craniosynostosis. *J Craniofac Surg.* 1996;**7**(3): 177–185.

5. Babaei AH, Inaloo S, Basiratnia M. Schimke immuno-osseous dysplasia: A case report. *Indian J Nephrol.* 2019;**29**(4): 291–294.

6. Cerrato P, Baima C, Bergui M, et al. Juvenile vertebrobasilar ischaemic stroke in a patient with Camurati-Engelmann disease. *Cerebrovasc Dis.* 2005;**20**: 283–284.

7. Mijajlovic M, Mirkovic M, Mihailovic-Vucinic V, Aleksic V, Covickovic-Sternic N. Neurosarcoidosis: Two case reports with multiple cranial nerve involvement and review of the literature. *Biomed Pap Med Fac Univ Palacky Olomouc Czech Repub.* 2014;**158**(4): 662–667.

8. Dardiotis E, Aloizou AM, Markoula S, et al. Cancer-associated stroke: Pathophysiology, detection and management (review). *Int J Oncol.* 2019;**54**(3): 779–796.

9. Ploumis A, Liampas A, Angelidis M, et al. Multiple exostoses syndrome and basilar artery aneurysm: A case report. *J Vasc Interv Neurol.* 2018;**10**(2): 28–32.

10. Minhas SV, Goyal P, Patel AA. What are the risk factors for cerebrovascular accidents after elective orthopaedic surgery? *Clin Orthop Relat Res.* 2016;**474**(3): 611–618.

# Eagle Syndrome

Anita Arsovska, Vida Demarin, Patrik Michel

## Case Presentation

A 37-year-old female was admitted due to transient right-sided hemiparesis and motor dysphasia that lasted several minutes. She was previously healthy, without any known risk factors. Laboratory blood analysis and magnetic resonance imaging (MRI) of the brain were normal, as well as her neurological examination, so the patient was discharged in a stable condition. After 10 months, a persistent pulsatile tinnitus in her left ear appeared. Otherwise, her neurological examination, laboratory blood analysis (including total peripheral blood count, biochemical screen, Fe, HbA1c, vitamin B12, folic acid, erythrocyte sedimentation rate, C-reactive protein, thyroid functions, renal and hepatic functions) and MRI of the brain were normal. Computed tomography (CT) angiography of the brain blood vessels was performed (Figure 10.2.1), which showed dissection in the distal half of the extracranial segment of the left internal carotid artery (ICA), 22 mm long, with intramural hematoma and two focal protuberances in the thrombotic part, mostly located in the media.

Reduction of the lumen in this segment, with stenosis up to 65% was registered. Also, the extracranial segment of the right ICA was widened by up to 7 mm, along its length of 30 mm, with wall irregularity in this part. After the diagnosis of carotid dissection was confirmed, further tests were ordered to search for its etiology. Physical examination, electrocardiogram (ECG), blood pressure and pulse were all within the normal range. Inflammatory and coagulopathy panel, antinuclear antibody, rheumatoid factor, anti-neutrophil cytoplasmic antibody, lupus anticoagulant, antithrombin, protein S, protein C, factor VIII levels, homocysteine levels, antiphospholipid antibodies, factor V Leiden mutation and activated protein C resistance were negative. Coagulation studies and D-dimer were normal, as was a skin biopsy. Treatment with acetylsalicylic acid (ASA) 100 mg/day was recommended and a second opinion was sought regarding the interpretation of the CT angiography images. What was missed in the initial interpretation was the elongated styloid process, part of the temporal bone (Figure 10.2.2).

Its length was measured to be 3 cm on the right and 4 cm on the left side. The styloid process interferes with the functioning of neighboring structures; it may compress the carotid arteries, especially during neck movements and can be a cause of carotid dissection and structural wall changes. Therefore a diagnosis of vascular Eagle syndrome was confirmed. Although an operative treatment was suggested for the elongated styloid, it was not accepted by the patient. She continued treatment with ASA 75mg/day. After three years, follow-up brain MRI and magnetic resonance angiography (MRA) showed the presence of a carotid dissection with low-grade stenosis in the left ICA. Her neurological examination had been normal and she did not have any other vascular events.

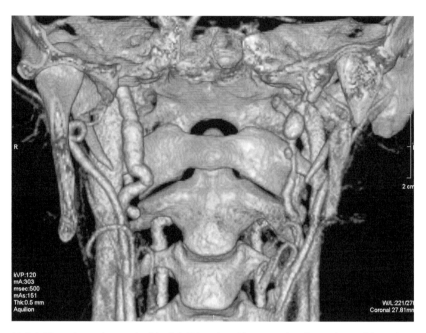

**Figure 10.2.1** Dissection and stenosis of the left ICA, widened lumen and wall irregularity of the right ICA

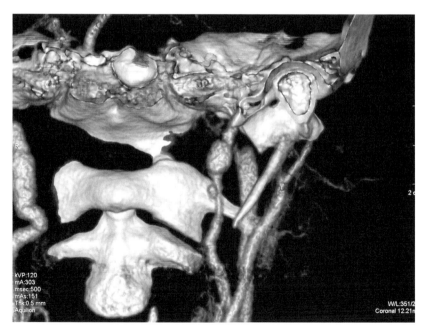

**Figure 10.2.2** Elongated styloid process, part of the temporal bone.

## Clinical suspicion of Eagle syndrome

Eagle syndrome – rare condition caused by elongated/disfigured styloid process, which interferes with the functioning of neighboring structures

**"Classic Eagle syndrome"** – pain in the distribution areas of V, VII, VIII, IX and X cranial nerves, sensation of a foreign body in the pharynx (55%), dysphagia, painful swallowing, otalgia, headache, pain along internal/external carotid arteries (ICA/ECA), pain on cervical rotation or mastication, facial pain and tinnitus; usually occurs after pharyngeal trauma or tonsillectomy

**"Vascular Eagle syndrome" (stylocarotid syndrome)** – occurs as a consequence of ICA/ECA compression by the elongated styloid process; can cause transient ischemic attack (TIA), stroke, vertigo and syncope. Symptoms occur by direct vascular compression (hemodynamic mechanism), or by dissection and thromboembolism resulting from injury to the carotid artery wall

## Diagnosis of Eagle syndrome

- Optimal medical history, physical examination
- Neuroimaging:
- CT is the most accurate method for the diagnosis of the elongated styloid process, allows precise measurement of the length of the styloid process and the ossified stylohyoid ligament, which is made with 3D CT reconstruction.
- CT angiography or catheter angiography should be obtained if carotid dissection is suspected, or if mechanical vascular compression is potentially the cause of ischemic symptoms, with the patient's head appropriately positioned to reproduce symptoms which may demonstrate mechanical stenosis of the carotid artery

## Management of Eagle syndrome

- Conservative treatment of Eagle syndrome: analgesics, antidepressants, anticonvulsants, transpharyngeal injection of steroids and lidocaine, diazepam, non-steroidal anti-inflammatory drugs and application of topical heat
- Management of carotid dissection: anticoagulation or antiplatelet therapy, sometimes carotid stenting.
- Surgical shortening of the styloid process via intraoral or external approaches

# Discussion

Eagle syndrome is caused by an elongated/disfigured styloid process, which interferes with the functioning of neighboring structures and causes orofacial and cervical pain, often triggered by neck movements. It was named after Watt Weems Eagle (1898–1980), an American otorhinolaryngologist, who described his first case in 1937. He described the combination of pain associated with an abnormal stylohyoid complex and later reported a case series of over 200 patients. Andreas Vesalius (1514–1564), a Belgian anatomist, first identified abnormalities in the stylohyoid complex of animals in 1543. Pietro Marchetti (1589–1673), an Italian surgeon, anatomist and doctor, provided the first description in humans in 1656. There are three types of Eagle syndrome, depending on whether or not the styloid process is continuous (Langlais' classification)[1]:

Type 1: there is no interruption in the continuity of the styloid process.

Type 2: there is a pseudo articulation between the styloid process and stylohyoid ligament.

Type 3: there are multiple interruptions of the styloid process continuity or of the calcified stylohyoid ligament, creating a multiple pseudo joint.

## Etiology

Eagle found that 4% of patients that have abnormalities with their stylohyoid complex have pain. He described two different presentations: classic type and carotid artery syndrome. Eagle proposed that surgical trauma (tonsillectomy) or local chronic irritation causes osteitis, periostitis or tendonitis of the styloid process and the stylohyoid ligaments, which result in reactive, ossifying hyperplasia. Further studies examined the relationship between tonsillectomy and Eagle syndrome and did not find the same relationship. Epifanio (1962) thought that ossification of the styloid process corresponds to endocrine disorders in menopausal women and ossification of other ligaments. Lentini (1975) thought that persistent mesenchymal elements could undergo osseous metaplasia in traumatic or stressful events. Gokce (2008) found out that patients with end-stage renal disease had abnormal metabolism of calcium, phosphorus and vitamin D and had heterotopic calcification, which caused elongation of the styloid process. Sekerci (2015) analyzed 3D CT scans of 542 patients and indicated a relationship between the presence of an arcuate foramen and an elongated styloid process.[2]

## Epidemiology

Eagle reported that a normal styloid process was ~2.5 cm, therefore, any process 2.5 cm was considered abnormally elongated. In a postmortem study of 80 cadavers, the length of the styloid process ranged 1.52–4.77 cm. Of the population, 4% have an elongated styloid process, and only 4% of these have symptoms. The true incidence is 0.16%, with a female-to-male ratio of 3:1. Patients are usually >30 years of age, and the process is usually bilateral, although unilateral cases have also been described.[3]

## Pathophysiology

There are several proposed mechanisms for Eagle syndrome:

- Compression of cranial nerves, most commonly the glossopharyngeal nerve, with throat and neck pain
- Compression of the ICA, which can cause a TIA or compression of sympathetic nerves along the artery, leading to symptoms
- Reactive hyperplasia and metaplasia after trauma
- Abnormal angulation associated with an abnormally lengthy styloid process causing irritation of adjacent musculature or mucosa
- Stretching and fibrosis involving the V, VII, IX and X cranial nerves after tonsillectomy
- Normal process of aging.

There are two types of Eagle syndrome:

"Classic Eagle syndrome" – usually occurs after pharyngeal trauma or tonsillectomy. Symptoms include pain in the distribution areas of V, VII, VIII, IX and X cranial nerves, sensation of a foreign body in the pharynx (55%), dysphagia, painful swallowing, otalgia, headache, pain along the ECA and ICA, pain on cervical rotation or mastication, facial pain and tinnitus.

"Vascular Eagle syndrome" (stylocarotid syndrome) occurs as a consequence of ICA/ECA compression (along with their perivascular sympathetic fibers) by a laterally or medially deviated styloid process and can lead to TIA, stroke, vertigo and syncope. These cerebrovascular symptoms are considered to be caused by direct vascular compression (hemodynamic mechanism), or by dissection and thromboembolism resulting from injury to the wall of the carotid artery. When patients meet the definition of having an elongated styloid process, they are four times more likely to develop a carotid artery dissection.[4]

Diagnosis of Eagle syndrome is established based on optimal medical history, physical examination and pain in the throat that radiates to the neck, ear or face. The characteristic pain is dull, throbbing and aggravates with deglutition; it can be duplicated by palpation of the tonsillar fossa. Upper aerodigestive tract malignancies, neuralgia and temporomandibular joint dysfunction should be excluded. Diagnosis of an elongated styloid process is confirmed by imaging, with CT being the most accurate method. Precise measurement of the length of the styloid process and the ossified stylohyoid ligament is made with 3D CT reconstruction. If mechanical vascular compression is potentially the cause of ischemic symptoms, angiographic examination (CT angiography or catheter angiography) should be obtained with the patient's head appropriately positioned to reproduce symptoms which may demonstrate mechanical stenosis of the carotid artery.

## Management

Conservative treatment of Eagle syndrome includes analgesics, antidepressants, anticonvulsants, transpharyngeal injection of steroids and lidocaine, diazepam, non-steroidal anti-inflammatory drugs and application of topical heat. There is no general consensus regarding the optimal management of carotid dissection in vascular Eagle syndrome. Anticoagulant therapy should be initiated when a thrombus is detected. For prevention of thromboembolic complications, anticoagulation with IV heparin followed by warfarin is recommended. If systemic anticoagulation is contraindicated, antiplatelet therapy should be started. Carotid artery stenting can be another option for the treatment of stylo-carotid symptoms of Eagle syndrome, but the efficacy of stenting for this syndrome is not well established. Intrastent thrombosis and thromboembolism of the distal cerebral artery after carotid artery stenting has been described, requiring subsequent surgical resection of the styloid process.[5] Thus, close follow-up is necessary for patients with vascular Eagle syndrome treated by carotid artery stenting. The choice among medical, endovascular and surgical options depends on the type of injury, anatomic location, mechanism of injury, coexisting injuries and comorbid conditions. It is important to determine the risk-to-benefit ratio for antithrombotic therapy and obtain vascular surgery or interventional radiology consultations. Patients who fail to respond to multiple medications may require surgical manipulations. Transpharyngeal manipulation with manual fracture of the elongated styloid process does not relieve symptoms and risks damage to adjacent neurovascular structures. Surgical shortening of the styloid process can be performed via intraoral or external approaches. Advantages of the intraoral approach are: simplicity of the technique, reduced operation time, achievability under local anesthesia, absence of any visible external scar. Disadvantages of the intraoral approach are: lack of access, particularly if there is subsequent hemorrhage and deep neck infection, poor visualization of the surgical field, especially in patients with significantly reduced jaw opening, risk of iatrogenic injury to major neurovascular structures and alterations of speech and swallowing from postoperative edema. Advantages of the external approach are: enhanced exposure of the styloid process and the adjacent structures, which overshadow all other benefits; this approach also aids the removal of a partially ossified stylohyoid ligament. Disadvantages of the external approach are: it is more time consuming, there is a risk of injury to the facial nerve and its branches, a disfiguring neck scar can possibly remain and a longer recovery period is required. Surgical failures in up to 20% of patients have been reported.[6]

## Conclusion

Diagnosis and management of vascular Eagle syndrome is not easy. Eagle syndrome should be considered an important cause of carotid dissection and subsequent cerebrovascular complications. It is important to understand the diagnostic work-up, adequate imaging and best treatment options. Treatment is complex and best undertaken with a multidisciplinary team. Surgery to excise the elongated styloid is recommended but is fraught with complications such as injury to the facial nerve. Clinicians should always consider conservative therapies first.

## References

1. Langlais RP, Miles DA, Van Dis ML. Elongated and mineralized stylohyoid ligament complex: A proposed classification and report of a case of Eagle's syndrome. *Oral Surg Oral Med Oral Pathol.* 1986;**61**(5): 527–532.

2. Medscape, Rinaldi V, Faiella F, Casale M, et al. Eagle Syndrome. https://emedicine.medscape.com/article/1447247-overview#a7 (accessed February 2022).

3. Aravind WS, Nanthini KC, Subadra K, Dhivya MH. Eagle's syndrome: A case report of a unilateral elongated styloid process. *Cureus.* 2019;**11**(4): e4430.

4. Raser JM, Mullen MT, Kasner SE, et al. Cervical carotid artery dissection is associated with styloid process length. *Neurology.* 2011;**77**: 2061–2066.

5. Ogura T, Mineharu Y, Todo K, Kohara N, Sakai N. Carotid artery dissection caused by an elongated styloid process: Three case reports and review of the literature. *NMC Case Rep J.* 2015;**2**(1): 21–25.

6. Balde D, Do Santos ZA, Ndiaye C, et al. Intra oral versus external approach in the surgical management of Eagle's syndrome. *Int J Otorhinolaryngology.* 2019;**5**(1): 9–14.

# Index

acute bacterial meningitis
(ABM) and stroke
case presentation, 125–129
cerebral spinal fluid
(CSF), 130
cerebrovascular event
frequency, 129
clinical features, 130
neuropathology, 130
stroke frequency, 129–130
treatment, 131
Alzheimer's disease (AD),
acute bacterial meningitis
(ABM) and stroke,
103–105
amphetamines. *See* illicit drug-
related stroke
anabolic steroids. *See* illicit
drug-related stroke
angiography
computed tomography
angiography (CTA), 5
digital subtraction
angiography (DSA), 5–6,
8, 9
fibromuscular dysplasia, 218
flat detector CT angiography
(FDCTA), 6, 7
MR angiography (MRA), 5
anticholinergic medication and
stroke, 188
antidepressants and stroke,
188–189
antiphospholipid antibody
syndrome (APS) and
stroke
case presentation, 151–152
clinical manifestations, 154
definition and clinical
features, 154
diagnosis, 155
diagnostic algorithm, 152
differential diagnosis, 155
therapy, 155–156

Behçet's syndrome (BS) and
stroke
case presentation, 72–73
clinical presentation, 75

defined, 74–75
diagnostic algorithm, 74
neurological
manifestations, 75
prognosis, 77
treatment, 77–78
Behçet's syndrome (BS) and
stroke, classification
parenchymal (p-NBS), 76
vascular involvement, 76–77
bone disorders and stroke
case presentation, 336–339
epidemiology, 339
bone disorders and stroke
complications
fat embolism syndrome, 341
fibrocartilaginous
embolism, 341
orthopedic procedures, 341
bone disorders and stroke,
types
bone tumors, 340–341
osteochondromas, 340
osteoporosis, 339
osteosarcoma, 341
skeletal abnormalities,
340
skull disorders, 339

CADASIL (cerebral autosomal
dominant arteriopathy
with subcortical infarcts
and leukoencephalopathy)
background, 237
case presentation, 234–236
definitions, 236–237
Call–Fleming syndrome. *See*
retinal vasculopathy with
cerebral
leukoencephalopathy and
systemic manifestations
(RVCL-S) and stroke
Camurati–Engelmann disease
and stroke, 340
cancer and stroke
case presentation, 179–180
clinical features, 182–183
diagnostic algorithm, 181
imaging, 182

treatment, 182
cannabis. *See* illicit drug-
related stroke
CARASIL (cerebral
autosomal recessive
arteriopathy with
subcortical infarcts and
leukoencephalopathy)
background, 238
case presentation,
234–236
definitions, 236–237
cardioembolism types
infective endocarditis (IE),
287–291
patent foramen ovale (PFO),
281–286
carotid artery dissection and
stroke
case presentation, 326–328
clinical presentation, 329
epidemiology, 328–329
imaging, 329
risk factors, 329
treatment, 329–330
cerebral amyloid angiopathy
(CAA), 103–105
cerebral amyloid angiopathy
(CAA) and stroke
case presentation, 314
classification, 316
clinical presentation and
imaging, 316
diagnostic criteria, 317,
318–319, 320
epidemiology and risk
factors, 318
imaging, 319–320
management, 318, 320
cerebral amyloid-related
disease types
Alzheimer's disease (AD),
103–105
cerebral amyloid angiopathy
(CAA), 103–105
cerebral amyloid-related
diseases
case presentation, 99–101
diagnostic algorithm, 101

cerebral venous sinus
thrombosis (CVST) and
stroke
case presentation, 331–332
classification stages, 334
clinical features, 334
clinical presentation, 334
diagnostic criteria, 334
epidemiology, 333–334
risk factors, 335
treatment, 335
cerebral venous thrombosis
during pregnancy, 303
cervical artery
dissection (CAD)
and migraine diagnosis,
308
and migraine
mechanisms, 308
Chagas disease and stroke
case presentation, 147–148
defined, 148
diagnostic algorithm, 148
etiology, 149
incidence, 148–149
treatment, 149
childhood arterial ischemic
stroke (CASCADE)
classification, 142
Churg–Strauss syndrome. See
eosinophilic
granulomatosis with
polyangiitis (EPGA) and
stroke
cocaine. See illicit drug-related
stroke
Cogan syndrome (CS) and
stroke
case presentation, 60–61
clinical features, 64
clinical presentation,
61, 64
defined, 63–64
diagnosis, 64
differential diagnosis, 63, 64
laboratory tests, 62
neurological
manifestations, 64
treatment, 63, 64–65
computed tomography
angiography (CTA), 5
computed tomography (CT)
Eales disease, 59
isolated central nervous
system vasculitis
(ICNSV), 5

craniosynostosis and
stroke, 339
cysticercotic encephalitis, 135

digital subtraction angiography
(DSA), 5–6, 8, 9
disseminated intravascular
coagulation (DIC) and
stroke. See also
Moschowitz syndrome
and stroke
clinical features, 171
defined, 171
diagnosis, 171
neurological manifestations,
171–172
pathogenesis, 171
treatment, 172
dolichoectasia, 324
DREAM center, 145
drug-related stroke
illicit, 190
medication, 185–189

Eagle syndrome and stroke
case presentation, 343
classification, 345, 346
diagnosis, 345, 347
epidemiology, 345, 346
etiology, 346
management, 345, 347–348
pathophysiology, 346
types, 346–347
Eales disease and stroke
case presentation, 54–55
clinical presentation, 58
defined, 57–58
diagnosis, 58
diagnostic algorithm, 56
imaging, 59
treatment, 59
eclampsia during pregnancy
and stroke
case report, 299–300
cerebral venous
thrombosis, 303
clinical presentation, 301
defined, 301
epidemiology, 300
imaging, 301–302
intracerebral hemorrhage
(ICH), 303
ischemic stroke, 302
pre-eclampsia, 301–302
stroke rate, 302
stroke risk, 302

Ecstasy. See illicit drug-related
stroke
Ehlers–Danlos syndrome and
stroke
case presentation, 199–200
clinical presentation, 201
complications, 201–202
defined, 201
diagnostic criteria, 201–202
differential diagnosis,
202–205
treatment, 202
vascular complications,
201
eosinophilic granulomatosis
with polyangiitis (EPGA)
and stroke
case presentation, 28–30
classification, 32
clinical features, 30–31
complications, 31
diagnosis, 31–32
evolving phases, 31
five-factors-score for
assessment of
prognosis, 32
treatment, 32–33
essential thrombocytopenia
(ET) and stroke, 165
extraparenchymal
neurocysticercosis, 135

Fabry disease and stroke
case presentation, 246–248
diagnosis delay, 250–251
diagnostic criteria, 249–250
epidemiology, 249
treatment, 250
fat embolism syndrome, 341
fibrocartilaginous
embolism, 341
fibromuscular dysplasia and
stroke
case presentation, 212–213
clinical presentation, 218
diagnosis, 218
epidemiology, 217–218
follow-up, 219
treatment, 218–219
five-factors-score for
assessment of prognosis of
eosinophilic
granulomatosis with
polyangiitis (EPGA), 32
flat detector CT angiography
(FDCTA), 6, 7

fusiform aneurysms and stroke
case presentation, 321–323
clinical presentation, 324
defined, 324
diagnostic criteria, 324
management, 325

genetic conditions and stroke, types
CADASIL and CARASIL, 234–238
Ehlers–Danlos syndrome, 199–205
Fabry disease, 246–251
fibromuscular dysplasia, 212–219
hereditary hemorrhagic telangiectasia (HHT), 228–233
Marfan syndrome, 206–211
Menkes disease, 262–266
mitochondrial diseases (MELAS), 253–261
neurofibromatosis type 1, 220–226
organic acid disorders, 271–278
retinal vasculopathy with cerebral leukoencephalopathy and systemic manifestations (RVCL-S), 240–245
Tangier disease, 267–270
giant cell arteritis (GCA) and stroke
case presentation, 10–12
clinical features, 12
diagnosis, 12
management, 13–14
treatment, 13
glutaric aciduria type 1 (GAI) and stroke
clinical presentation, 275–276
pathophysiology, 276–277
granulomatosis with polyangiitis (GPA) and stroke
case presentation, 34–35
clinical features, 38
complications, 38
incidence, 38
mortality rate, 38
treatment, 38

Henoch–Schönlein purpura. *See* immunoglobulin A vasculitis and stroke
hereditary hemorrhagic telangiectasia (HHT) and stroke
case presentation, 228–229
clinical features, 232
clinical presentation, 230, 232
diagnosis, 232
epidemiology, 231
genetic testing, 231
prognosis, 232
therapy, 231, 233
heroin. *See* illicit drug-related stroke
HIV disease in sub-Saharan Africa and stroke
case presentation, 141–142
differential diagnosis, 143
DREAM center, 145
education and training, 145
geography, 142–143
hypertensive patient percentage, 144
incidence, 143
prevalence, 144–145
treatment, 145
hormone replacement therapy (HRT) and stroke, 187
hyperhomocysteinemia and stroke
case presentation, 157–158
clinical features, 160
clinical presentation, 157–158
defined, 159–160
diagnosis, 157–158
homocysteinemia, 160
incidence, 160
management, 157–158
stroke frequency, 160
hyperviscosity syndrome (HVS) and stroke
case presentation, 162–163
clinical features, 166
clinical manifestations, 166
defined, 164
diseases associated with, 165
elevated blood viscosity, 164–165
essential thrombocytopenia (ET), 165
leukemias, 165
polycythemia vera (PV), 165

sickle cell disease (SCD), 165–166
treatment, 166–167

illicit drug-related stroke
case presentation, 190
imaging and diagnostic work-up, 197
incidence, 192–197
therapy, 197
immunoglobulin A vasculitis and stroke
background, 176
case presentation, 174
clinical presentation, 177
clinical symptoms, 176–177
diagnosis and treatment algorithm, 175–176
imaging, 177
management, 177–178
neurological manifestations, 177
outcomes, 178
pathophysiology, 176
infectious and postinfectious vasculitis, types
acute bacterial meningitis (ABM), 129–131
Chagas disease, 148–149
HIV disease, 142–145
Lyme disease (LD), 113–117
meningovascular syphilis, 108–110
neurocysticercosis (NCC), 134–136
tuberculosis meningitis (TBM), 121–124
varicella zoster virus (VZV), 137–139
infective endocarditis (IE) and stroke
case presentation, 287–288
diagnosis, 290
epidemiology, 290
neurological complications, 290
risk factors, 290
treatment, 290–291
inflammatory bowel diseases (IBD) and stroke
case presentation, 92–93
defined, 97
diagnostic algorithm, 93
gastrointestinal manifestations, 97
TAK, 97–98

inflammatory conditions and stroke, case presentation, 1–2

inflammatory conditions and stroke, types of
Behçet's syndrome (BS), 74–78
cerebral amyloid-related diseases, 101–105
Cogan syndrome (CS), 61–65
Eales disease, 56–59
eosinophilic granulomatosis with polyangiitis (EPGA), 30–33
giant cell arteritis (GCA), 12–14
granulomatosis with polyangiitis (GPA), 38–39
inflammatory bowel diseases (IBD), 93–98
isolated central nervous system vasculitis (ICNSV), 4–7
lymphomatoid granulomatosis (LG), 41–43
polyarteritis nodosa (PAN), 26–27
sarcoidosis, 87–91
Sjögren syndrome, 80–83
Susac syndrome (SS), 47–48
systemic lupus erythematosus (SLE), 69–70
Takayasu arteritis (TAK), 19–22
Vogt–Koyanagi–Harada disease (VKH), 51–53

intracerebral hemorrhage (ICH) and stroke during pregnancy, 303

intraparenchymal neurocysticercosis, 135

ischemic stroke in pregnancy
eclampsia, 302
etiology, 302
peripartum cardiomyopathy, 302
postpartum benign angiopathy, 302
risk factors, 302

isolated central nervous system vasculitis (ICNSV) and stroke
clinical features, 4
mortality causes, 4
pathogenesis and etiology, 4

isolated central nervous system vasculitis (ICNSV) imaging
biopsy evaluation, 6
computed tomography (CT), 5
CT angiography (CTA), 5
diagnostic criteria, 6
digital subtraction angiography (DSA), 5–6, 8, 9
flat detector CT angiography (FDCTA), 6, 7
magnetic resonance imaging (MRI), 4–5, 8
MR angiography (MRA), 5
MR venography (MRV), 5
treatment, 6–7
vessel-wall imaging (VWI) MR technique, 5, 8

leukemias and stroke, 165

LSD. See illicit drug-related stroke

Lyme disease (LD) and stroke
antibiotic treatment, 114
case presentation, 112–113
defined, 114
diagnosis, 116
diagnostic algorithm, 113
pathophysiology, 114–115
treatment, 116–117

Lyme disease (LD) stages
early, 115
late, 115–116

lymphomatoid granulomatosis (LG) and stroke
case presentation, 40
classification, 42
clinical features, 42
clinical presentation, 41, 42
diagnostic algorithm, 41
histological analysis, 42
imaging, 43
management, 43
physiopathology, 42

magnetic resonance imaging (MRI)
Eales disease, 59
isolated central nervous system vasculitis (ICNSV), 4–5, 8

lymphomatoid granulomatosis (LG), 43

Moschowitz syndrome, 170

organic acid disorders and stroke, 276

tuberculosis meningitis (TBM), 123

marble bone disease, 339

Marfan syndrome and stroke
case presentation, 206–207
clinical features, 208–209
defined, 207–208
diagnosis, 209–211
differential diagnosis, 209
epidemiology, 209
pathophysiology, 209
prognosis, 211
treatment, 211

medication and stroke
anticholinergic, 188
antidepressants and non-steroidal anti-inflammatory (NSAIDs), 188–189
case presentation, 185–186
controversial nature of, 187
hormone replacement therapy (HRT), 187
testosterone replacement (TRT), 187–188

meningovascular syphilis and stroke
case presentation, 107
cerebral spinal fluid (CSF), 109
clinical presentation, 109
diagnosis, 109–110
diagnostic algorithm, 108
imaging, 109
incidence, 108–109
treatment, 110

Menkes disease and stroke
case presentation, 262
diagnostic algorithm, 263
diagnostic criteria, 263–266
epidemiology, 263

methylmalonic aciduria (MMA) and stroke
clinical presentation, 277
etiology, 277

migraines and stroke
background, 306–307
case presentation, 305–306
cervical artery dissection (CAD) diagnosis, 308

cervical artery dissection
    (CAD) mechanisms, 308
mitochondrial diseases
    (MELAS) and stroke
    case presentation, 253–256
    clinical presentation,
        259–260
    diagnosis, 259
    diagnostic criteria, 259
    epidemiology, 258–259
    pathogenesis, 260
    pathophysiology, 259
    treatment, 260–261
Moschowitz syndrome and
    stroke. See also
        disseminated
        intravascular coagulation
        (DIC) and stroke
    case presentation, 168–171
    clinical features, 173
    clinical presentation, 172
    defined, 172
    imaging, 172–173
    neurological
        manifestations, 172
    pathophysiology, 172
    plasmapheresis, 173
moyamoya disease (MMD) and
    stroke
    case presentation, 309
    in children, 225
    classification and diagnosis,
        312–313
    clinical presentation, 312
    epidemiology, 312
    etiology, 312
    pathophysiology, 312
    treatment, 313
MR angiography (MRA), 5
MR venography (MRV), 5

neuroborreliosis. See Lyme
    disease (LD) and stroke
neurocysticercosis (NCC) and
    stroke
    case presentation, 132–133
    clinical manifestations,
        134–135
    diagnostic algorithm,
        133
    diagnostic criteria, 135
    differential diagnosis, 135
    etiology, 134
    incidence, 134
    treatment, 134, 135
    types, 135

neurofibromatosis type 1 and
    stroke
    case presentation, 220–222
    clinical features and
        incidence, 223
neurofibromatosis type 1 and
    stroke diagnosis
    algorithm, 223
    central nervous system
        abnormalities, 224–225
    clinical presentation, 224
    epileptic seizures, 225
    genetics, 225–226
    imaging, 226
    management, 226
    ophthalmologic features, 224
    vascular abnormalities, 225
non-steroidal anti-
    inflammatory drugs
    (NSAIDs) and stroke,
    188–189

ocular neurocysticercosis, 135
organic acid disorders and
    stroke
    case presentation, 271
    clinical features, 273
    diagnosis, 273–274
    epidemiology, 273
    imaging, 275–276
    metabolic stroke and, 273
organic acid disorders and
    stroke, treatment
    acute decompensation, 278
    acute decompensation
        prevention, 277–278
    chronic monitoring, 278
organic acid disorders, types of
    glutaric aciduria type 1
        (GAI), 275–277
    methylmalonic aciduria
        (MMA), 277
    propionic aciduria, 277
osteochondromas and
    stroke, 340
osteopetrosis and stroke, 339
osteoporosis and stroke, 339
osteosarcoma and stroke, 341

Paget's disease and stroke, 339
patent foramen ovale (PFO)
    and stroke
    case presentation, 281–285
    clinical features, 285
    diagnosis, 286
    diagnosis difficulties, 285

hemorrhage, 285
    imaging, 285
    paradoxical embolism
        (PDE), 285–286
    patent foramen ovale (PFO),
        285–286
    role of, 286
    treatment, 286
peripartum cardiomyopathy
    and stroke, 302
plasmapheresis
    HVS, 166–167
    Moschowitz syndrome,
        173
polyarteritis nodosa (PAN) and
    stroke
    case presentation, 24–25
    classification, 27
    clinical features, 27
    diagnostic algorithm, 27
    manifestation, 27
    treatment, 27
polycythemia vera (PV) and
    stroke, 165
postpartum benign
    angiopathy, 302
pre-eclampsia during
    pregnancy and stroke
    clinical presentation,
        301
    defined, 301
    imaging, 301–302
    intracerebral hemorrhage
        (ICH), 303
primary systemic vasculitis,
    types
    giant cell arteritis (GCA),
        12–14
    granulomatosis with
        polyangiitis (GPA), 38–39
    lymphomatoid
        granulomatosis (LG),
        41–43
    polyarteritis nodosa (PAN),
        26–27
    Susac syndrome (SS),
        47–48
    Takayasu arteritis (TAK),
        19–22
    Vogt–Koyanagi–Harada
        disease (VKH), 51–53
propionic aciduria and
    stroke, 277

retinal periphlebitis. See Eales
    disease and stroke

retinal vasculopathy with
    cerebral
    leukoencephalopathy and
    systemic manifestations
    (RVCL-S) and stroke
    case presentation, 240–243
    diagnosis, 244
    diagnostic criteria, 243–244
    treatment, 244–245
reversible cerebral
    vasoconstriction
    syndrome (RCVS) and
    stroke
    case presentation, 293–295
    clinical presentation, 296
    complications, 296
    differential diagnosis, 297
    etiology, 295
    imaging, 296–297
    pathophysiology and triggers
    for, 295–296
    postpartum benign
    angiopathy, 302
    treatment, 297

sarcoidosis and stroke
    case presentation, 85–86
    clinical features, 89
    clinical presentation, 89
    defined, 89
    diagnosis, 90
    diagnostic algorithm, 86
    treatment, 90
sickle cell disease (SCD) and
    stroke, 165–166
Sjögren syndrome and stroke
    case presentation, 79–80
    classification, 80
    defined, 82
    diagnosis, 83
    diagnostic algorithm, 80
    imaging, 83
    neurological
    manifestations, 82
    neurological symptoms,
    82–83
    pathogenesis, 82
    therapy, 83
skeletal abnormalities and
    stroke, types
    Camurati–Engelmann
    disease, 340
    spondyloepiphyseal
    dysplasia congenita, 340
skull disorders and stroke,
    types

craniosynostosis, 339
    osteopetrosis, 339
    Paget's disease, 339
spinal neurocysticercosis and
    stroke, 135
spondyloepiphyseal dysplasia
    congenita and stroke, 340
Susac syndrome (SS) and
    stroke
    case presentation, 45–47
    classification, 47–48
    defined, 47
    diagnosis, 48
    diagnostic algorithm, 47
    etiology, 47
    treatment, 48
systemic lupus erythematosus
    (SLE) and stroke
    case presentation, 66–67
    defined, 69–70
    diagnostic algorithm, 67
    pathogenesis, 70
    stroke and CNS related to, 70

Takayasu arteritis (TAK) and
    stroke
    case presentation, 17–19
    diagnostic algorithm, 19
    diagnostic criteria, 19–21
    differential diagnosis, 21–22
    imaging, 21
    inflammatory bowel diseases
    (IBD) and, 97–98
    therapy, 22
Tangier disease and stroke
    case presentation, 267
    clinical presentation, 269
    diagnostic algorithm,
    267–269
    differential diagnosis, 270
    pathophysiology, 269
    research findings, 269
    therapy, 269–270
testosterone replacement
    therapy (TRT) and stroke,
    187–188
thrombotic thrombocytopenic
    purpura (TTP). *See*
    Moschowitz syndrome
    and stroke
transesophageal
    echocardiography
    (TEE), 286
tuberculosis meningitis (TBM)
    and stroke
    case presentation, 119–120

diagnosis, 123
    diagnostic algorithm, 121
    incidence and mortality, 122
    neurological
    manifestations, 123
    stroke frequency, 122–123
    treatment, 123

varicella zoster virus (VZV)
    and stroke
    case presentation, 137
    clinical features, 139
    stroke and cerebral venous
    thrombosis complications
    from, 137–138
    treatment, 139
vasculitis secondary to systemic
    disease, types
    Behçet's syndrome (BS),
    74–78
    inflammatory bowel diseases
    (IBD), 93–98
    sarcoidosis, 87–91
    Sjögren syndrome, 80–83
    systemic lupus
    erythematosus (SLE),
    69–70
vasculitis with prominent eye
    movement, background,
    57
vasculitis with prominent eye
    movement, types
    Cogan syndrome (CS),
    61–65
    Eales disease, 56–59
    Susac syndrome (SS),
    47–48
    Vogt–Koyanagi–Harada
    disease (VKH), 51–53
vasculopathies, non-
    inflammatory and stroke,
    moyamoya disease
    (MMD), 309–313
vasculopathies, non-
    inflammatory and stroke
    carotid artery dissection,
    326–330
    cerebral amyloid angiopathy
    (CAA), 314–320
    dolichoectasia and fusiform
    aneurysms, 321–325
vasospastic conditions and
    stroke
    eclampsia during pregnancy,
    299–303
    migraines, 305–308

reversible cerebral
vasoconstriction
syndrome (RCVS),
293–297
venous occlusive conditions
and stroke
bone disorders, 336–341
cerebral venous sinus
thrombosis (CVST),
331–335

Eagle syndrome, 343–348
vessel-wall imaging (VWI) MR
technique, 5, 8
Vogt–Koyanagi–Harada
disease (VKH) and
stroke
background, 51
case presentation,
50
classification, 52

diagnostic algorithm,
51
stages, 52
treatment, 51,
52–53

Wegener's granulomatosis. *See*
granulomatosis with
polyangiitis (GPA) and
stroke